Timescapes of Health, Illness and Care

"This is a wonderful collection. Contributors all bring a wealth of fresh and diverse insights on the chronologies of health, caring and the body. They bring cutting edge humanities and social science perspectives from semiotics, philosophy, sociology, health services research, literacy criticism and more to unsettle normative conceptions of linear clock time, and to suggest a renewed chronopolitics of multiple timescapes. Drawing on rich empirical material spanning diverse everyday and clinical sites, from epidemics to medical teaching, and doctors' waiting rooms to ADHD – these chapters show how embodied and social time resists, complicates, stretches and haunts other chronologies. Essential reading for scholars of health, medicine and care."

— Judith Green, *Professor of Sociology, Centre for Cultures and Environments of Health, University of Exeter, UK*

"This important and exciting book demonstrates how much we can learn about illness, health and care (and indeed life itself) by adopting temporal perspectives. While the significance of time to experiences such as chronic illness is well-established, this collection is groundbreaking in its attentiveness to the diverse operations and considerations of time that shape our sense of everyday life, embodiment and duration. The chapters are wide-ranging in topic and location, from ADHD in Chilean schools to the burden of patient waiting in UK National Health Service. However they are unified by an exciting conceptual richness and a critical sensibility: themes such as chrononormativity, viral temporalities, deep time and temporal recursivity combine to challenge ideas of time as 'incremental, unidirectional, linear and smooth'."

— Helen Keane, *Professor of Sociology, Research School of Social Sciences, The Australian National University. Australia*

Katherine Kenny
Mia Harrison • Anthony K J Smith
Editors

Timescapes of Health, Illness and Care

palgrave
macmillan

Editors
Katherine Kenny
Sydney Centre for Healthy Societies
The University of Sydney
Sydney, NSW, Australia

Mia Harrison
Centre for Social Research in Health
UNSW Sydney
Sydney, NSW, Australia

Anthony K J Smith
Centre for Social Research in Health
UNSW Sydney
Sydney, NSW, Australia

ISBN 978-981-96-7054-3 ISBN 978-981-96-7055-0 (eBook)
https://doi.org/10.1007/978-981-96-7055-0

Cover illustration: Joaquin Corbalan pastor / Alamy Stock Photo

This Palgrave Macmillan imprint is published by the registered company Springer Nature Singapore Pte Ltd.
The registered company address is: 152 Beach Road, #21-01/04 Gateway East, Singapore 189721, Singapore

Acknowledgements

We would like to thank all the contributors who wrote chapters for this volume, as well as the many individuals who contributed to the research that appears in these pages. We also acknowledge that the idea for this collection developed in part following our work on a special issue titled "Matters of time in health and illness" published in the journal *Health Sociology Review*, which received enormous interest and included proposals from some of the contributors to this collection (Harrison et al., 2024). In particular, we acknowledge the work of Sophie Adams, who co-edited the issue with Mia Harrison and Anthony K J Smith.

Katherine Kenny would like to acknowledge the financial support of the Australian Research Council through her Discovery Early Career Research Award (DE220101498) as well as The University of Sydney's SOAR Program. She would also like to acknowledge the ongoing support of the Sydney Centre for Healthy Societies in the Faculty of Arts and Social Sciences at The University of Sydney and its Director, Professor Alex Broom. Mia Harrison and Anthony K J Smith acknowledge that the Centre for Social Research in Health at the University of New South Wales (UNSW Sydney) is supported by funding from the Australian Government Department of Health.

The Afterword to this volume—*Between deep time and Indigenous well-being*—by Susie Anderson originally appeared in 2021 as part of The University of Melbourne exhibition *Emu Sky* at Old Quad, curated by Zena Cumpston. We are grateful to be able to republish it here.

Contents

Notes on Contributors

Samanta Alarcón-Arcos is a Sociologist with a master's degree in public policy, specializing in childhood studies through both quantitative and qualitative methods. She also focuses on care research, particularly children's and caregivers' and children needs, education and environments, and is a co-researcher on the Fondecyt grant "Caring Cities." She currently works on public policy from a civil society perspective.

Susie Anderson is a Wergaia/Wemba Wemba writer from Western Victoria whose poetry, non-fiction and criticism is published widely in print and online. Her debut poetry collection the body country was shortlisted for the Victorian and NSW Premier's Literary Awards. More info at www.susan.fyi

Alex Broom is Professor of Sociology in the School of Social and Political Sciences, Faculty of Arts and Social Sciences, and Director of the Sydney Centre for Healthy Societies at The University of Sydney, Australia. He is recognised as an international leader in sociology, with a specific interest in health, illness and care. His work takes a person-centred approach, qualitatively exploring the intersections of individual experience and social, political and economic context.

Fernanda Bywaters-Collado is Psychologist by the Universidad de Santiago de Chile, currently studying for a master's degree in Psychology, mention in Psychoanalytic Theory and Clinic at the Universidad Diego Portales. Her main research interests are linked to the social studies of medicine and health. She is currently developing a research project on temporality in psychoanalytic work with terminal cancer patients in institutional contexts.

Amanda M. Caleb is Professor of Medical Humanities at Geisinger Commonwealth School of Medicine, having previously served as the founding director of the Medical and Health Humanities program at Misericordia University. Her research interests include the medical and public health humanities, health communication, health narratology, narrative medicine, and bioethics and the Holocaust. She is co-editor (with Dougals A. Vakoch and John C. Pollock) of Covid Communication: A Case Study in Pandemic Discourse (Springer, 2023) and author of the forthcoming Global Inequities: Differing Health Experiences (Cambridge University Press, 2025).

Jorge Castillo-Sepúlveda is Assistant Professor at the School of Psychology of the Universidad de Santiago de Chile. His interests include the epistemic and technological aspects of health politics, informed by material-semiotics approaches, being developed case studies mainly centred on Chilean health reforms. He is author of articles and book chapters addressed from STS and have responsible of different research projects, currently studying the socio-material composition of time in political, clinical and experiential health care settings.

Johannes Deutschbein is a Sociologist at Charité-Universitätsmedizin Berlin whose expertise encompasses the sociology of medicine, the sociology of architecture, and both qualitative and quantitative research methods. His main areas of research have been healthcare structures for vulnerable patients, patient-centered healthcare, emergency departments, professionalization, and nutrition.

Michael J. Flexer is Co-Director for Public Engagement at the Wellcome Centre for Cultures and Environments of Health at the University of Exeter. His forthcoming monograph–The Madness of Meaning—is a semiotic dissection of 'psychosis.' He is currently collaborating with people who see, hear and sense things others don't, using creative methodologies to disrupt 'disruptive' technologies like AI and their use in mental health diagnostics and therapeutics.

Mariana Gálvez-Ramírez is Psychologist at the University of Santiago de Chile, currently a student in the master's programme in Adult Clinical Psychology at the University of Chile. She works as a clinical psychologist at the Women's Mental Health Unit of the San José Hospital. Member of the Inter-American Research Network on Psychoanalysis and Politics (RedIPPol), and member of the Working Group Psychoanalysis and Maternities, her main research interests are linked to the social studies of medicine and health. Her work has developed from psychoanalysis, biopolitical studies, public health, maternity and violence, and the intersections between these fields.

Imogen Harper is a Postdoctoral Research Associate at the Sydney Centre for Healthy Societies and Charles Perkins Centre at The University of Sydney. Imogen's research focuses on experiences surrounding chronic illness and disability, health inequality, embodiment, and youth, and she uses person-centred qualitative methods to situate these experiences in social and political narratives and power structures.

Mia Harrison is a transdisciplinary Research Fellow at the Centre for Social Research in Health (CSRH) at UNSW. Her work is informed by approaches in science and technology studies (STS), critical medical humanities, and sociology of health and illness. Mia's research explores the temporalities, places, materials, and affects of situated practices and complex social assemblages. Her work is characterised by critical and creative qualitative methodologies that extend across and beyond disciplinary conventions.

Katherine Kenny is Associate Professor of Sociology, Australian Research Council DECRA Research Fellow, and Deputy Director of the Sydney Centre for Healthy Societies at The University of Sydney, Australia. Her work draws on social and cultural theory and a range of qualitative methods to better understand how health, illness and care are understood, governed, 'treated' and made meaningful in clinical contexts and in everyday life.

Daniela Krüger is a Sociologist interested in the social study of emergency care, its professions, patients and current developments and changes. She conducts both quantitative and qualitative research, with a particular interest in combining the two.

Martin Möckel is Professor of Medicine, Medical Director of Emergency and Acute Medicine and Vice Dean for Education at Charité. His research comprises of emergency medical care with the focus on acute coronary syndromes and heart failure, cardiovascular and infectious diseases diagnostic biomarkers and digital health solutions. He has led a number of multicenter trials, research consortia and published more than 300 full papers listed in PubMed.

Kelly Moes is a Doctoral Candidate at Curtin University. She holds a master's degree in Disability Studies, alongside extensive professional background in disability and mental health community services. Broadly interested in Critical Disability Studies, Kelly's PhD research foregrounds the collective knowledge and experiential expertise of those who live with Intracranial Hypertension. Her research seeks to extend the narrative about Intracranial Hypertension, and radically reconfigure the way this condition—and chronic illness disability more broadly—is researched and managed. Kelly's research interest has been shaped and informed by her lived experience with Intracranial Hypertension, which has fueled her passion to engage and empower her community.

Roberta Pala is a Postdoctoral Research Fellow in the Sydney Centre for Healthy Societies at The University of Sydney. Her research draws on feminist science and technology studies, multispecies studies and sociology of health. Her work looks at the entangled nature of social and scientific events and considers biological interventions and technological artefacts as material sites of political investigations of the body. She is currently researching human–microbial relations in family settings and ideas of more-than-human health.

Mara Pieri is Associate Researcher at the Center for Social Studies at the University of Coimbra. A sociologist with a PhD in Human Rights, she works on queer theory, crip studies, and sociology of health and illness. She recently published "LGBT+ people with Chronic Illness:

Chroniqueers in Southern Europe" (Palgrave). She leads the project "DIVERS—Diversity and inclusion in access to health" on access to health care for the LGBTQ+ population.

Sarah Riley is a Professor in Critical Health Psychology at Massey University. Her award-winning, interdisciplinary research focuses on health identities and the relationships between discourse, affect, technology, and materiality that shape them. Recent co-authored books include Postfeminism and Health (Routledge, 2019), Postfeminism and Body Image (Routledge, 2022); and Digital Feeling (Palgrave, 2023).

Martine Robson is a Lecturer in psychology at Aberystwyth University. Her research focuses on the ways that people negotiate individualistic health discourses and uses poststructural theories to examine the ways that people adopt and resist healthism. Recent co-authored books include Postfeminism and Health (Routledge, 2019), Postfeminism and Body Image (Routledge, 2022).

Sebastián Rojas-Navarro is Associate Professor at Universidad Andres Bello, Chile and a dedicated scholar and researcher specializing in the intersections of urban environments, care practices, and social inequality. His work spans multiple disciplines, including medical sociology, urban studies, and Science and Technology Studies (STS). Sebastian's research focuses on how urban spaces shape experiences of health and illness, with a particular emphasis on childhood development, parental care, and the impact of city environments on marginalized groups.

Marsha Rosengarten is Visiting Professor at King's College London and Professor Emerita at Goldsmiths, University of London. She is the author of HIV Interventions: Biomedicine and the Traffic in Information and Flesh, co-author with Mike Michael of Innovation and Biomedicine: Ethics, Evidence and Expectation in HIV and co-editor with Alex Wilkie and Martin Savransky of Speculative Research: The Lure of Possible Futures. Her work explores the contributions that speculative modes of thought can make to transforming our understanding of the microorganisms we live and die with, including the limits and unsuspected potentials of how biomedicine strives to know them.

Liane Schenk is a Professor of Health Services Research with a focus on vulnerable populations. Her research focuses on diversity-sensitive health care in hospitals and nursing homes, the health care of vulnerable populations in various care settings and methodological issues of diversity-oriented health services research.

Anna Schneider is a Public Health Scientist at Charité-Universitätsmedizin Berlin with a focus on quantitative research on healthcare structures in emergency departments and the impact of psychosocial working conditions on the mental well-being of hospital physicians and nurses.

Aimee Sinclair is a Doctoral Candidate at the School of Allied Health at Curtin University, Australia. Her academic interests include Mad theorising and methodologies, activism, lived experience work, and the limits of inclusion. She teaches and provides supervision for lived experience (peer) workers in the Australian mental health sector.

Anthony K J Smith is a Research Fellow at the Centre for Social Research in Health, UNSW Sydney. His work draws on the sociology of health, gender, and sexuality, with a focus on HIV, sexual health, and LGBTQ+ communities. Anthony specialises in qualitative methodologies, and he draws on sociological theory, data justice, critical bioethics, and science and technology studies to understand health workforces, community well-being, and how biomedical technologies shape social life.

Jianni Tien is a Postdoctoral Research Fellow in the Sydney Centre for Healthy Societies at The University of Sydney. Jianni works at the intersection of science and technology studies, the feminist environmental humanities, and sociology of health. She researches a range of topics including human-microbial relations; sustainable technological innovation and the material ontologies of pollution. Her current book project examines the ontologies and epistemologies at work in our Anthropocene era and the power structures that underpin them, including questions of situated and enforced Western knowledges.

Francisco Tirado is Senior Lecturer in the Social Psychology Department of Universitat Autònoma de Barcelona. He is now full member of STS-b

(Barcelona Science and Technology Studies Group) and was its director for the preceding five years. His research interests are related with four topics: (a) Science and Technology Studies, (b) power relationships and political action in new sociotechnical contexts, (c) citizen participation in technoscientific controversies; (d) artificial intelligence and its relation with new forms of power. He is the author of several articles and books on STS and Power Relationships in new sociotechnical contexts.

Andreas Wagenknecht is a Sociologist at Charité-Universitätsmedizin with a focus on theory and qualitative methodology. His research focuses on disability studies and medical sociology. He is particularly interested in the study of communication, as well as physical and technological phenomena.

Peter Winter is a Sociologist of science and technology and a Senior Research Associate at the University of Bristol, United Kingdom. His research explores expertise, expert authority, and the critical role of experts in shaping debates on the testing, safety, and regulation of digital technologies, with a specific focus on AI systems.

List of Figures

List of Images

1

Introduction

Katherine Kenny, Mia Harrison, and Anthony K J Smith

Academic explorations of time and temporality are very 'of the moment'. But the flurry of social science scholarship over the last few decades belies an enduring human concern with time—its inescapability, its generative and destructive potentials, its capriciousness and so on—since time immemorial (see Adam, 1990, 1998; Elias, 1992; Hochschild, 2001; Giddens, 1991; Grosz, 2005, 2020; Rosa, 2013; Samuels, 2017; Yunkaporta, 2023; McGrath et al., 2023). Human societies have made sense of time in relation to the natural world and social practices across cultures and societies as far back as the historical record extends, and likely much further. In Aboriginal and Torres Strait Islander cultures

K. Kenny (✉)
Sydney Centre for Healthy Societies, The University of Sydney, Sydney, NSW, Australia
e-mail: katherine.kenny@sydney.edu.au

M. Harrison • A. K. J. Smith
Centre for Social Research in Health, UNSW Sydney, Sydney, NSW, Australia
e-mail: mia.harrison@unsw.edu.au; anthony.smith@unsw.edu.au

K. Kenny et al. (eds.), *Timescapes of Health, Illness and Care*,
https://doi.org/10.1007/978-981-96-7055-0_1

dating back 65,000 years or more in Australia, 'deep time' is central to stories of Country, in which past, present and future are interwoven with holistic understandings of people and place across time (see Anderson, this volume; also Yunkaporta, 2023, 2024; McGrath et al., 2023). Other cultural and faith traditions around the world have featured temporal deities, such as the Ancient Greek gods of cyclical or eternal time (*Aion*), chronological time (*Chronos*) and fortuitous moments (*Kairos*), or espoused temporally structured beliefs such as notions of eternity and life everlasting (see Deng, 2024). More recently, Benjamin Franklin's much-quoted aphorism 'time is money', positioned time as a daily sacrifice at the altar of capitalism (see Weber, 1972). Across societies and throughout history, time is consistently recognised as a fundamental dimension of human existence, providing the temporal backdrop to life's beginning, progression and ending.

Perhaps nowhere is time experienced more acutely than in relation to instances of ill health and the need for care. These are key sites for understanding the operation of time—how it is felt, lived, managed and made meaningful both in healthcare settings and in everyday life. The steady march of incremental 'clock' time that was accelerated by the proliferation of quantified and commodified logics of industrialised capitalism now structures both the operation of daily life in many places and, often, our expectations of how the future may unfold, in an omnipresent way (see Thompson, 1967). In tension with this, instances of illness and the need for care can render time non-linear, discontinuous, and qualitatively and relationally different to 'well' or 'productive' time, profoundly disrupting our anticipated futures (see Adams et al., 2009). It is in the tension between these two registers of time—clock time on the one hand and experiential time on the other—that we propose *timescapes* as a useful way of understanding and studying the temporal dimensions of health, illness and care. Building on the work of scholars such as Barbara Adam (1990), we adopt the idea of timescapes as both a conceptual framing and a methodological approach for better understanding temporal experience in health, illness and care, how time is institutionalised with respect to healthcare, its normative functioning and its lived multiplicity. Drawing on research across a number of international contexts, across a variety of disciplinary and interdisciplinary traditions, and across different empirical settings, the chapters contained here each seeks to better understand how *considerations* of time—its ontological standing, normative value, and embodied and intersubjective experience—are vital to understanding the phenomenology of health and illness, and the governance of both the institutions that provide formal (health)care and the cultures that circulate around (and often obscure) informal care. Our main objective for this collection was to explore and theorise the tensions that emerge between how time is typically 'treated' and how it is experienced in relation with moments (of whatever duration) of illness and care.

Measuring and Experiencing Time

Time constitutes an often-taken-for-granted backdrop to almost every social process, interaction and institution, a 'fact of life' that doesn't obviously require further consideration or interrogation (Adam, 1990). In daily conversation, time is invoked in (at least) two distinct registers: as the abstract quantified units that structure and coordinate everyday schedules, meeting times and workdays, and as the more ineffable quality of every moment's passage. In the first register, reference to time through the quantified units of time-keeping devices reigns supreme. From the sundials and water clocks of ancient civilisations to the modern precision of quartz and atomic clocks, these keepers of time demarcate its linear unfolding through uniform and sequential units that can be universally validated and coordinated through their 'objective' measurement (Adam, 2008). These measurable units of clock time have become integral to Western science and biomedicine, and an essential organising mechanism of health, illness and care (Harrison et al., 2024).

Whether in minutes and hours or the weeks and months of the calendar year, these units of time shape how we come to know, experience and care for health and illness. In clinical settings, appointment systems, work rosters and care schedules all shape who receives care, from whom and when. Opening hours, visiting hours and 'quiet time' all variously structure how care is delivered and experienced not only by patients and healthcare providers but also by all of those entangled in the relational webs that coalesce around formal and informal care. Treatment regimens define the precise scheduling of care and, often, the time of and between the administration of pharmaceutical interventions. Health surveillance devices monitor bodily signals and carefully calibrate them in relation to 'healthy' times. Anticipated timelines of prognosis and recovery present estimates of 'time left' (until death or the return of 'good' health). Measurements of time also produce the boundaries of health in different ways, be that through articulating sequential stages of 'normal' development (and decline), identifying temporal thresholds in diagnosis (e.g. the point when illness becomes 'chronic') or determining the rate of prevalence or deterioration at which a health issue becomes a 'crisis' requiring 'urgent' response (e.g. Harrison et al., 2022).

Alongside the pervasiveness and institutional and cultural dominance of clock time, its inability to characterise the lived experience of temporality has long drawn criticism. It is here that the second register in which time is often discussed emerges: in the common refrain that 'you can't rush recovery', for example, or in the directive to 'take it one day at a time' or that 'today is the first day of the rest of your life.' In the nostalgic aphorism 'the days are long, but the years are short'. Or in the puzzling experience of 'lockdown time', which was at once both fleeting and interminable and required various forms of temporal reorganisation and recalibration (van Emmerik et al., 2025). Both the tyranny of clock time and its shortcomings in attempts to fully account for temporal experience are particularly evident in illness and care, perhaps all the more so in the wake of COVID-19.

One prominent alternative that has attempted to grapple with the inadequacies of the clock for capturing the lived experience of time emerged out of the tradition of process philosophy (e.g. Bergson, 1889, 1911; Whitehead, 1967,1978). In particular, and in reaction to what he characterised as the (linearly) spacialised approach to time that underpins Newtonian mechanics (as well as Western Enlightenment thinking, more generally), French philosopher Henri Bergson introduced the idea of *durée* or 'duration' as a contextualised, experiential counterpart to abstracted quantified clock time. Durational or process time has variously been proposed as fundamentally enmeshed in social relations, inextricably intertwined with social context and as unfolding through processes—like care—that do not easily yield to the kind of metrification often demanded by the external yardstick of clock time (Davies, 1994). Instead of *keeping* time, experiences and practices like illness and care *take* the time they need. Durational time can be experienced as quick *and* slow, short *and* long, and unfolding through overlapping and criss-crossing pathways. Thus, two people can experience the same two moments in time according to the clock and measure the same length of time between these two points, but their lived experiences of time between them—their experience of duration—will never be precisely the same.

Another important line of criticism of the cultural dominance of clock time comes from feminist thought, which has illustrated how the industrial capitalist origins of clock time has led to the systematic exclusion of those whose work operates primarily outside of the economic realm—namely, women performing the unpaid work of caring (Walby, 1984; Adkins, 2009; Kristeva, 1981). For example, feminist philosopher Nancy Fraser (2016, p. 100) points out the contradiction inherent in every capitalist society whereby,

> on the one hand, social reproduction is a condition of possibility for sustained capital accumulation; on the other, capitalism's orientation to unlimited accumulation tends to destabilize the very processes of social reproduction on which it relies.

One manifestation of the resulting crisis of care, argues Fraser, is a type of 'time poverty' whereby the relentless productivity demanded of financialised capitalism increasingly encroaches on the time once preserved for the work of care (see also Hochschild, 2001).

This same encroachment of 'productive' time can be seen through the lens of the (temporally delimited) Parsonian sick role (Parsons, 1975), in which experiences of illness are circumscribed by normative expectations around accomplishing a 'timely' recovery and return to 'productive' citizenship. The orientation towards recovery, or at least progress in that direction, also inflects narratives of 'biographical disruption' (Bury, 1982) and narrative reconstruction in the face of ill-health (Bury, 1982; Charmaz, 1990; Hydén, 1997; Frank, 2013). On the one hand, such ideas challenge the incremental unfolding of linear 'clock' time by highlighting the temporally disruptive nature of illness (Bury, 1982; Charmaz, 1990). But positioning illness as 'disruption' to the status quo, or illness narratives as 'wrecked' insofar as they invariably depart from the conventional flow of narrative temporality and the expectation of 'a past that leads into a present that sets in place a foreseeable future' (Frank, 2013, p. 55), ultimately does little to disrupt the cultural dominance of clock time. Instances of illness and the need for care are positioned as exceptions rather than as the norm, and thus inadvertently reinforce the construction of linear clock time continuously marching on.

The normative conflation of time and productivity, which elides the inevitability of embodied vulnerability, frailty and disability, has been resisted by scholars across a number of fields. Importantly, feminist and disability scholars have proposed the idea of 'crip time' as both theory and practice—as a way of both understanding and experiencing a non-normative relationship to linear clock time and creating alternative ways of navigating an ableist world. Thus, Alison Kafer (2013, p. 27) explains, 'rather than bend disabled bodies and minds to meet the clock, crip time bends the clock to meet disabled bodies and minds' (see also Ehlers et al., 2024; Ahmed, 2006; Halberstam, 2005; McRuer, 2006; Garland-Thomson, 2011; Pieri, 2023; Samuels, 2017; Sheppard, 2024). This idea of 'bending' or otherwise remoulding time to better accommodate the lived experience of 'less-than-perfect' health is aided in many ways, we argue, by the idea of 'timescapes'.

Spatialising and Situating Time

In contrast to the abstracted yardstick and perpetual motion of normative clock time, Barbara Adam's (1990) idea of 'timescapes' affords a multidimensional conceptualisation that aligns more closely with the experiential register of time, including experiences of illness and the need for care. In a similar vein to Bergson (1889), Adam critiques the (linearly) spatialised nature of clock time that underpins classical Newtownian mechanics and the associated principles of abstraction, objectivity and universalisability. Instead, Adam presents a (multidimensionally) spatialised conceptualisation of timescapes that aligns more closely with the quantum rendering of time, as discussed by scholars such as feminist theorist Karen Barad (e.g. 2010, 2013). On this view, the positionality of the observer matters significantly in how time is experienced and materialised. Adam usefully provides a set of orienting dimensions through which timescapes might be understood, including the following: *time frames* that are imposed externally—such as years, generations or historical/geographic epochs; *timing, tempo and sequence*, including the synchronisation and coordination of time, its velocity and rate of change, and its order and succession; *temporality*, the irreversible unfolding of time internal to systems and processes such as ageing; *duration*, the temporal distance or horizon that gives rise to an extent of time; and the *temporal modalities* of past, present and future that are associated with memory, experience and anticipation.

Imagining time as a multidimensional plane rather than a unidirectional line along which clock time steadily progresses offers a useful framework not only for conceptualising time but also for studying it in action, too (see also Neale, 2021, 2022). In particular, attuning to the timescapes of health, illness and care requires that we attend also to different dimensions of how time plays out. For example, in healthcare, *time frames* structure medical practice, from appointment schedules and hospital shifts to treatment plans and recovery periods. Set and held in motion by timekeeping devices and imposed by healthcare systems, institutions and policies alike, time frames meaningfully shape how care is delivered and experienced. For instance, the prescribed duration of a hospital stay, the timing of medication administration and the length of a rehabilitation program are all made to fit within externally determined periods, often imposed with considerations other than wellness (cost, for example) front of mind. However, these frames are not inherently fixed; they shift based on evolving medical knowledge, individual patient needs, resource availability and political will—all of which are also subject to the temporal cycles of annual budgets and political terms (see Kenny et al., 2024).

Temporality, the second dimension of timescapes that Adam articulates, speaks to the inner experience of time that is fundamental in understanding illness and care. The body operates on its own biological rhythms, from circadian cycles to the slow progression of birth, growth, degeneration and death. Healing, ageing and disease progression occur as part of a larger natural temporality—one that cannot be easily compressed or controlled. Thus, Adam explains:

> [A] focus on temporality… confronts us with the realisation that change is inescapable and that both sameness and reversibility are impossible. Importantly, focus on the temporality feature of time shows us that we are time, that we embody and have all of time encoded within us. It demonstrates that we live, use, know and create time in interaction. And it reveals that the world is irrevocably and irreversibly different with every action, interaction and transaction. (2021, p. xx)

For patients, time is experienced and lives are transformed through waiting for diagnoses, enduring prolonged treatments, or facing the irreversible progression of terminal conditions. Health professionals and informal care providers, too, engage with this temporality as they witness the gradual impact of interventions, the ebb and flow of symptoms, and the body's capacity for resilience and deterioration.

Timing, tempo and sequencing are critical in (health)care, as well. Whether it is administering medication at the right moment, adhering to 'workflows' and scheduling procedures, or synchronising team-based care, healthcare systems aim to operate with precise coordination. The contrast between the speed of medical advancements and the slow adaptation of healthcare systems highlights the tension between urgency and systemic inertia. Medical technology and drug development, and, increasingly, digitised health move at their own tempo, often faster than healthcare infrastructure can accommodate. Similarly, the tempo of patient care can be dictated by the speed of administrative processes, insurance approvals, access to medical professionals and whether care is delivered through public or privatised healthcare systems. Importantly, Adam points out that in lived time, tempo is context-specific and variable—unlike the unrelenting uniform tempo of clock time that equates speed and efficiency, ultimately, with economic productivity (Adam, 2021, p. *xx*), setting up the forms of chrononormativity that instances of illness and the need for care frequently jar against (Freeman, 2010).

Lastly, the modalities of *past, present and future* shape experiences of health and illness at individual, local and global levels. People live in a continuum of health histories, present conditions and future anticipations. Whereas clock time exists as a succession of incremental moments—an interminable 'now' with little connection to the past or future—past experiences of illness and future anticipations of either wellness or mortal horizons leave physical and emotional traces, influencing present well-being. Medical records, family histories and genetic predispositions anchor individuals in a temporal framework where past experiences inform future risks and decisions. Unlike clock time, which 'progresses' unrelentingly in a uniform forward direction, the human experience of time in health is constantly being reworked in relation with memories past and anticipated futures.

Explicit attention to timescapes broadens our focus on time beyond the temporal efficiencies of medical systems or health gains afforded by care, measured in days, months or years. Instead, it requires we pay closer attention to the multidimensional qualities and lived experience of illness and care. Addressing healthcare inequalities requires understanding the different temporal logics at play—how time is experienced by patients, structured by institutions and constrained by economic and political forces. Solutions cannot simply involve adding more time to existing structures but require a fundamental rethinking of how time is valued and managed in health and care. By recognising the complexities of time in illness and recovery, we might move toward a more compassionate, patient-centred healthcare system—one that acknowledges the irreversibility of time, the unique tempos of healing and the deeply personal experience of waiting, enduring and hoping as we all, at moments, occupy positions of vulnerabilities upon the timescapes of health, illness and care.

Overview of Chapters

Duration and the Governance of Time

The chapters in the first part of this collection present varied methods and cases for analysis but all theoretically build on and from Henri Bergson's concept of *durée* (e.g. Bergson, 1889). In the first two chapters, Marsha Rosengarten and Amanda Caleb explore the viral temporalities of the COVID-19 pandemic in relation with other viral outbreak events: for Rosengarten, the West African Ebola epidemic of 2014–2016, and for Caleb, the Great Influenza pandemic of 1918–1920 as recounted through Virginia Woolf's *Mrs. Dalloway*. Yet an important caveat we must make here—one that Rosengarten and Caleb's analyses render unavoidable—is that even our naming of these three viral events constitutes time in ways that are open to political and philosophical scrutiny. When we talk about COVID-19, West African Ebola, and the Great Influenza, we are not merely describing the emergence of a virus in the world but locating that virus in time and with time. Moreover, understanding viral events *as* events requires us to accept that they have a beginning and an end, and a before and an after.

Both Rosengarten and Caleb's chapters problematise the beginnings and endings of viral 'events' in different ways. Rosengarten brings Bergson's philosophical writing on time together with that of other scientific thinkers, most notably Alfred North Whitehead (1967, 1978) and William James (1996). Her chapter explores how conceptualising time as something that is divisible—that can be described in terms of discrete moments, units or events—remakes these temporal divisions as static and thus observable, while obfuscating the connections that hold them together. Following this, to identify a viral 'outbreak' is not merely to describe the presence and replication of a virus, it is a declaration that the virus has broken out from the expectations of how that virus *should* behave within the boundaries of a particular time and place (e.g. who the virus affects, how many are affected, how quickly that is changing, and so on). Identifying 'epidemics', 'pandemics' and 'endemics' (or describing them as 'ended') are similarly temporal practices that recast viral replication as not merely a problem of geography and scale but an articulation of how viral geographies and scales locate in time.

Caleb's chapter is also concerned with how viral events demarcate time. It takes as its case Virginia Woolf's 1925 novel *Mrs. Dalloway*—in particular, how it has been read as a pandemic novel in 2020. Caleb argues that both Woolf's eponymous character and her contemporary readers experience (to use Woolf's language) 'an indescribable pause', wherein the heterogeneous temporalities of illness, viral contagion, isolation, social connection, war and much more enfold and disrupt linear time. These twin temporal moments that take place almost a century apart can, in one sense, be measured by the clock—as an hour marked by the chime of Big Ben in post-World War I London or as days and months of lockdown across the world in 2020. Caleb emphasises that the embodied experiences of such moments cannot be quantified by the clock, but she also calls our attention to the ways in which the clock interrupts, distracts from and reframes *durée*. The chime of the clock asserts itself and momentarily aligns our temporal experiences and perceptions to clock time, before dissolving away.

Also like Rosengarten, Caleb's analysis highlights uncertainties regarding COVID-19's classification as still a 'pandemic' (or something other) and questions how we can 'move forward' through ambivalently defined temporalities. Caleb argues that for many the experience of COVID-19 has remade the time before and after into 'pre-COVID' and 'post-COVID' time. The chapter pairs Bergson's concept of *durée* with his work on memory to explore the making of this pandemic juncture as a temporal *dis*junction enacted through the collision of 'shared' (but also incommensurable) pandemic temporalities that situate experiences of pandemic time in 2020 not only in relation with the COVID-19 pandemic at large but also as part of a much longer pandemic history of illness, death, survival and health governance (including the Great Influenza, AIDS and more). This, too, resonates with Rosengarten's analysis, which reframes historical learning and foresight in public health governance as a kind of temporal curation, where past events and possible futures are included or excluded to produce explanatory narratives of science.

Francisco Tirado, Jorge Castillo-Sepúlveda, Fernanda Bywaters-Collado and Mariana Gálvez-Ramírez also take *durée* as a starting point for conceptualising time in their chapter. They build upon critiques of time as something singular and stable, and especially how these critiques have been applied through analyses of clinical and mundane practices of care in the field of science and technology studies (STS), such as by Maria Puig de la Bellacasa (2017), Bruno Latour (2008) and Stefan Timmermans (1998). Their chapter develops a concept they call 'sensitive trajectories' to describe the situations in healthcare through which time itself is cared for, is problematised and becomes a matter of care. Applying their concept to ethnographic work conducted in clinical and government sites across the Chilean health system, they explore the materials and practices that configure temporal flows in health political design.

Tirado and colleagues' framework of 'sensitive trajectories' emphasises that health temporalities are multiple and are constituted through practices. Moreover, these constitutions are fragile and vulnerable to disruption and, so, must be 'cared for'. The case study of the Chilean health system enables Tirado and colleagues to empirically trace these caring practices and their effects and thereby develop an understanding of how health interventions reorganise the temporal experiences and practices of health by delimiting time. They therefore distinguish *time* as a (precariously) coherent object that materialises with care, from *temporality* as a scheme of relations between messy and motile human and non-human elements in healthcare assemblages.

Though each of the three chapters in this part work with the concept of *durée* in health in different ways, all call attention to how the mess, multiplicity and ongoing and interfolding nature of lived time becomes problematic in health response. Time must be cut up, (re)arranged and given beginnings and endings that produce an aesthetic of order and function. The authors' analyses point to the limits of this constitution of time; from multi-year pandemics to the scheduled minutes of clinical care, what is described as 'time' is a particular rendering that can only make sense in isolation. Importantly, this rendering of time is not universally experienced, and thus can always be made otherwise.

Institutionalised Temporalities

Another key theme of this volume is how time is made within healthcare institutions—as medical time, clinical time, hospital time—in ways that can be alien and hostile to those working and receiving care within them. The chapters in this part locate how institutionalised temporalities are practised by people in ways that attempt to resist or rework standardised rigidity (Ihlebæk, 2021; van Pijkeren et al., 2024). While there are limits to how people can rework these systems to better address workforce and lived experience, the chapters here make visible the rhythms of waiting and anticipation, the temporal structure of consultations and clinical education, and how different actors attempt to reform institutionalised temporalities to better accommodate a multiplicity of timescapes.

Andreas Wagenknecht, Johannes Deutschbein, Anna Schneider, Daniela Krüger, Martin Möckel and Liane Schenk draw on rhythm and practice theory to understand the temporalities of emergency departments in Berlin, Germany. This ethnographic work focuses on the patient journey and interactions with health staff amongst older adults, and their analysis focuses on duration, waiting, events, schedules and body time. While staff perceived an overarching rhythm to the patient flow, patients experienced an overwhelming sense of obscure unpredictability. The stressful environment results in patients being at the behest of hospital time, and in a state of anticipation and waiting for information about the next step in the course of their care, with little predictability and transparency about the length of their stay. A perennial set of questions emerge from this analysis: How can the hospital rhythm be improved to reduce the burden of waiting, and how can patients be provided with more transparency about the predicted length of their stay?

The burden of being patient and waiting for care is central in Michael Flexer's chapter, who attends to the spatio-temporal semiotics of general practice (GP) waiting rooms in the United Kingdom. The waiting room is presented as a hierarchical space-time through which the patient is not attended *with*, but rather *against*: as an object for others. This liminal, transitory space is comprised of key spatial features—chairs, brochures, posters, partitions, distance from the clinician—that structure how time is enacted and felt. The waiting room perhaps best exemplifies how health institutions structure care and the ways in which patient agency is ultimately confined through these structuring processes. Equally, Flexer observes that the waiting room became an apt metaphor for the experience of much of the world between 2020 and 2022 during physical lockdowns in response to COVID-19.

The spatio-temporal practices of demarcating boundaries continue into clinical teaching, in which medical students must be efficiently taught increasingly complex medicine in time-poor institutions. Peter Winter draws on video ethnographic work in the United Kingdom to examine the temporal demands and boundary work practices of educating medical students to interpret x-ray imagining. Here, clinical educators develop a strategy of containing image teaching interpretation into 'structured reviews' and 'spot diagnoses'. These 'whistle stop' teaching practices not only shape the hierarchy of junior doctors and radiologists, instilling these respective boundaried roles, but also, as Winter cautions, potentially reduce the interpretative work afforded to medical students, in which diagnosis is prioritised over a more well-rounded understanding of interpreting medical imaging.

The tensions of institutionalised temporalities are perhaps best exemplified through the conflicts over time made visible with the introduction of mental health peer support within mental health systems. Aimee Sinclair draws on Mad theorising to trouble the gap between Mad temporalities and institutionalised temporalities amongst peer workers in Western Australia. Here, peer support workers are disciplined to enact normative temporalities and a 'curative futurity', with an expectation that recovery with the goal of neoliberal citizenship is normative and desirable, which runs counter to supporting people to live with mental ill health in the present. Sinclair argues that peer support relations hold the potential to disrupt these stifling temporalities, and to value Mad existences, knowledges and practices, offering a valuable introduction to the thinking in the next part.

Challenging Chrononormativities

Chrononormativity refers to the regulatory force of normative timelines and rhythms that are internalised to be a productive neoliberal citizen (Freeman, 2010). The work across this volume critiques the normative aspects of measuring and living time, but the contributions in this part focus particularly on how disabled people and people living with chronic illnesses challenge all too common ableist chrononormativities. The entries here also draw particularly on crip theory and its theorising of 'crip time', which expose the normative and ableist assumptions underlying how cure and recovery are framed (Sheppard, 2023; Clare, 2017).

Mara Pieri provides a critical reflection on the chronopolitics of chronic illness, arguing that chrononormativity imposes many of the modes of oppression that structure the lives of people living with chronic illnesses.

Here, time is fundamentally political: a matter of fitting into others' schedules and ultimately being a productive citizen. A 'failure' to live up to these standards, while often a source of friction, also offers the potential to live life, and time, differently. The chapter provides an excellent synthesis of both queer and crip temporalities, and Pieri suggests that these temporalities enable possibilities not only for resisting institutionalised temporalities but also to reimagine futures not predicated on cisheteronormative and able-bodied health norms.

The ways that disabled people, neurodivergent people and people with chronic illness make sense of their time and energy have been well captured by the popular 'spoon theory'. Coined by Christine Miserandino (2003), spoon theory posits that a person has a finite but not always predictable number of 'spoons' in each day (each representing energy to complete a task), and that disruptions or oversights can unexpectedly use up these spoons. Imogen Harper's chapter draws on a digital ethnography to consider what spoon theory offers to conceptualising time and chronic illness. Spoon theory has endured and resonated online with so many people as a way to articulate a defining aspect of life and galvanise community solidarity and support through sharing a common language of experience. As Harper suggests, the metaphor of spoons offers a different way of doing time that centres the contingencies of living with chronic illness, challenging the expectation of being consistently 'productive' as a citizen and disrupting the normative idea that all time (and energy) is equally distributed for each day.

The day-to-day living of time is often contrasted with anticipations of future, and challenging the chrononormativities structured between present and future is vital. Kelly Moes focuses on the lives of people with an uncommon chronic illness-disability, intracranial hypertension. Drawing on mixed methods, Moes argues that people living with intracranial hypertension live life with two competing temporalities: a medicalised and curative framework, and uncertainty and hopelessness about the future. Understanding the contradictory effects generated by the temporal dissonance between these two temporalities is vital to ensuring epistemic justice and validating people living with this condition. That is, while there are possibilities for crip joy, it is also important to acknowledge experiences of grief and bitterness tied to the temporal dissonance brought on by living with an uncertain future. Methodologically, Moes's chapter highlights that being inclusive and reflexive about these different temporal modes of being is important to doing meaningful research with people living with chronic illness.

Temporal Recursivity

One of the main threads of this volume is the inadequacies of dominant Western notions of clock time for making sense of lived experiences of illness and care. In challenging this temporal hegemony, the chapters contained in this part variously illustrate how time is constantly renegotiated, with the past and future reworked through the ever unfolding present (Barad, 2013). These contributions foreground the multiplicity of lived time across a diverse set of illness and care contexts, highlighting the tensions between the normative construction of linear time as singular, definitive and smooth and its lived experience as multiple, tentative and recursive.

Martine Robson and Sarah Riley draw on Giles Deleuze's (1988, 1994) philosophy of time and the case of couples living with coronary heart disease to argue that the temporal is an under-theorised dimension of critiques of lifestyle change. Normative constructions of linear time contribute to the individualising and responsibilising effects of much lifestyle advice. Instead of a smooth trajectory towards 'healthy' futures, achieved by 'rational' individuals making 'healthier' lifestyle 'choices', their chapter demonstrates how engaging with lifestyle change involves multiple temporal selves within relationally enacted plural timeframes. These shifting temporalities afford multiple subject positions and legitimise a range of practices that can variously work for and against engagement in lifestyle change. While the linear discourses of healthy living could be experienced as oppressive and alienating, recognising the multiplicity of participants' experiences opened up new possibilities and hopeful effects, such as an acceptance of illness, ageing and death as natural processes, which buffered against fear, self-blame and uncertainty.

Shifting from lifestyle advice oriented towards materialising 'healthy' futures to the consequences of diagnostic categories for *how* the future is materialised, Sebastian Rojas Navarro and Samantha Alarcón-Arcos examine the case of mental health diagnoses in children. Drawing on ethnographic research in Chilean schools and Jacques Derrida's (1994) ideas on hauntology, they show how a diagnosis of attention deficit/hyperactivity disorder (ADHD) imposes a certain recursivity whereby children's future possibilities become delimited by their pasts. Within institutional care settings (in this case schools) that incentivise diagnoses as a pathway to increased funding and enhanced service provision, diagnoses take on a spectral presence haunting both how children are perceived and how they are cared for and supported in ongoing ways.

If diagnosis continues to haunt experiences well into the future, so too does prognosis, especially when that prognosis calls into question the very time one might have left to live. The chapter by Katherine Kenny, Jianni Tien, Roberta Pala and Alex Broom takes the case of life-limiting illness to examine the recursive tensions between the statistical projections and lived experiences of cancer prognoses. Drawing on work by Karen Barad (2010, 2013) and interviews with people living with cancer and those that care for them, Kenny and colleagues investigate how time is rearranged and reconfigured in the experience of cancer diagnosis, treatment and care, especially for those who *outlive* their prognosis and exist in the uncertain terrain of living 'on borrowed time'. The chapter asks: How does the certainty of one's impending mortality shape the temporal landscapes that come into view? Moreover, what futures are imposed upon one's present and how does terminality imbue whatever time is left?

Each of the chapters in this part, in its own way, illustrates the shortcomings of dominant notions of time as incremental, unidirectional, linear and smooth. Together, they help build a better understanding of time as a constant process of repatterning past and future in the present, as it recursively unfolds across multiple bodies, in multiple directions and always in relation.

Afterword

The volume concludes with an Afterword by Wergaia/Wemba Wemba woman Susie Anderson reflecting on Indigenous notions of well-being and their connections to deep time. In stark contrast to dominant Western notions of clock time, Aboriginal and Torres Strait Islander peoples—the First Nations peoples of Australia—have long conceptualised a cosmology in which time is lived and felt not in relation to the ticking clock but with/in an interwoven web of people, place and time that stretches millions of years into the past and millions of years into the future. This mode of being with time reminds us that care—in reciprocal ways with Country, culture and community—is enacted holistically across timescapes.

In taking seriously the interconnectedness of time, people and place, we are urged to consider that time is something which carries responsibilities that transcend the here and now and the institutional forces that often dominate our attention. By contending with timescapes of health, illness and care, we might imagine how life, death and the apprehension of 'ill' and 'well' health might be enacted differently.

Competing Interests Katherine Kenny is supported by an Australian Research Council Discovery Early Career Research Award (DE220101498). The authors have no conflicts of interest to declare that are relevant to the content of this chapter.

References

Adam, B. (1990). *Time and social theory*. Polity Press.

Adam, B. (1998). *Timescapes of modernity: The environment and invisible hazards*. Routledge.

Adam, B. (2008). The timescapes challenge: Engagement with the invisible temporal. In R. Edwards (Ed.), *Researching lives through time: Time, generation and life stories. Timescapes working paper series, no 1*. University of Leeds.

Adam, B. (2021). Academic timescapes in focus. In F. Vostal (Ed.), *Inquiring into Academic Timescapes*. Emerald Publishing.

Adams, V., Murphy, M., & Clarke, A. E. (2009). Anticipation: Technoscience, life, affect, temporality. *Subjectivity, 28*, 246–265.

Adkins, L. (2009). Sociological futures: From clock time to event time. *Sociological Research Online, 14*(4), 88–92.

Ahmed, S. (2006). *Queer phenomenology: Orientations, objects, others*. Duke University Press.

Barad, K. (2010). Quantum entanglements and Hauntological relations of inheritance: Dis/continuities, SpaceTime Enfoldings, and justice-to-come. *Derrida Today, 3*(2), 240–268.

Barad, K. (2013). Ma(r)king time: Material entanglements and re-memberings: Cutting together-apart. In P. R. Carlile, D. Nicolini, A. Langley, & H. Tsoukas (Eds.), *How matter matters: Objects, artifacts, and materiality in organization studies* (p. 0). Oxford University Press.

Bergson, H. (1889). *Time and free will: An essay on the immediate data of consciousness*. George Allen & Unwin.

Bergson, H. (1911). Matter and memory (N. M. Paul & W. S. Palmer, Trans.). George Allen & Unwin.

Bury, M. (1982). Chronic illness as biographical disruption. *Sociology of Health & Illness, 4*(2), 167–182.

Charmaz, K. (1990). "Discovering" chronic illness: Using grounded theory. *Social Science & Medicine (1982), 30*(11), 1161–1172.

Clare, E. (2017). *Brilliant imperfection: Grappling with cure*. Duke University Press.

Davies, K. (1994). The tensions between process time and clock time in care-work. *Time & Society, 3*(3), 277–303.

Deleuze, G. (1988). *Bergsonism*. Zone Books.

Deleuze, G. (1994). Difference and repetition (P. Patton, Trans.). : Columbia University Press.

Deng, N. (2024). Eternity in Christian thought. In E. N. Zalta & U. Nodelman (Eds.) *The Stanford encyclopedia of philosophy* (Fall 2024 Edition) https://plato.stanford.edu/archives/fall2024/entries/eternity

Derrida, J. (1994). *Spectres of Marx* (P. Kamuf, Trans.). Routledge.

Ehlers, N., Broom, A., & Kenny, K. (2024). Living and dying in shadow times. *Sociology*, Online first.

Elias, N. (1992). *Time: An Essay*. Blackwell.

Frank, A. (2013). *The wounded storyteller: Body, illness, and ethics*. University of Chicago Press.

Fraser, N. (2016). Contradictions of capital and care. *New Left Review, 100*(Jul/Aug.), 99–117.

Freeman, E. (2010). *Time binds: Queer temporalities, queer histories*. Duke University Press.

Garland-Thomson, R. (2011). Misfits: A feminist materialist disability concept. *Hypatia, 26*(3), 591–609.

Giddens, A. (1991). *Modernity and self-identity: Self and Society in the Late Modern age*. Stanford University Press.

Grosz, E. (2005). *Time travels: Feminism, nature, power*. Duke University Press.

Grosz, E. (2020). *The nick of time: Politics, evolution and the untimely*. Routledge.

Halberstam, J. (2005). *In a queer time and place: Transgender bodies, subcultural bodies*. New York University Press.

Harrison, M., Lancaster, K., & Rhodes, T. (2022). "A matter of time": Evidence-making temporalities of vaccine development in the COVID-19 media landscape. *Time & Society, 31*(1), 132–154.

Harrison, M., Smith, A. K. J., & Adams, S. (2024). Matters of time in health and illness. *Health Sociology Review, 33*(1), 1–9.

Hochschild, A. (2001). *The time bind*. Metropolitan Books.

Hydén, L.-C. (1997). Illness and narrative. *Sociology of Health & Illness, 19*(1), 48–69.

Ihlebæk, H. M. (2021). Time to care—An ethnographic study of how temporal structuring affects caring relationships in clinical nursing. *Social Science & Medicine, 287*, 114349.

James, W., (1996). A pluralistic universe: Hibbert lectures at Manchester college on the present situation in philosophy (New Ed edition). University of Nebraska Press.

Kafer, A. (2013). *Feminist, queer, Crip*. Indiana University Press.

Kenny, K., Broom, A., Peterie, M., Bennett, J., & Broom, J. (2024). *Cultures of activity, cultivating resistance*. Qualitative Health Research.

Kristeva, J. (1981). Women's time. *Signs, 7*(11), 13–35.

Latour, B. (2008). What is the style of matters of concern? In N. Gaskill & A. J. Nocek (Eds.), *The lure of Whitehead* (pp. 92–126). University of Minnesota Press.

McGrath, A., Troy, A., & Rademaker, L. (2023). *Everywhen: Australia and the language of deep history*. University of Nebraska Press.

McRuer, R. (2006). *Crip theory: Cultural signs of queerness and disability*. New York University Press.

Miserandino, C. (2003). The spoon theory. But you don't look sick? https://butyoudontlooksick.com/articles/written-by-christine/the-spoon-theory/

Neale, B. (2021). *The craft of qualitative longitudinal research*. Sage.

Neale, B. (2022). Time and the Lifecourse. In N. Worth & I. Hardhill (Eds.), *Researching the Lifecourse*. Cambridge University Press.

Parsons, T. (1975). The sick role and the role of the physician reconsidered. The Milbank Memorial Fund quarterly. *Health and Society*, 257–278.

Pieri, M. (2023). *LGBTQ+ people with chronic illness: Chroniqueers in southern Europe*. Springer International Publishing.

Puig de la Bellacasa, M. (2017). *Matters of care: Speculative ethics in more than human worlds*. University of Minnesota Press.

Rosa, H. (2013). *Social acceleration: A new theory of modernity*. Columbia University Press.

Samuels, E. (2017). Six ways of looking at crip time. *Disability Studies Quarterly, 37*(3), Article 3.

Sheppard, E. (2023). *Chronic pain, BDSM and crip time*. Routledge.

Sheppard, E. (2024). *Chronic pain, BDSM and crip time*. Routledge.

Thompson, E. P. (1967). Time, work-discipline, and industrial capitalism. *Past & Present, 38*, 56–97.

Timmermans, S. (1998). Mutual tuning of multiple trajectories. *Symbolic Interaction, 21*(4), 425–440.

van Emmerik, C., Coleman, R., & Lyon, D. (2025). Towards a minor sociology of futures: Shifting futures in mass observation accounts of the COVID-19 pandemic. *Journal of Sociology, 61*(1).

Van Pijkeren, N., Schuurmans, J., Wallenburg, I., & Bal, R. (2024). "The night is for sleeping": How nurses care for conflicting temporal orders in older person care. *Health Sociology Review, 33*(1), 10–23.

Walby, S. (1984). *Patriarchy at work*. Polity Press.

Weber, M. (1972). *The Protestant ethic and the spirit of capitalism* (S. Kalberg, Trans.). Routledge.

Whitehead, A. N. (1967). *Science and the modern world* (Reissue edition). Free Press.

Whitehead, A. N. (1978). *Process and reality* (2nd ed.). Free Press.

Yunkaporta, T. (2023). *Sand talk: How indigenous thinking can save the world*. Text Publishing.

Yunkaporta, T. (2024). *Right story, wrong story: Adventures in indigenous thinking*. Text Publishing.

Part I

Duration and the Governance of Time

2

The Winged Power of Time in Outbreak Science

Marsha Rosengarten

> The only certainty is that it [a viral pandemic] will present extraordinary challenges. Many … are asking the multiple research and logistical questions needed to develop an appropriate response. Clearly, there is much to be accomplished, and *time is of the essence*. (My italics; Fauci, 2005, p. 423)

> With an outbreak like this, it's *a race against time*. One Ebola patient with symptoms can infect several people every day. (My italics; Jawor, 2018)

Refrains such as 'time is of the essence' and 'it's a race against time' have become almost mantra-like for the global health response to life-endangering infectious disease outbreaks. Time enables us to structure our thinking and acting—unquestionably, as it seems, with urgency when identifying an outbreak. Yet it is especially curious, separated from the events that make it matter. I am referring here to the self-evidency of linear, sequential, calculable time, achieved by the mechanical (now

M. Rosengarten (✉)
King's College London, London, UK

Department of Sociology, Goldsmiths, University of London, London, UK
e-mail: marsha.rosengarten@kcl.ac.uk

K. Kenny et al. (eds.), *Timescapes of Health, Illness and Care*,
https://doi.org/10.1007/978-981-96-7055-0_2

digital) clock. And, as stories go, the inspiration for mechanistic thought on which modern medicine was founded (Mumford, 1955). It remains the core explanatory mode for bodily infection—irrespective of whether it is 'communicable' or not. But do outbreaks of infectious diseases conform? And if they do, what makes them appear so? Or, to pose this another way, what exclusions does time require for its claim on reality?

For Catherine Houlihan (a specialist in virology and infectious diseases) and James Whitworth (a professor of international public health), an 'outbreak is defined as more cases of a disease than expected in a specific location over a specific time period' (2019, p. 140). This simple and altogether neat definition applies to all infectious disease outbreaks, including those regarded as repeats (for example, Ebola) and those said to be novel because they are new to biomedicine (for example, COVID-19). Houlihan and Whitworth follow their expert claim with stepwise principles for action: 'establish the presence of an outbreak, verify the diagnosis, make a case definition, find cases and contacts, conduct basic epidemiology, test hypotheses, institute control measures, communicate the situation and establish ongoing surveillance' (Houlihan & Whitworth, 2019, p. 141). These undertakings and also modes of anticipatory surveillance instituted to prevent or mitigate outbreaks are matched to a singular cause of urgency: the time-measured temporality of a replicating microbial substance. Mostly, the microbe is a virus that has 'jumped the species barrier' at a point in time which defines the infection as zoonotic.

The typical biomedical explanation for zoonotic infections is that they arise from 'molecular mechanisms driving … [microbial] emergence in animals,' which are then 'spread to humans' (Fauci, 2005, p. 423). This spread is achieved by 'chains of transmission' in and against sequences of time (Faye et al., 2015; Villandré et al., 2019; Bart et al., 2021). To be sure, without the locational affordance of time, it is difficult to imagine the biomedical and biomedically informed epidemiological facts sought to contain, if not eradicate, an infectious disease. Without this concept of time, it is also hard to imagine the politically potent evidence of our 'modern civilising ways' understood to be amplifying the rate and scale of zoonotic infectious diseases (Morens & Fauci, 2020; Chakrabarty, 2020; Gandy, 2022). Yet it is also evident that time is no neutral player. The idea of a forward-driving calculable time orients modes of health governance toward the future as if what is known of the past can foretell what will become (Savransky et al., 2017). This selective framing of an outbreak constitutes time-bound objects and events with the promise of an endgame (Lancaster & Rhodes, 2023). While critiques of time put to the test the response to outbreaks (see, for example, Adams et al., 2009; Leach et al., 2022), my hunch is that similar and further concerns about time can be applied to the prestated mechanistic formulation of infectious disease.

In what follows, I draw on aspects of process philosophy to show that there is a coterminous relationship between linear sequential time and mechanistic scientific thought. In the first part of this chapter, I set out what is meant by 'the winged power of time' and, by way of a brief historico-cultural background, the founding of a mechanistic science. While I do not suggest that this should lead us to reject scientific endeavours to mitigate infectious disease, it raises the question of what is presupposed as the materiality of objects and events. The strange power of what is evidenced as a fabricated notion of time is argued to naturalise a time-bound reality. In the second part, I shift focus from what may be regarded as a metaphysical argument to the decided actuality of COVID-19 and the infamy of Ebola achieved by the West African Ebola epidemic. I take up the provocation of COVID-19 as a 'wake-up' to our 'modern' civilising ways, which are leading to planetary destruction and exacerbating the emergence of zoonotic diseases. Not unlike what I go on to show as a problematic reliance on time in the biomedical formulation of COVID-19 and also Ebola, the same co-terminus relationship of linear time and spatially oriented mechanistic thought is central to planetary 'time running out.' I conclude that because clock (digital) time is a fabrication of human thought, it is within our powers of thought to situate it and, thus, the response to outbreaks differently.

Time as Space and the Curious Play of Stasis

It is possible to find numerous examples of how the word 'time' is deployed and what may be understood as its commonsense meaning. However, it is the last definition provided by the *Long Oxford Dictionary* that is most encompassing of what informs the definition of outbreaks and underpins the formulation of infection: 'a limited stretch or *space* of continued existence, as the *interval* between two successive events or acts, or the period through which an action, condition, or *state* continues; a finite portion of "time" (in its infinite sense)' (my italics). In light of this conception of time, it may not surprise that Henri Bergson, arguably most well-known for his philosophy of time, was provoked to observe: 'When we evoke time, it is space that answers our call' (Bergson, 1946, p. 4). His appraisal is directed chiefly at the intellectualism of philosophy, which he viewed as overly abstract and, thus, unable to consider the heterogeneous creative flow and flux of existence. By contrast, he makes an allowance for the natural sciences because, unlike philosophy, its mistaking of space for time is consistent with what it presupposes as its objects of inquiry. It fits the scientific mission to foresee, according to which the spatialisation of time enables objects and events to be imagined as if 'repetitious and calculable'(1946, pp. 1, 2). Nevertheless, this does not exempt it from critique.

Writing in agreement with Bergson on the spatialisation of time and the inspiration for the title of this chapter, the pluralist and pragmatic philosopher William James says the idea that time can be divided into serial periods and points (spaces) omits the creative connection between things: 'with our faculty of abstracting and fixing concepts we are there in a second, almost as if we controlled a fourth dimension, skipping the intermediaries as by *a divine winged power*, and getting at the exact point we require without entanglement with any context' (1996, pp. 247/8; my italics). By trading what James proposes as felt time, which he says comes in 'drops' likened to the duration of pulses that 'compenetrate each other,' for discrete points and periods, we are able 'to harness up reality in our conceptual system in order to drive it better' (1996, pp. 232 and 247/8). However, when accepted without question, we are led to believe that, at some point, things are 'absolutely static' (1996, p. 234).

Although this critique of time can be traced to Ancient Greek thought, more immediately pertinent to the focus of this chapter is the legacy of the European Enlightenment when the workings of the mechanistic clock inspired the scientific imaginary. Early sundials for tracking solar time were matched to the variability in the Earth's rotation due to events such as earthquakes and, now more so, global warming (Agnew, 2024;

France-Presse, 2022; Public Health England, 2020), whereas contained time became possible with the use of devices such as water clocks, sandglasses, and candles. These devices no longer tracked to solar time. Nevertheless, they were concrete in their direct measure. Needless to say, none were so proficient nor so abstract in their claim of time as the mechanical clock. According to the conceptual historian Reinhardt Koselleck, by the thirteenth century, the clock 'had already affected a new organisation of the human division of time over the long term.' By the sixteenth century, it could indicate minutes and, by the seventeenth century, seconds (Koselleck, 2002, pp. 103, 104). Paradoxically, the more precise, the more apart from the happenings that informed its relevance. As Lewis Mumford (1955, p. 15) says in his historical study of technology and material culture: 'by its essential nature [the mechanistic clock during the period of the Enlightenment] … disassociated time from human events and helped create the belief in an independent world of mathematically measurable sequences: the special world of science.'

Of the many mathematical 'geniuses' whose legacy continues to prevail in 'the special world of science' and, no less, a mechanistic spatial imaginary, René Descartes and Isaac Newton have earned particular acclaim. Having distinguished human reason as a feature of the mind, Descartes was able to conceive of bodies as composed of obtuse mechanistic parts: 'I know that animals do many things better than we do, but this does not surprise me. It can even be used to prove they act naturally and mechanically, like a clock which tells the time better than our judgement does' (Descartes, 1989, p. 64). Precisely what he meant by this statement is contested. Jessica Riskin stresses that we should not mistake his mechanistic thought to mean that bodies were analogous to a clockwork mechanism but that they, like all of nature, function as a machine: 'clockwork represented a mode of intelligibility rather than the particular machinery of life' (2018, p. 55). Nevertheless, 'while not advocating a cogged machine per se,' Stephen Snobelen (2012, p. 152) notes that Descartes was 'fond of describing animals as clocks and humans as clocks with souls.' Although some have mistakenly attributed Newton with the idea that God was the clockmaker of a regular and predictable universe, he remains famed for having devised a closed mechanistic system whereby all of existence could be explained by predictive laws (Newton et al., 2016).

In the words of the theoretical biologist Stuart Kauffman (2016, p. xii): 'Descartes unleashed the scientific objective worldview, culminating somewhat more than a century later with Newton and the creation of classical physics.... [according to which] all could be, in principle known and mastered, mystery gone.' While Kauffman is careful to acknowledge that the mechanistic mode of scientific thought may provide answers to some of its questions, his research leads him to align his critique of mechanistic thought with Alfred North Whitehead's speculative philosophy. Although there are clear resonances with the thought of Bergson and James, as outlined above, one statement by Whitehead may suffice at this stage for encapsulating the problem inherited from the likes of Descartes and Newton: 'There is no holding nature still and looking at it' (Whitehead, 1920, p. 10). It is precisely what is at stake in what Bergson says of the scientific mission to foresee and James' superbly eloquent account of the stasis making by a 'divine winged power.'[1] Nonetheless, some readers might well ask: How, then, does the aspiration to know nature and, as pertains to this chapter, to mitigate infectious disease succeed even if only in degree?

On this score there is no mystery, although due to a different kind of reasoning to that of Descartes and Newton. According to Whitehead, all things engage in modes of abstraction. For instance, a plant abstracts water from the soil, a rock abstracts heat from the sun, and scientific inquiry abstracts objects and events from an insistent flux and flow of creativity: '[w]e cannot think without abstractions' (Whitehead, 1967, p. 73). Indeed, it is the mode of abstraction that provides a situation with purpose and effectivity (Halewood, 2011, p. 6). Since abstractions cannot be avoided, they are not for refuting. Rather, they require care for what they are. Which is to say, we should not mistake what they vectorise as if concreteness, as can be said of scientific abstractions that vectorise closed conceptions of time, nature, and, thus, infection (Whitehead,

[1] It is beyond the scope of this chapter to elaborate the overlaps and divergences between Whitehead, Bergson, and James. However, to avoid confusion, although Whitehead agrees with Bergson's claim that we mistake space for time, he does not share Bergson's rejection of intellectualism, and this is evident in many other aspects of his cosmological approach, including what I shall come to of the work of abstraction. By contrast, Whitehead's appreciation for the creativity of feeling or 'prehending' along with his pragmatism aligns with James. See *Process and Reality* (Whitehead, 1978), or, for a lucid account of his philosophy with reference to Bergson and James, see Debaise (2017).

1967, p. 51; Rosengarten & Savransky, 2018). Amongst the few who have applied Whitehead's philosophy to infectious disease and specifically in reference to COVID-19, John Dupré and Sabina Leonelli (2022, p. 19) state: 'Any attempt to stabilise viral infections enough to be able to study them requires procedures that we call "reification" consisting in the identification and treatment of relevant features of the world as stable things for the purposes of inquiry.' They continue, 'thus disregarding their 'volatile, changeable nature.'

In the remainder of this chapter, I pursue this critique by asking: What are the consequences of assuming non-human entities share our compliance in thought and action with what is known in the name of time? Which is to also ask: What is the price paid for assuming our human endurance and perishing conforms 'to getting at the exact point we require without entanglement with any context' (James, 1996, pp. 247/8)?

COVID-19 Time

A striking feature of the early phase of the COVID-19 pandemic was the call for new modes of scientific thinking to generate biological and epidemiological facts (Ghebreyesus & Swaminathan, 2020). More expansively, others saw the pandemic as a wake-up call to our 'modern' civilising modes that are wreaking planetary destruction. As many of us watched the global count of lives lost to COVID-19 infection clocked on a John Hopkins University website,[2] the political theorist/social commentator Dipesh Chakrabarty (2020) wrote: 'Our history in recent decades has been that of the Great Acceleration and expansion of the global economy … From the point of view of the virus, however, the environmental disturbance this has caused, and the fact of human global mobility have been welcome developments.' Situating COVID-19 as representative of a moment in the history of biological life when humans are acting as the 'amplifiers of a virus,' Chakrabarty joined a growing number of scholars and institutions who share the view that the recorded rise in outbreaks of

[2] John Hopkins University tracker map https://coronavirus.jhu.edu/map.html. Data collection ceased on 3rd October 2023.

infectious diseases cannot be separated from the ills of modernity: poverty, deforestation, agricultural intensification and the commodification of animals, urbanisation, and global mobility (Gandy, 2022; Hinchliffe, 2015; Wolf, 2016).

Tackling the refrain 'When can we return to normal?' frequently asked in response to modes of social containment intended to mitigate the spread of COVID-19, the novelist Arundhati Roy (2020) proposed that COVID-19 presented a 'portal': 'even while the virus proliferates, who could not be thrilled by the swell of birdsong in cities, peacocks dancing at traffic crossings and the silence in the skies? … unlike the flow of capital, this virus seeks proliferation, not profit, and has, therefore, inadvertently, to some extent, reversed the direction of the flow.' Having described in horrific detail the tragic US situation under the Trump regime and that in India under Modi with its colonial past, Roy continued in a somewhat optimistic mode, '[i]n the midst of this terrible despair, [the COVID-19 pandemic] offers us a chance to rethink the doomsday machine we have built for ourselves. Nothing could be worse than a return to normality.'

Whether there can be a return to a before may be a moot point, but what should we make of the sentiment that it should be possible? Insofar as we might mock those who ask for a return to a before, is it so out of kilter with the abstraction of time which enables clocks to go back to maximise sunlight in summer or, as is now familiar, the future forecasting of events on the presupposition that objects and events repeat, as if conformal to the spatial points and periods of linear time? While we can appreciate Chakrabarty's mention that humans are acting as amplifiers of the virus, and, as Roy captures it, 'the doomsday machine we have built for ourselves,' might we consider that the image of time is a key player while, paradoxically, excluding itself from critique?

In *The Nick of Time: Politics, Evolution, and the Untimely*, published prior to the pandemic, Elizabeth Grosz (2004, p. 4) noted how our strangely settled conception of time provokes thought only 'when we are jarred out of immersion in its continuity, when something untimely disrupts expectations.' The observation resonates with the frequent COVID-19 phrase, 'we've all lost track of time' and, as the journalist George Dillard (2021) also wrote: 'We feel like we are swimming in an ocean of time—while being surrounded by machines that make us acutely aware of it—and we weren't prepared.' Having exposed how the rule of mechanistic time and capitalism that orders our everyday lives was disrupted by modes of social containment, Dillard's pithy article suggests that the fabricated order of time has become so naturalised that it not only infects our expectations but, without it, we feel oddly out of sync. Our cultural investment in the continuity of 'clock' time—the abstraction of objects and events without entanglement—leads us to expect a return to a 'before' and, no wonder, because life is merely a matter of spatial repeats until, simply put, we die.

Yet, whatever has been known and continues to be learnt of COVID-19 and, as I shall come to with Ebola, its ever-evolving volatile nature has exceeded its fact in 'winged time.' Of the many stories that can be told of COVID-19, arguably the most prominent is its origin in the Chinese city of Wuhan and due to a (still-to-be-identified) 'species jump.' It emerged from the identification of unusual pneumonia cases, which were later linked to the morphology of a virus that resembled a previously classified coronavirus known to cause contagious respiratory disease. This reification of the virus, presented as a spatial entity with spikes, laid the ground for what could be expected of its consequences. Nevertheless, this has been of little guide to what a body may do with it (Stein et al., 2022; Rosengarten, 2021). Questions continue on the significance of its asymptomatic infection for ongoing transmission (Escandón et al., 2021, p. 15), who is most calculably at risk for severe and possibly fatal consequences (Bristow & Borthwick, 2020; Public Health England, 2020), and what enables it to endure for many more days than the statistical norm correlated with the morphology (in one case, 220 days) (Stein et al., 2022). The debilitating 'after' of 'Long COVID' in the absence of the virus also continues to confound biomedicine (see Callard, 2020; Michelen et al., 2021).

While these uncertainties have furnished a growing field of scientific inquiry, they were put aside by public health authorities whose primary task was to contain viral spread at a population level. Epidemiological models of R_0 (the basic reproduction number) and R (the effective reproduction rate) as guides to 'flatten the curve' (of an epidemic spread by 'chains of transmission') over a set period became 'ubiquitous as tools of anticipatory governance' (Rhodes et al., 2020, p. 253). Although many countries relied on these models to determine the timing and length of circuit-breaking social lockdowns, those producing them were acutely aware that their predictive calculation was never precise (Rhodes & Lancaster, 2022). It is now evident that the aim of 'foreseeing' required excluding the unforeseeable consequences of lockdowns (see, for example, the British Academy, 2021; Buheji et al., 2020). In short, the accuracy of R_0 was always contingent on a nexus of dynamic factors but taken as a politically expedient 'fact' for policymaking (Adam, 2020). Which is to say, the mathematic models were often adopted as an accurate determination, as if evidence of what is known (from the past) could be mathematically synthesised to enable acting in the present on the presupposition that the future will conform (Rhodes et al., 2020; Savransky et al., 2017). Needless to say, despite the continuing questions about the infection, the reified notion of a replicating morphological substance has not been questioned.

Parallel with social lockdowns, an armoury of research pursued an effective vaccine. While no scientist promised a magic bullet, the public was assured that vaccination against the virus would end the pandemic and a return to 'normal' life. To the surprise of vaccine advocates, the arrival of vaccines was not uniformly welcomed. Indeed, there was an irony to the reliance on measures of linear time to verify their research. In a study of how public media enacted COVID-19 vaccine development, Mia Harrison et al. (2021) argue that time became an 'ontopolitical concern' among public assessments of vaccines. For those who had conducted time-bound 'gold standard' randomised control trials, there was no doubt that vaccines were statistically efficacious and safe (Bhide et al., 2018; Michael & Rosengarten, 2013). However others, sharing the same concept of time, questioned the validity of the findings because it was seen as 'too short.' To date, the global health view is that vaccination is generally safe, although its timed efficacy remains uncertain. Recorded 'adverse events' following vaccination have been excluded according to the future forecasting probability that the benefit of vaccination outweighs its risk. Growing evidence of mutating virus thought to undermine vaccine efficacy is addressed by the provision of repeatedly adjusted vaccine 'boosters.' Yet, here again, the drive to certainty affixed to the causality of a distinct morphological substance appears to be unravelling.

The current hope of health governance is that while 'boosters' may not prevent infection, they may reduce the potential for long COVID and fatalities (Català et al., 2024).

If we accept Houlihan and Whitworth's (2019) epidemiological definition of outbreaks 'as more cases of a disease than expected in a specific location over a specific period,' the declaration in May 2023 by WHO that the pandemic has ended is correct. Nevertheless, it is not gone. The accompanying statement by WHO Director-General Ghebreyesus acknowledged this, although only in part: 'It is still killing and it is still changing. The risk remains of new variants emerging that cause new surges in cases and deaths.' Nevertheless, a downward trend in the time-reckoning of numbers was seen to justify a 'return to life as we knew it before COVID-19' (UN News, 2023). The fact that COVID-19 is now regarded as endemic may lead us to assume that what is not gone is the reified virus. However, as Kari Lancaster and Tim Rhodes (2023) remind us, the spatial presence of the virus is not all that should concern us. What *has* happened cannot be erased from what becomes. While the image of objects and events—presented as conforming to a fabricated reality—allows us to view the world as composed of locatable entities that move, mutate, and come to a finite end, it refutes their potentiality and possibilities (Debaise, 2017). Undoubtedly, the reification of distinct substances (viruses, bodies, vaccines, social lockdowns) as if correlative with spaces of time has enabled science to make a difference, the 'new variants' are isolated features of mechanistic reductionism. As if we exist in a first order of static 'things,' as James says, without intermediaries and, as Whitehead says, can be mythically held for view.

Ebola Time

The 'race against time' expressed by Paul Jawor at the beginning of this chapter was made during an Ebola outbreak in the Democratic Republic of Congo. However, the refrain gained earlier currency due to the West African Ebola epidemic, when approximately 28,600 people were infected or suspected of being infected with the Ebola virus, and 11,325 died during the official dating of 2014–2016 (WHO Ebola Response Team, 2016).

Many factors are said to have contributed to the number of cases and the geographical scope of the epidemic. The World Health Organisation (WHO) has since acknowledged its failure 'to act in time.' It assumed Ebola would repeat the pattern of previous outbreaks thought to conform to prior time-designated events: short-lived, geographically confined to a specific area and, hence, a predictable limited number of fatalities. Consequently, the outbreak reached an unprecedented scale across the porous boundaries of Guinea, Liberia, and Sierra Leone (Medecins Sans Frontieres, 2015). In their review of the epidemic, anthropologist Melissa Leach and colleagues (2021, pp. 3, 4) state: 'Initially ignored by the international community – based on assumptions that Ebola is "too deadly" to generate large outbreaks – the social circumstances of the outbreak [regional conflicts, fragile health systems and postcolonial mistrust] soon showed that complacency was unwise.' Indeed, a complacency that stemmed from 'linear assumptions and predictions of epidemiological models [which] did not align with the region's embedded entanglements.'

I will not attempt to rehearse Leach and colleagues' detailed commentary and those of many others who witnessed first hand the extreme militarised strategies of containment and mass anonymous burials entangled with and amplified by gross health and socio-economic inequities (see, for example, Fairhead, 2016; Kutalek et al., 2015; Medecins Sans Frontieres, 2015; Mullan, 2014). It is unlikely that any person who lived through the hellishness of the epidemic would dispute that many of the deaths resulted not from the awfulness of the disease but from the efforts to contain it. Yet the demand for containment by health authorities took precedence, claiming those who did not conform as ignorant due to 'premodern' beliefs (Chandler et al., 2015; Richards, 2016). In a review of the Ebola epidemic, the WHO Ebola Response Team (2016, p. 594) stated: 'In the long tail of the epidemic, foci of transmission persisted for many months … where symptomatic patients were unwilling to seek medical care, where contacts of patients fled quarantine, and where deaths from EVD were followed by unsafe burials.' Based on this perspective, they concluded that future efforts to mitigate Ebola would need to focus on achieving compliance with biomedical and epidemiological facts that the article itself acknowledged were incorrect.

Earlier, I asked whether non-human entities share our compliance with periodised, spatial time or, for that matter, whether our human endurance and perishing conform 'to getting at the exact point we require without entanglement with any context' (James, 1996, p. 247/8). I have endeavoured to show how the premise of serial time and the mechanistic explanatory mode that is its fit delimited an appreciation of the processual (flow and flux) nature of COVID-19 infection. While modes of containment are surely necessary to sever the connections that enable infectious disease, the starting premise is that connections are epiphenomenal to a world whose first order is composed of distinct entities. Here, I will be more explicit about the consequences of this premise and but also where new imaginings might emerge from the interstices of scientific research and epidemiological dating.

As noted above, the official period of the West African Ebola epidemic is 2014–2016. However, reaching this finite claim required two revisions due to the emergence of new infections after 42 days, twice the maximum amount of time expected for incubation of Ebola Viral Disease (EVD) (Centers for Disease Control and Prevention, 2019). These cases overturned the assumption that infection is restricted to chains of transmission from someone with EVD. The *New Scientist* reported that 'researchers have now discovered how the virus …completely *shuts down and doesn't even replicate* – something never seen before in this type of virus.' Further on, the same article referred to the genetic structure of Ebola: 'Analysing 294 more sequences, the [researchers] … found 15 that were similarly *out of sync with their times*' (Mackenzie, 2016; my italics). The expression 'out of sync' was undoubtedly used colloquially but the same conclusion appeared in peer-reviewed scientific publications (Blackley et al., 2016; Jacobs et al., 2016). It underscores the unwitting epistemic violence that arises from presupposing our fabricated reality of time as fact and not merely as provisional and, thus, questionable affordance. Not surprisingly but no less worrying, the finding that Ebola has not conformed to the locational work of time parallels the finding that COVID-19 has not behaved as expected.

As is usual, the biomedical and epidemiological facts of Ebola have been reviewed. It is now known to be transmitted from 'immune-privileged' sites, notably semen, the eye, breast milk, urine, and vaginal secretions, all without necessarily showing expression as EVD (Racine & Kobinger, 2017). Yet, although the facts of Ebola have been subject to biomedical revision—as can also be said of COVID-19—they have not provoked scientists to question a tenuous morphological ontology hitched to the wings or, to be more specific, dated/spatial time. Nor, I add, has it provoked reflection on how a delimited biomedical conception of Ebola disqualified other modes of knowing judged as mistaken or ignorant.

I will finish this albeit brief discussion with two further accounts of Ebola. The first is the official story of Ebola's dated beginning, said to have begun in December 2013 when a two-year-old boy contracted the virus (possibly from contact with bats) and died two days later, having passed the virus on in his Guinean village located close to the porous borders of Libera and Sierra Leone (WHO, n.d.). It resembles the conventional narrative of zoonotic origins to explain all infectious disease outbreaks (see Wald, 2008). Which is to say, it renders the world to fit the scientific mission to foresee. The species jump and the originary tale of the boy's death precisely 'two days' after infection conformed to and confirmed what was prestated of Ebola—now shown to be worryingly insufficient. The second story was relayed to the anthropologist James Fairhead (2019) by a local health worker from the same village as the 'ground zero' boy. According to the health worker, before the boy's death, a woman called Fanta came and went on two occasions with months in between to visit a healer for a rash (rashes are now included in the list of symptoms). She was healed and went back to Sierra Leone, and then returned for more treatment. She lived with the boy's family and died of Ebola sometime later. Fairhead says it is not the only story circulating among village members. I introduce it, having primarily focused on what I call 'top-down' knowledge-making, because it goes to the heart of what I have sought to dramatise about time.

Like Fairhead, I do not want to privilege the second story over others that might be told by the many witnesses of Ebola. However, when contrasted with the official story of origins, it tells us that there may be other ways of knowing, having drawn from the actuality of what an infection can do. It offers an otherwise to the time-bound conception of Ebola that led to the surprise of biomedicine. Indeed, it might have furnished biomedicine with an awareness of what it only later came to realise after immense suffering and loss. While infectious disease in the general is an intractable problem, we are left with the question of whether there might be an otherwise to the authorised approach decided by what has been claimed of time.

Conclusion

Refrains such as 'acting in time,' 'racing against time,' and 'time is of the essence' as well as 'time is running out' call for action. However, if time were truly a transcendent linear passage apart from happenings that nevertheless conform to its sequential spatial points and periods, surely assuaging infectious diseases would be more straightforward. Their zoonotic origin, amplified by our civilising ways, would demand very little if, at some point, cause (microbe) and effect (disease) were 'absolutely static' and replicable. Indeed, it is hard to imagine their happening or that of our human-engineered 'planetary doom.' In contradistinction, I return to Whitehead (1920, pp. 43, 44). Having made clear that while scientific theory relies on measurable time, it also limits our awareness of the creativity of experience—a continuity of the difference arising from enduring and perishing; he offers his readers a decision: 'We have first to make up our minds whether time is to be found in nature or nature is to be found in time? The difficulty of the latter alternative – namely of making time prior to nature – is that time then becomes a metaphysical enigma. What sort of entities are its instants or its periods?' To this, he proposes: 'There is time because there are happenings, and apart from happenings there is nothing.'

Those invested in the scientific mission to foresee might rightly ask: What would this mean for the spatial facts of their evidence-making and the effective, at least by degrees, interventions that help to alleviate our ills? Indeed, we may recall that although James condemns the obfuscation of connections by the 'divine winged power' of time, he also recognises its affordance for thinking and acting. Hence, rather than presume that time should or can be jettisoned, Whitehead's proposal leads me to ask whether we might appreciate time for what it is: more akin to a tool or technology.

As with any technology, the fit of 'winged time' to the task remains an open question. However, more so than other technologies whose faltering at a task may be more conspicuously *out of line*, what I have endeavoured to dramatise in this chapter is how *it* decides the line. When mistaken as a mirror of existence, its indiscriminate determinations and disqualifications render other realities extraneous or merely false. By attending to its 'divine' powers and its winged transcendence over us, we have within our powers of thought the affordance of becoming more attuned to the challenge of our inquiries. At the very least, we have the affordance of becoming more attuned to the perceptible and imperceptible *potential* of what time 'on our hands'—an especially odd little refrain, but perhaps the point of this chapter—currently elides or disqualifies: the immanent connections that make possible infection for severing and the now-made-possible planetary destruction amplifying it.

Acknowledgements I would like to thank Mia Harrison as an editor of the collection, Amanda Caleb as a contributor, and my valued colleague Nele Jensen, for their instructive comments on an earlier version of this chapter.

Competing Interests The author has no conflicts of interest to declare that are relevant to the content of this chapter.

References

Adam, D. (2020). Special report: The simulations driving the world's response to COVID-19. *Nature, 580*, 316–318. https://doi.org/10.1038/d41586-020-01003-6

Adams, V., Murphy, M., & Clarke, A. (2009). Anticipation: Technoscience, life, affect, temporality. *Subjectivity, 28*, 246–265. https://doi.org/10.1057/sub.2009.18

Agnew, D. C. (2024). A global timekeeping problem postponed by global warming. Nature 1–4. https://doi.org/10.1038/s41586-024-07170-0.

Bart, S. M., Flaherty, E., Alpert, T., Carlson, S., Fasulo, L., Earnest, R., White, E. B., Dickens, N., Brito, A. F., Grubaugh, N. D., Hadler, J. L., & Sosa, L. E. (2021). Multiple transmission chains within COVID-19 cluster, Connecticut, USA, 2020. *Emerging Infectious Diseases, 27*, 2669–2672. https://doi.org/10.3201/eid2710.211196

Bergson, H. (1946). *Creative mind: An introduction to metaphysics*. Dover Publications, Inc.

Bhide, A., Shah, P. S., & Acharya, G. (2018). A simplified guide to randomized controlled trials. *Acta Obstetricia et Gynecologica Scandinavica, 97*, 380–387. https://doi.org/10.1111/aogs.13309

Blackley, D. J., Wiley, M. R., Ladner, J. T., Fallah, M., Lo, T., Gilbert, M. L., Gregory, C., D'ambrozio, J., Coulter, S., Mate, S., Balogun, Z., Kugelman, J., Nwachukwu, W., Prieto, K., Yeiah, A., Amegashie, F., Kearney, F., Wisniewski, M., Saindon, J., ... Palacios, G. (2016). Reduced evolutionary rate in reemerged Ebola virus transmission chains. *Science Advances, 2*, e1600378. https://doi.org/10.1126/sciadv.1600378

Bristow, I. R., & Borthwick, A. M. (2020). The mystery of the COVID toes—Turning evidence-based medicine on its head. *Journal of Foot and Ankle Research, 13*, 1–2. https://doi.org/10.1186/s13047-020-00408-w

Buheji, M., da Costa Cunha, K., Beka, G., Mavrić, B., do Carmo de Souza, Y.L., Souza da Costa Silva, S., Hanafi, M., & Chetia Yein, T. (2020). The Extent of COVID-19 Pandemic Socio-Economic Impact on Global Poverty. A Global Integrative Multidisciplinary Review. *American Journal of Economics, 10*, 213–224. https://doi.org/10.5923/j.economics.20201004.02

Callard, F. (2020). Very, very mild: Covid-19 symptoms and illness classification. *Somatosphere*. Retrieved June 5, 2020, from http://somatosphere.net/2020/mild-covid.html

Català, M., Mercadé-Besora, N., Kolde, R., Trinh, N. T. H., Roel, E., Burn, E., Rathod-Mistry, T., Kostka, K., Man, W. Y., Delmestri, A., Nordeng, H. M. E., Uusküla, A., Duarte-Salles, T., Prieto-Alhambra, D., & Jödicke, A. M. (2024). The effectiveness of COVID-19 vaccines to prevent long COVID symptoms: Staggered cohort study of data from the UK, Spain, and Estonia. *The Lancet Respiratory Medicine, 12*, 225–236. https://doi.org/10.1016/S2213-2600(23)00414-9

Centers for Disease Control and Prevention (CDC). (2019). History of Ebola virus disease [WWW Document]. Retrieved January 23, 2021, from https://www.cdc.gov/vhf/ebola/history/summaries.html/

Chakrabarty, D. (2020). An era of pandemics? What is global and what is planetary about COVID-19. *In the Moment*. Retrieved June 11, 2020, from https://critinq.wordpress.com/2020/10/16/an-era-of-pandemics-what-is-global-and-what-is-planetary-about-covid-19/

Chandler, C., Fairhead, J., Kelly, A., Leach, M., Martineau, F., Mokuwa, E., Parker, M., Richards, P., & Wilkinson, A. (2015). Ebola: Limitations of correcting misinformation. *The Lancet, 385*, 1275–1277. https://doi.org/10.1016/S0140-6736(14)62382-5

Debaise, D. (2017). *Nature as event: The lure of the possible*. Duke University Press.

Descartes, R. (1989). Animals are machines. In *Animal rights and human obligations*. Pearson.

Dillard, G. (2021). How the clock came to rule modern life [WWW Document]. *Medium*. Retrieved December 24, 2021, from https://historyofyesterday.com/how-the-clock-came-to-rule-modern-life-837fba795920

Dupré, J., & Leonelli, S. (2022). Process epistemology in the COVID-19 era: Rethinking the research process to avoid dangerous forms of reification. *European Journal for Philosophy of Science, 12*, 20–20. https://doi.org/10.1007/s13194-022-00450-4

Escandón, K., Rasmussen, A. L., Bogoch, I. I., Murray, E. J., Escandón, K., Popescu, S. V., & Kindrachuk, J. (2021). COVID-19 false dichotomies and a comprehensive review of the evidence regarding public health, COVID-19 symptomatology, SARS-CoV-2 transmission, mask wearing, and reinfection. *BMC Infectious Diseases, 21*, 710. https://doi.org/10.1186/s12879-021-06357-4

Fairhead, J. (2016). Understanding social resistance to the Ebola response in the forest region of the Republic of Guinea: An anthropological perspective. *African Studies Review, 59*, 7–31. https://doi.org/10.1017/asr.2016.87

Fairhead, J. (2019). Is the Ebola Reservoir in people? The idea of "Patient Zero" in the narration and comparative analysis of (Ebola) epidemic origins. Paper delivered at London School of Hygiene and Tropical Medicine.

Fauci, A. S. (2005). Race against time. *Nature, 435*, 423–424.

Faye, O., Boëlle, P.-Y., Heleze, E., Faye, O., Loucoubar, C., Magassouba, N., Soropogui, B., Keita, S., Gakou, T., Bah, E. H. I., Koivogui, L., Sall, A. A., & Cauchemez, S. (2015). Chains of transmission and control of Ebola virus disease in Conakry, Guinea, in 2014: An observational study. *The Lancet Infectious Diseases, 15*, 320–326. https://doi.org/10.1016/S1473-3099(14)71075-8

France-Presse, A. (2022, November 18). Do Not Adjust Your Clock: Scientists Call Time on the Leap Second. *The Guardian*. https://www.theguardian.com/world/2022/nov/18/do-not-adjust-your-clock-scientists-call-time-on-theleap-second

Gandy, M. (2022). The Zoonotic City: Urban political ecology and the pandemic imaginary. *International Journal of Urban and Regional Research, 46*, 202–219. https://doi.org/10.1111/1468-2427.13080

Ghebreyesus, T. A., & Swaminathan, S. (2020). Scientists are sprinting to outpace the novel coronavirus. *The Lancet.* https://doi.org/10.1016/S0140-6736(20)30420-7

Grosz, E. (2004). *The nick of time: Politics, evolution, and the untimely.* Duke University Press Books.

Halewood, M. (2011). *A.N. Whitehead and social theory: Tracing a culture of thought.* Anthem Press.

Harrison, M., Lancaster, K., & Rhodes, T. (2021). 'A matter of time': Evidence-making temporalities of vaccine development in the COVID-19 media landscape. *Time & Society,* 0961463X211032201. https://doi.org/10.1177/0961463X211032201

Hinchliffe, S. (2015). More than one world, more than one health: Re-configuring interspecies health. *Social Science & Medicine, 1982*(129), 28–35. https://doi.org/10.1016/j.socscimed.2014.07.007

Houlihan, C. F., & Whitworth, J. A. (2019). Outbreak science: Recent progress in the detection and response to outbreaks of infectious diseases. *Clinical Medicine (Lond),* 19, 140–144. https://doi.org/10.7861/clinmedicine.19-2-140.

Jacobs, M., Rodger, A. Bell, D. J., Bhagani, S., Cropley, I., Filipe, A., Gifford, R. J., Hopkins, S., Hughes, J., Jabeen, F., Johannessen, I., Karageorgopoulos, D., Lackenby, A., Lester, R., Liu, R. S. N., MacConnachie, A., Mahungu, T., Martin, D., Marshall, N., Thomson, E. C. (2016). Late Ebola virus relapse causing meningoencephalitis: a case report. *The Lancet, 388,* 498–503. https://doi.org/10.1016/S0140-6736(16)30386-5

James, W. (1996). A pluralistic universe: Hibbert lectures at Manchester college on the present situation in philosophy (New Ed.). University of Nebraska Press.

Jawor, P. (2018). Fighting Ebola in DRC: A race against time [WWW Document]. Retrieved March 8, 2019, from https://www.msf.org.uk/article/fighting-ebola-drc-race-against-time

Kauffman, S. A. (2016). *Humanity in a creative universe.* OUP USA.

Koselleck, R. (2002). *The practice of conceptual history: Timing history, spacing concepts* (Illustrated edition). Stanford University Press.

Kutalek, R., Wang, S., Fallah, M., Wesseh, C. S., & Gilbert, J. (2015). Ebola interventions: Listen to communities. *The Lancet Global Health, 3,* e131. https://doi.org/10.1016/S2214-109X(15)70010-0

Lancaster, K., & Rhodes, T. (2023). Problematising the emergence of outbreak science in the governance of global health: Making time for slow dis-ease. *Critical Public Health, 33,* 838–847. https://doi.org/10.1080/09581596.2023.2232523

Leach, M., MacGregor, H., Scoones, I., & Wilkinson, A. (2021). Post-pandemic transformations: How and why COVID-19 requires us to rethink development World Development. *World Development, 138*, 105233. https://doi.org/10.1016/j.worlddev.2020.105233

Leach, M., MacGregor, H., Ripoll, S., Scoones, I., & Wilkinson, A. (2022). Rethinking disease preparedness: Incertitude and the politics of knowledge. *Critical Public Health, 32*, 82–96. https://doi.org/10.1080/09581596.2021.1885628

Mackenzie, Deborah. (2016). Ebola virus does a total shutdown to hide before a fresh strike [WWW Document]. *New Scientist*. Retrieved March 22, 2018, from https://www.newscientist.com/article/2086498-ebola-virus-does-a-total-shutdown-to-hide-before-a-fresh-strike/

Medecins Sans Frontieres. (2015). *Ebola pushed to the limit and beyond*. https://www.msf.org.uk/sites/uk/files/ebola_-_pushed_to_the_limit_and_beyond.pdf

Michael, M., & Rosengarten, M. (2013). *Innovation and biomedicine: Ethics, evidence and expectation in HIV* (1st ed.). Palgrave Macmillan.

Michelen, M., Manoharan, L., Elkheir, N., Cheng, V., Dagens, A., Hastie, C., O'Hara, M., Suett, J., Dahmash, D., Bugaeva, P., Rigby, I., Munblit, D., Harriss, E., Burls, A., Foote, C., Scott, J., Carson, G., Olliaro, P., Sigfrid, L., & Stavropoulou, C. (2021). Characterising long COVID: A living systematic review. *BMJ Global Health, 6*(9), e005427. https://doi.org/10.1136/bmjgh-2021-005427

Morens, D. M., & Fauci, A. S. (2020). Emerging pandemic diseases: How we got to COVID-19. *Cell, 182*, 1077–1092. https://doi.org/10.1016/j.cell.2020.08.021

Mullan, Z. (2014). Ebola: The missing link. *The Lancet Global Health, 2*, e550. https://doi.org/10.1016/S2214-109X(14)70278-5

Mumford, L. (1955). *Technics and civilization*. Routledge and Kegan Paul Ltd.

Newton, I., Cohen, I. B., Whitman, A., & Budenz, J. (2016). The principia: The authoritative translation: Mathematical principles of natural philosophy (Illustrated edition). University of California Press.

Public Health England. (2020). Disparities in the risk and outcomes from COVID-19. https://www.gov.uk/government/publications/covid-19-review-of-disparities-in-risks-and-outcomes

Racine, T., & Kobinger, G. P. (2017). Viral pathogenesis: Unlocking Ebola persistence. *Nature Microbiology, 2*, 1–2. https://doi.org/10.1038/nmicrobiol.2017.124

Rhodes, T., & Lancaster, K. (2022). Making pandemics big: On the situational performance of Covid-19 mathematical models. *Social Science & Medicine, 301*, 114907. https://doi.org/10.1016/j.socscimed.2022.114907

Rhodes, T., Lancaster, K., & Rosengarten, M. (2020). A model society: Maths, models and expertise in viral outbreaks. *Critical Public Health*. https://doi.org/10.1080/09581596.2020.1748310

Richards, P. (2016). *Ebola: How a people's science helped end an epidemic*. Zed Books.

Riskin, J. (2018). The restless clock: A history of the centuries-long argument over what makes living things tick (Reprint edition). University of Chicago Press.

Rosengarten, M. (2021). COVID-19 diagnoses: A source of immanent value and novelty. *Medicine Anthropology Theory, 8*, 1–10.

Rosengarten, M., & Savransky, M. (2018). A careful biomedicine? Generalization and abstraction in RCTs. *Critical Public Health, 29*, 181–191. https://doi.org/10.1080/09581596.2018.1431387

Roy, A. (2020). The pandemic is a portal [WWW Document]. *Financial Times*. Retrieved May 25, 2020, from https://www.ft.com/content/10d8f5e8-74eb-11ea-95fe-fcd274e920ca

Savransky, M., Wilkie, A., & Rosengarten, M. (2017). The lure of possible futures on speculative research. In A. Wilkie, M. Savransky, & M. Rosengarten (Eds.), *Speculative research: The lure of possible futures*. Routledge.

Snobelen, S. (2012). The myth of the clockwork universe: Newton, Newtonianism, and the enlightenment. In C. L. Firestone & N. Jacobs (Eds.), *The persistence of the sacred in modern thought*. University of Notre Dame Press.

Stein, S. R., Ramelli, S. C., Grazioli, A., Chung, J.-Y., Singh, M., Yinda, C. K., Winkler, C. W., Sun, J., Dickey, J. M., Ylaya, K., Ko, S. H., Platt, A. P., Burbelo, P. D., Quezado, M., Pittaluga, S., Purcell, M., Munster, V. J., Belinky, F., Ramos-Benitez, M. J., Boritz, E. A., Lach, I. A., Herr, D. L., Rabin, J., Saharia, K. K., Madathil, R. J., Tabatabai, A., Soherwardi, S., McCurdy, M. T., Peterson, K. E., Cohen, J. I., de Wit, E., Vannella, K. M., Hewitt, S. M., Kleiner, D. E., & Chertow, D. S. (2022). SARS-CoV-2 infection and persistence in the human body and brain at autopsy. *Nature, 612*, 758–763. https://doi.org/10.1038/s41586-022-05542-y

The British Academy. (2021). The COVID Decade: Understanding the long-term societal impacts of COVID-19. https://www.thebritishacademy.ac.uk/publications/covid-decade-understanding-the-long-term-societal-impacts-of-covid-19/

UN News. (2023). WHO chief declares end to COVID-19 as a global health emergency | *UN News* [WWW Document]. Retrieved February 8, 2023, from https://news.un.org/en/story/2023/05/1136367

Villandré, L., Labbe, A., Brenner, B., Ibanescu, R.-I., Roger, M., & Stephens, D. A. (2019). Assessing the role of transmission chains in the spread of HIV-1 among men who have sex with men in Quebec, Canada. *PLoS One, 14*, e0213366. https://doi.org/10.1371/journal.pone.0213366

Wald, P. (2008). *Contagious: Cultures, Carriers, and the Outbreak Narrative*. Duke University Press. https://doi.org/10.1215/9780822390572

Whitehead, A. N. (1920). *The concept of nature* (Reprint edition). Cambridge University Press.

Whitehead, A. N. (1967). *Science and the modern world* (Reissue edition). Free Press.

Whitehead, A. N. (1978). *Process and reality* (2nd ed.). Free Press.

WHO. (n.d.). Origins of the Ebola epidemic [WWW Document]. Retrieved February 6, 2024, from https://www.who.int/news-room/spotlight/one-year-into-the-ebola-epidemic/origins-of-the-2014-ebola-epidemic

WHO Ebola Response Team. (2016). After Ebola in West Africa—Unpredictable risks, preventable epidemics. *New England Journal of Medicine, 375*, 587–596. https://doi.org/10.1056/NEJMsr1513109

Wolf, M. (2016). Rethinking Urban Epidemiology: Natures Networks and Materialities. *International Journal of Urban and Regional Research, 40*, 958–982. https://doi.org/10.1111/1468-2427.12381

3

"An Indescribable Pause": Reading Pandemic Time Through Virginia Woolf's *Mrs. Dalloway*

Amanda M. Caleb

A month into the COVID-19 pandemic, Evan Kindley wrote an article for the *New Yorker* which recounted the appearance of *Mrs. Dalloway*-inspired tweets, beginning on March 16 with "Mrs. Dalloway said she would disinfect the doorknobs herself," escalating to "Mrs. Dalloway said she would have the flowers delivered because they were [a] non-essential need, but she would make sure to tip the delivery guy at least 30% herself," and, finally "Mrs. Dalloway said she would make the mask herself" (Kindley, 2020, para 1). This comical take on the opening line of Woolf's novel demonstrates an affinity between a collective pandemic experience of many social media users and Clarissa Dalloway's historical (and literary) experience, underscored by both the desire for autonomy in the face of social and medical restrictions and the sense of lingering time, marked by the linguistical construction of the line and the novel's attention to lost time. Clarissa's decision to "buy the flowers herself" at the onset of

A. M. Caleb (✉)
Department of Medical Education, Geisinger Commonwealth School of Medicine, Scranton, PA, USA
e-mail: acaleb@geisinger.edu

K. Kenny et al. (eds.), *Timescapes of Health, Illness and Care*,
https://doi.org/10.1007/978-981-96-7055-0_3

Woolf's novel is underscored by what she labels "an indescribable pause," reflective of both the anticipation of Big Ben striking the hour and the eponymous character's lingering symptoms of influenza (Woolf, 1925/2000, pp. 3, 4). This temporal moment, marked by chronological time and increased awareness of philosophical theories of time and historical events, intersects with the geographical space and emotional place of post–World War I London and the corporeal space of Clarissa's body. This moment is one to which many contemporary readers can relate: the "indescribable pause" of 2020 was one delineated by chronological time but understood through and disrupted by the chronoception of the pandemic experience (whereby 2020 seemed to drag because of the loss of temporal markers and feels both recent and ages ago) and historical echoes (i.e., both a pandemic and parallels between the war in Ukraine and World War I).

One of the most compelling accounts of illness disruption to linear time is that of viral temporality, which describes "what happens when there is a colliding or unfolding of these temporal disjunctions: in illness, to name one of the phenomena caused by the human-pathogen interaction, humanist linear time collides with nonhuman, cellular, pathogenic, and epidemiological temporal framings" (Clemens & Casey, 2023, p. 64). While this framing allows for a more expansive understanding of time, one that challenges chrononormativity and the capitalist focus on productivity (Freeman, 2010, p. 3), it also relies on temporal framings that are inherently tied to spatial representation, such as the progression of the pathogen in the body/community, flattening the curve, and so on (Clemens & Casey, 2023, pp. 65–66). Applying the framework of both philosophical conceptions of time—specifically the theories of Henri Bergson, a twentieth-century philosopher who was also referenced during the COVID-19 pandemic—and viral temporality, I argue that Woolf's novel engages with pandemic temporality: the heightened sense of temporal experience that is defined by the contagion of illness and shared experience.

Woolf's stream of consciousness novel follows one day in the life of the upper-class Clarissa Dalloway in June 1923 as she moves across London to prepare for and eventually host a party. Throughout the narrative, Clarissa slips into memories of the past, including her youth in the country, her decision to marry Richard Dalloway (a Member of Parliament), and her past relationships. Clarissa's memories are paired with those of her rejected lover Peter Walsh, who is critical of social structures even as he adheres to them. He still loves Clarissa and visits her during the day, later attending her party. Finally, the novel shifts to Septimus Warren Smith, a World War I veteran who suffers from "shell shock" and hallucinations, eventually committing suicide near the end of the novel. While not much happens in the novel per se, it engages with important questions about agency and meaning in a post-pandemic and postwar world.

Academics and bloggers alike noted a shared affinity with Woolf's novel during the height of the COVID-19 pandemic, recognizing the loss of the banality of life coupled with the loss of time and lives (Clark, 2021, pp. 45–46; Dickey, 2021, para 3) and implicitly countering claims that "the pandemic appears to be incidental to the novel's preoccupation with war and death" (Honigsbaum, 2014, p. 221). Woolf's novel—and what I think appealed to readers during the COVID-19 pandemic and even after—describes and distorts the concept of lived time, revealing the tensions of spatial-temporal markers of time, singled by the chiming of a clock, with the experience of lived time, in which time is experienced through sensations that challenge quantified clock time. Thus, the novel engages with philosophical debates about time and lived experiences within the context of viral temporalities, one that acknowledges both the unquantifiable experience of time and the disruption to human time caused by the influenza virus.

Before COVID-19, *Mrs. Dalloway* was rarely read as a pandemic novel, though, as Elizabeth Outka (2020, p. 104) contended, Woolf had centered influenza, "crafting innovative ways to write about illness that embody the pandemic's effects as well as exposing (paradoxically) the way it hides in plain sight," which represents the pandemic experience for Woolf's contemporaries. It is exactly because influenza is simultaneously present and obscured—along with the novel's setting of a single day in June 1923—that readers both overlook and accept the lingering impact of the Great Influenza. It is this single day during which the novel is set that demonstrates the tensions of time as characters' subjective experience of time as a merging of temporalities (past, present, and future) is interrupted and intersected by clock time. More than that, the shadows of the pandemic—which represent a merging of past, present, and future—shape the temporality of the novel. As Clemens and Casey (2023, p. 75) argued in their analysis of Woolf's "On Being Ill" (1926), illness prompts "different temporal frameworks [that] evoke other times, one which exist concurrently despite their different timescales." In this chapter, I will explore pandemic temporality that can be framed as the tension between *durée* and clock time, which both shape the novel and help to explain the draw to it during the COVID-19 pandemic.

Theorizing the Experience of Time: Clock Time and Subjective Time

The aforementioned social media alignment of the COVID-19 pandemic with Woolf's novel suggests some affinity between 2020 and 1923, connected through a shared perception of time as changed. Ungirding this affinity are nineteenth-century theories of time perception that both influenced Woolf and continue to influence how time is understood today. Not surprisingly, Woolf's father Leslie Stephen espoused theories on time that subsequently influenced his daughter's own work. In his 1889 essay "On Some Kinds of Necessary Truth" (the first of two with this title), Stephen explored the relationality of time: that of one point of time to another and that of chronological time as an agreed-upon measure between people's otherwise subjective experiences of time. To the latter, chronological time requires an external measurement precisely to allow for comparison: one cannot judge the passage of time based on the grumblings of one's stomach (Stephen's example) because another person does not know when that grumbling occurs (Stephen, 1889, p. 60). To the former, our understanding of time is dependent on fixed moments: one knows the passage of an hour because one marked the beginning and end of an hour with a clock. To this point, Stephen posited an axiom: "if our experience coincides now and coincided at another fixed point, the interval has been the same for both" (Stephen, 1889, p. 61).

What complicates these objective measurements of time is how individuals experience them. To continue with Stephen's example: "We parted and met; you have been reading *Ivanhoe* and I have been reading *MIND*. The time, therefore, must have been the same, although, judging from our sensations, it has seemed long to you and short to me" (Stephen, 1889, p. 61). Stephen's example leads to the error of qualifying a fixed measurement: a minute is neither quick nor slow because what is being evaluated is not the minute itself but rather what can be accomplished in that minute. Here the conflation of chronological time with the sensation of time leads to a judgment of time that is no longer standardized. What Stephen describes is what thinkers such as Herbert Spencer (1873, pp. 207–215) were struggling to understand for two decades previous: How does the mind experience time differently than the body in space and in relation to a fixed measurement?

At the same time Stephen was theorizing about the perception of time in England, Henri Bergson was doing the same in France. In 1889, he published his doctoral dissertation, which was subsequently translated into English and published in 1910 under the title *Time and Free Will: An Essay on the Immediate Data of Consciousness*, followed quickly by *Creative Evolution* (1910) and *Matter and Memory* (1911). This explosion of translated publications of Bergson's work marked his status as one of the great thinkers of the time, popular in intellectual circles and England more broadly (Ardoin et al., 2013, p. 4). While Woolf denied having read Bergson, his popularity and press about his works in periodicals to which she regularly contributed indicates she was certainly aware of and was even influenced by his ideas (Douglass, 2013, p. 116).

Like Woolf and *Mrs. Dalloway*, Bergson's theorization of time became a topic of blogs about COVID-19 experiences, used to help conceptualize changes to the experiences of time during the COVID-19 pandemic and the relationship to human agency, stymied by a sense of an indeterminant end to the COVID-19 pandemic, particularly in the first year (Moravec, 2020, paras 8–12). The appeal for both Woolf and her contemporaries and for the COVID-19 audience was Bergson's philosophical undertaking of how time is experienced. In *Time and Free Will*, Bergson describes our quantification of time (i.e., conventional time or clock time) as spatialized time through the juxtaposition of "successive images [set] alongside each of the new units which we picture to ourselves" (Bergson, 1910, p. 77). This quantification of time is contrasted with qualified time, what Bergson terms *durée* (duration). Using the example of a chiming bell, Bergson concluded that upon hearing the bell:

> Either I retain each of these successive sensations in order to combine it with the others and form a group which reminds me of an air or rhythm which I know: in that case I do not count the sounds, I limit myself to gathering, so to speak, the qualitative impression produced by the whole series. Or else I intend explicitly to count them, and then I shall have to separate them, and this separation must take place within some homogeneous medium in which the sounds, stripped of their qualities, and in a manner emptied, leave traces of their presence which are absolutely alike. (Bergson, 1910, pp. 86–87)

The latter is conventional time, quantified through homogenous spaces between events, such as that between minutes defined by a clock. The former is *durée*, the heterogenous and subjective qualified experience of time that defies the limitations of spatial construction, which "forms both the past and the present states into an organic whole, as happens when we recall the notes of a tune, melting, so to speak, into one another" (Bergson, 1910, p. 100). As a qualified multiplicity, *durée* comes with the emotions associated with how time is experienced; as Bergson (1910/1911a, pp. 9–10) described in *Creative Evolution*, waiting for sugar to melt in water

> is not that mathematical time which would apply equally well to the entire history of the material world, even if that history were spread out instantaneously in space. It coincides with my impatience, that is to say, with a certain portion of my own duration, which I cannot protract or contract as I like. It is no longer something thought, it is something lived.

Emotion, then, informs experience of time and therefore the conception of how it passes.

Like Stephen, Bergson distinguished the chronology of time and the sensation of time, one that accounts for our perception of how time passes as distinct from quantified time, arguing that tensions exist between clock time and *durée*. One of these tensions is the contrast between the reflective consciousness of clock time and the immediate consciousness of *durée*. The former is "goaded by an insatiable desire to separate, substitutes the symbol for the reality, or perceives the reality only through the symbol," which Bergson argued is "much better adapted to the requirements of social life" (Bergson, 1910, p. 128). *Durée* is the impetus for clock time, just as clock time is the means by which we position the simultaneity of *durée* (Scott, 2006, p. 186). For Bergson (1965, p. 62), "Real duration is experienced; we learn that time unfolds and, moreover, we are unable to measure it without converting it into space and without assuming all we know of it to be unfolded." The marginalization of the immediate consciousness is a product of not only the social pressure of defining experience by clock time but also the inability to describe *durée* because of the very limitations of language and of describing an experience without altering it—and making the internal external—by giving "a fixed form to fleeting sensations" (Bergson, 1910, p. 131). Thus, the immediate consciousness is "confused, ever changing, and inexpressible, because language cannot get hold of it without arresting its mobility or fit it into its common-place forms without making it into public property" (Bergson, 1910, p. 129). At the same time, undergirding the symbolic representation of *durée* (both linguistically and spatially through clock time) is "the psychical life unfolding beneath the symbols which conceal it [and which] readily perceive[s] that time is just the stuff it is made of" (Bergson, 1910/1911a, p. 4). In essence, Bergson' theory of time acknowledges the limitations of both clock time and *durée*; in doing so, however, he articulates that "thinking thus always occurs in time, knowledge is always in the process of being made and remade, and any system of thought or representation that suggests otherwise is [...] privileging the static product over the living process" (Ardoin et al., 2013, p. 22).

That living process of knowledge and self always becoming emerges from the continuity of lived experiences. Part of this process is memory, which, like time, Bergson separates into two types: habitual memory and pure memory. Using the example of studying a lesson, Bergson (1911b, pp. 89–93) demonstrated that habitual memory is the lesson itself, which is learned, repeated, and drawn up consciously and singularly in order to inform present action. Trying to recall how the lesson was learned requires pure memory, a "latent and unconscious" state that, once a memory-image is created, is no longer pure memory (Bergson, 1911b, pp. 89–91, 181). Thus, like *durée*, the act of accessing pure memory (or describing *durée*) impacts its existence

> from the moment that it becomes image, the past leaves the state of pure memory and coincides with a certain part of my present. Memory actualized in an image differs, then, profoundly from pure memory. The image is a present state, and its sole share in the past is the memory whence it arose. (Bergson, 1911b, p. 181)

The automatic preservation of past in pure memory thus continually informs our experiences and therefore *durée*; as Bergson (1910/1911a, p. 5) argued in *Creative Evolution*:

> all that we have felt, thought and willed from our earliest infancy is there, leaning over the present which is about to join it, pressing against the portals of consciousness that would fain leave it outside [...] even though we may have no distinct idea of it, we feel vaguely that our past remains present to us. What are we, in fact, what is our *character*, if not the condensation of the history that we have lived from our birth—nay, even before our birth, since we bring with us prenatal dispositions?

Here, Bergson conflates past with history, referencing both an individual past and a holistic history "based on a notion of the survival of the past" (Ter Shure, 2019, p. 155), in order to demonstrate "how the past is something lived" (Lundy, 2013, p. 24) and how it informs our present through *durée*.

Bergson's theories of time and memory help to contextualize how time was experienced during the pandemic, through both the passing of quantified days and the subjective *durée* of what folks did and the collective impressions of the day that constituted a qualitative experience, one that altered how folks perceived quantified time. Writers and journalists described the endless *durée* of the pandemic, aligning the lack of agency during lockdowns to the altered perception of past (e.g., the challenging of placing the timing of events as anything more than pre-COVID), present (e.g., the slow passing of a day), and future (e.g., the inability to plan vacations) (Moravec, 2020, paras 11–12). Such feelings are likely familiar to many readers, particularly in the early months of the COVID-19 pandemic: a questioning of how this happened, imagining the next pandemic, and feeling uncertain about protective measures and the integrity of one's bubble. This resulted in a "practical and epistemic reconfiguration of temporality [...creating] anxiety regarding an insecure past and apocalyptic futures and about a fragmented present dominated by disjunction and uncertainty" (Venkatesan & Joshi, 2022, para 9). Megan Craig (2020, para. 7) took this altered experience of time one step further, describing *durée* as "the unhinged time of labor or illness [...that] drifts from the reliable rhythm of counting or dates. Denied an organized past or an open future, the present thickens." This ceaseless misalignment with clock time leads to an overemphasis on the present, one that makes decisions all the weightier because the anchoring to past and future as previously known has been denied. Moravec (2020, para 15) suggested that as schedules and calendars were disrupted by the pandemic, *durée* took over as the only "real" experience of time; thus, the pandemic gave "everyone an insight into the fundamental nature of time." In contrast, Craig (2020, para. 9) argued for the inevitable return to clock time: "durée was never meant to last so long. Even Bergson [...] knew that a person abandoned to prolonged durée would be isolated and cut off from the social world." Here we might ask: Does the isolation of a pandemic (via lockdowns) create *durée*, or does *durée* create the sense of isolation? Or are the two mutually reinforcing? I would argue that pandemic temporality makes *durée* more present and makes us more attentive to it, thus engaging us to think more consciously about time.

While popular discussions of Bergon during COVID-19 stopped at *durée*, it is worth noting that his writing about memory is also relevant to how many folks collectively experienced the COVID-19 pandemic. The preservation of past in memory intimates the connections to previous pandemics such as AIDS and the Great Influenza, which were not simply about public health strategies (e.g., flattening the curve) but rather about a sense of a previous experience that informs our present being. Living in a pandemic can feel like a harkening back to past pandemics—even in the face of biomedical advances—and to anxieties about future pandemics, precisely because of the limitations of biomedicine. Thus, the turn to Bergson during COVID-19 was an attempt to make sense of this merging of experiences that are both *durée* and memory—just as turning to Woolf's *Mrs. Dalloway* was an attempt to make sense of COVID-19 *durée* as part of a longer pandemic history.

Mrs. Dalloway: "The Indescribable Pause" of a Pandemic

Woolf's novel begins with the oft-parodied sentence "Mrs. Dalloway said she would buy the flowers herself" (Woolf, 1925/2000, p. 5), a line that particularly resonated with many folks during COVID-19 as it represented the appeal of being able to leave one's home to complete the otherwise mundane act of running errands (Kindley, 2020, para. 2). This appeal is true for Clarissa as well, whose decision to run the errand herself suggests being healthy enough after her bout of influenza to venture out into the London crowds. Yet, as Elizabeth Winkler (2020, p. 16) notes, "she retains the perspective of the sickroom: the sense, as she watches the taxi cabs, 'of being out, out, far out to sea and alone,'" and her return home to rest in the attic room is a reminder of her lingering illness (Woolf, 1925/2000, p. 34). Her decision to walk into London is framed by movement from the interior to the exterior, marked by the anticipation of the house doors being "taken off their hinges" and her reminiscence of plunging into the open air at Bourton, her country childhood home (Woolf, 1925/2000, p. 3). The contrast of London to the countryside is repeated throughout the novel, specifically in relation to illness recovery, including Peter Walsh's claim that "if only for Clarissa's health it would have been better to live in the country. But Clarissa had always been fond of society" (Woolf, 1925/2000, p. 196). Yet Clarissa's fondness for both society and London is undermined by her feelings of isolation and of feeling "something not herself" (Woolf, 1925/2000, p. 187). Peter's recollection of her fondness for London and for society predates her influenza; in her post-influenza state, her relationship to the place is muddled by the conflation of the sickroom, her drawing room, and London itself, all three of which are reminders of past illness, present recovery, and potential relapse. While these rooms are spatially demarcated, the continuum of the three alongside the progression of her illness are reconfigured as *durée*, expressed through qualitative multiplicities, experienced yet not fully described by the characters.

The novel's *durée* is constantly in tension with quantified time, represented by the authoritarian time of clocks (Whitworth, 2009, pp. 120–22). This tension is fundamental to both the literal and literary pandemic experience: *durée* seeks to question the authority of clock time, seen in the delayed echoes of Big Ben by St. Margaret's clock (Woolf, 1925/2000, p. 54) and suggesting the "arbitrary measure" of clock time (Whitworth, 2009, p. 120). Clarissa's illness both informs and is informed by her experience of *durée*: "an indescribable pause, a suspense (but that might be her heart, affected, they said, by influenza) before Big Ben strikes" (Woolf, 1925/2000, p. 4). Embodied time, measured by the heart's literal and figurative experience with influenza and enclosed within the textual body in parentheses, disrupts time through this pause and suggests "the pandemic's spectral presence, paradoxically hidden and silenced and yet omnipresent" (Outka, 2020, p. 117). Clarissa's post-pandemic time is neither a return to the stability of clock time, nor truly post-pandemic, as the lingering effects of the Great Influenza create an ongoing pause in time, one that cannot be fully articulated. This pause is interrupted by Big Ben: "First a warning, musical; then the hour, irrevocable. The leaden circles dissolved in the air" (Woolf, 1925/2000, p. 4). Woolf's description echoes Bergson's example of the chiming bell; however, instead of distinguishing clock time from *durée*, she describes how the *durée* of the first chime becomes the clock time of the second, then both dissolve. It is this dissolution that speaks to a pandemic temporality, one that dissolves any time boundaries precisely because it relies on the inability of those boundaries to inoculate us against temporalities we cannot control and that do not function spatially or linearly. The bell's resonance moves fluidly between and around time, representing a dissolution of present suspense and uncertainty in the "indescribable pause" (Woolf, 1925/2000, p. 4), past illness anxiety set aside linguistically but present corporeally and temporally, and anticipation of the death knells that follow, which remind her of her past illness.

This ongoing pause is revisited in the echoed delay of St. Margaret's bell, which initially Peter constructs as clock time, marking 11:30 am and his position near the House of Commons. Yet almost immediately, Peter conflates the bell with Clarissa, describing how "the sound of St. Margaret's glides into the recesses of the heart and buries itself in ring after ring of sound, like something alive which wants to confide itself, to disperse itself, to be, with a tremor of delight, at rest—like Clarissa herself" (Woolf, 1925/2000, p. 54). The dissolution of the bell into a living being—and eventually Clarissa—suggests the potential for rejecting clock time as a sole definer of time and therefore life; Peter instead imagines *durée* that is defined by Clarissa herself, both in the act of living and in a state of rest, dissolving the two seemingly incompatibilities into a lived experience of multiplicities and temporal linearity. Peter also notes, "Some grief for the past holds it back; some concern for the present" (Woolf, 1925/2000, p. 54), suggesting the lingering effects of influenza that blur past infection with present anxieties of future relapse.

The bell allows for the dissolution of time and space, transporting Peter to memories that seemingly occur concurrently with his present. He reflects on the bell:

> It is Clarissa herself, he thought, with a deep emotion, and an extraordinarily clear, yet puzzling recollection of her, as if this bell had come into the room years ago, where they sat at some moment of great intimacy, and had gone from one to the other and had left, like a bee with honey, laden with the moment [...] Then, as the sound of St. Margaret's languished, he thought, She has been ill, and the sound expressed languor and suffering. It was her heart, he remembered; and the sudden loudness of the final stroke tolled for death that surprised in the midst of life, Clarissa falling where she stood, in her drawing-room. (Woolf, 1925/2000, p. 54)

On initial reading, the passage suggests the unexpected nature of illness, the surprise of death in the moment of fond memories; Elizabeth Outka (2020, p. 117) describes Peter as "a pandemic mourner, one who must witness the weakness and suffering of a loved one while coping with both denial and shock at a sudden death." Here, Peter moves from past joy to present recovery to the potential future relapse and death, and while these moments may appear distinct, they are blurred by the reverberations of the bell's ringing that echo Big Ben's, a paused marking of time. By likening the bell to both a pollinator moving from person to person and a death knell, Peter unknowingly imagines pandemic contagion in the past, making Clarissa's illness more predictable and her potential death less unexpected.

Read within the framework of pandemic temporality—the anxiety of past and future and the uncertainly of the present—the passage also reveals how influenza infects not only time but place as well: the undisclosed room of Peter's memory shifts into Clarissa's drawing room and the scene of her imagined death, smudging the lines of past happiness with future anxiety. In the echo of St. Margaret's bell to that of Big Ben, "Peter now finds the chime bringing the same thoughts of Clarissa's ailing heart as it did her, and without his realizing that he now carries this thought, which has passed on, disease-like, without notice or intention" (Fifield, 2020, p. 107). The movement from spatial to embodied time, represented in their shared thought of her ailing heart as a source of illness and contagion, speaks to how clock time is undermined within the context of illness and specifically a pandemic.

The parallels between Big Ben's chime and that of St. Margaret's mark not only pandemic temporality but also the isolation associated with it. Despite being in public space, both Clarissa and Peter are isolated, the former momentarily in the pause of her heart and the suspense of the bell and the later alone after Clarissa's imagined death. Once again, Woolf reminds the reader of the inability to fully—or at all—escape pandemic temporalities, as the reverberations of having lived through a pandemic echo, like the clock bells, across the continuum of past, present, and future.

Clocks both delineate through interruption and dissolve in the ring of their bells and in the interconnectivity of time and people. Woolf four times describes Big Ben's chime as "The leaden circles dissolved in the air": at the beginning (as previously described), when she invites Peter to her party, when Septimus Smith and his wife Rezia are walking to see Sir William Bradshaw (and as Clarissa is laying out her green dress), and when Clarissa is by herself before rejoining her party at the end of the novel (Woolf, 1925/2000, pp. 4, 52, 103, 204). While the first instance suggests Clarissa's isolation, the other instances clearly connect characters: Clarissa to Peter and Clarissa to Septimus. As Anne Fernihough (2007, p. 4) noted, "the same tolling of Big Ben is heard by the various characters (Clarissa, Septimus, Peter Walsh), but serves only to accentuate the way in which their situated individuality diverges from the commonality imposed by clock time." This divergence, I argue, is a product of pandemic temporalities, whereby the imposed measures of clock time are distractions from the *durée* of survival, which both is demarcated by a past and present and dissolves these very distinctions by the inability to be fully present in homogenous time.

Although Septimus's status as survivor is read almost exclusively as that of being a World War I veteran, Elizabeth Outka (2020, pp. 131–139) provided a compelling reading of "a composite Septimus" who embodies the psychological traumas of both war and pandemic. Outka (2020, p. 127) traced the neurological impact of influenza that paralleled the traumatic impact of war, include hallucinations, depression, and suicidal ideation, as well as a shared survivor's guilt. Notably, "sometimes it was difficult to distinguish between the depression that inevitably follows so many deaths and the depression left by the virus" (Outka, 2020, p. 128). With this context, Septimus can be read as part of the pandemic temporalties of the text, impacted by the conflation of war and influenza that resulted in previously unimaginable loss of life. This is illustrated in a passage in which Septimus imagines the return of his fallen friend Evans:

> The word 'time' split its husk; poured its riches over him; and from his lips fell like shells, like shavings from a plane, without his making them, hard, white, imperishable, words, and flew to attach themselves to their places in an ode to time; an immortal ode to Time. He sang. Evans answered from behind the tree. The dead were in Thessaly, Evans sang, among the orchids. There they waited till the War was over, now the dead, now Evans himself. (Woolf, 1925/2000, p. 76)

Septimus's hallucination is framed within the lived experience of *durée* that splits from its clock time, denying the linearity and finality of life as the dead soldiers turn to London, which "narrates how such inchoate fears were literally realized with the pandemic's arrival" (Outka, 2020, p. 136).

The ongoing anxiety and impact of the pandemic is further emphasized in Septimus's suicide. As with the clock bells that frame Peter imagining Clarissa's death, Septimus's death is followed by the sound of a clock: "The clock was striking—one, two, three: how sensible the sound was; compared with all this thumping, and whispering; like Septimus himself. She [Rezia] was falling asleep. But the clock went on striking, four, five, six" (Woolf, 1925/2000, p. 164). Woolf juxtaposes Rezia longing for the order of clock time against her falling asleep, a liminal state between awake and asleep that also suggests the *durée* of this post-pandemic world, one in which clock time tries to order what has the sensation of being unordered. Clarissa experiences something similar in her preparation for her party and in thinking about Septimus. As she greets guests, she has "this feeling of being something not herself, and that every one was unreal in one way; much more real in another" (Woolf, 1925/2000, p. 187). This illusionary feeling echoes Septimus's hallucinations of Evans and the broader awareness of having survived the pandemic, whereby not just time but experiences feel real and unreal. Shortly after this feeling, Clarissa is confronted with hearing of Septimus's death and thinks, "in the middle of my party, here's death" (Woolf, 1925/2000, p. 201). As Outka (2020, p. 139) has argued, "The phrase echoes how death had rippled through homes, first from afar—through the news of war—and then from within the home, erupting in the midst of Armistice celebrations."

The juxtaposition of life and death is echoed again in Clarissa's reflection on Septimus, which are framed by the striking of the clock:

> The young man had killed himself; but she did not pity him; with the clock striking the hour, one, two, three, she did not pity him, with all this going on [...] She felt somehow very like him—the young man who had killed himself. She felt glad that he had done it; thrown it away while they went on living. The clock was striking. The leaden circles dissolved in the air. But she must go back. (Woolf, 1925/2000, p. 204)

Although framed by the clock, Clarissa's thoughts go beyond the mechanistic construction of time: it is three in the morning, and the designation of that time is completed by the time she starts her reflection, yet the clock is still striking at the end of the passage. Experienced time, *durée*, temporarily denies the power of clock time as Clarissa contemplates what it means to be a survivor, a joy of being alive yet a closeness to death. The closeness of this reflection—she is in a room in her house by herself—changes the shape of the novel, "condens[ing] the novel's metropolitan panoramas and its enormous arc of historical time into the innermost spaces of Clarissa's home [and] allow[ing] Clarissa the apparently impossible experience of living and dying in a single moment" (Seshagiri, 2023, p. 21). Death, which lingers in the background throughout the novel in the chiming of bells, momentarily jolts Clarissa from the past, only to be reminded of the repetition of life by the clock striking and its "leaden circles dissolve[ing] in the air," a callback to the "indescribable pause" from the beginning of the novel (Woolf, 1925/2000, pp. 204, 4).

Mrs. Dalloway in the Time of COVID-19

The sense of repetition and continuation from pandemic to pandemic draws contemporary readers to pandemic literature to make sense of their pandemic experience. The attraction to fiction about the Great Influenza during the COVID-19 pandemic—despite the relative paucity of material—is guided by a perceived similarity of respiratory diseases, their severity, and public health responses—and the desire for pandemic closure. Yet what Great Influenza fiction like *Mrs. Dalloway* actually reveals is that the pandemic remains with us, not only through disease transmission but also in the continued experience of pandemic temporality that denies both the certainty of action in the present and the delineation of past, present, and future. Both spatial and social isolation have contributed to altered time perception—and arguably that altered time perception has further impacted responses to such isolation, including pandemic fatigue.

The entanglement of multiple temporalities helps to, in part, frame how the typical experience of time is altered by illness. In the case of the COVID-19 pandemic, this includes "disruptions to the chrononormative calendar of the working day and week, the time of holidays, festive time, and social time" and the emergence of new "temporal units of incubation, isolation, quarantine, lockdown, immunity, and recovery" (Clemens & Casey, 2023, pp. 65–66). While these temporal units existed before COVID-19, their widespread use outside of medicine and public health suggests the ways in which the pandemic has been internalized within us and by us and reminds us of the tension between clock time (e.g., period of isolation after testing positive) and by *durée* (the lived experience of how that time passes).

In discussing readers' draw to *Mrs. Dalloway* in the early days of COVID-19 and the momentousness of ordinary acts like shopping, Evan Kindley proclaimed, "We are all Mrs. Dalloway now" (Kindley, 2020, para. 1). I would counter, however, that many folks are more Mrs. Dalloway now, four years out from the onset of the pandemic and still subject to pandemic temporalities. They are able to return to many of their pre-pandemic activities, with few or no restrictions. Yet COVID-19 is still part of life, especially for folks with long COVID—a viral temporality that has changed the experienced time of disease progression (Clemens & Casey, 2023, p. 66). For many, time is described and remembered in broad strokes of pre-COVID and post-COVID and with a telescoping effect that compresses and stretches our memory of time (Wilson, 2024, para. 5) and that echoes Bergson's concepts of pure memory and *durée*.

We continue to wade through a period of uncertainty regarding the COVID-19 pandemic, including questions of classification (Is it still a pandemic? Is it endemic?), protocols (changing masking measures in healthcare facilities), and the concept of normalcy in living with COVID-19 variants (Ducharme, 2024, paras. 6, 18, 21–23). The appeal of *Mrs. Dalloway* is that it engaged with this uncertainty, asking the question of how one moves forward when elements of the past are still present—how does one throw a party in the face of death and survival? And how does one live in "the everyday, banal world of Before, shot through now with the dead and their ghosts—where everything is the same but all is changed, changed utterly" (Dickey, 2021, para. 4)? Winkler (2020, p. 16) argued that Woolf's novel demonstrates how "The virus itself is gone but the strange new perspectives it granted remain – a pandemic consciousness lingering in bodies and cities, language and literature." While the COVID-19 virus is not gone—and may never be—a pandemic consciousness, one tied inextricably to the temporal experience of COVID-19, continues to shape engagements with language, with space, and with time.

Acknowledgments A version of this chapter was presented at a panel sponsored by the International Virginia Woolf Society at the 2023 Modern Language Association annual conference. I am grateful for the feedback I received from the attendees, who helped to shape this chapter.

Competing Interests The author has no conflicts of interest to declare that are relevant to the content of this chapter.

References

Ardoin, P., Gontarski, S. E., & Mattison, L. (Eds.). (2013). *Understanding Berson, understanding modernism*. Bloomsbury Publishing.

Bergson, H. (1910). *Time and free will: An essay on the immediate data of consciousness* (F. L. Pogson, Trans.). George Allen and Unwin.

Bergson, H. (1911a). *Creative evolution* (A. Mitchell, Trans.). Henry Holt. (Originally published in 1910)

Bergson, H. (1911b). *Matter and memory* (N. M. Paul & W. S. Palmer, Trans.). George Allen and Unwin.

Bergson, H. (1965). *Duration and simultaneity* (H. Dingle, Ed.; L. Jackson, Trans.). Bobbs-Merrill (Original work published in 1922).

Clark, T. (2021). 'Still, life had a way of adding day to day': Revisiting *Mrs. Dalloway* in a global pandemic. *South Central Review, 38*(2–3), 42–46. https://doi.org/10.1353/scr.2021.0028

Clemens, R., & Casey, M. (2023). Viral temporalities: Literatures of disease and posthuman conceptions of time. In B. Ağin & S. Horzum (Eds.), *Posthuman pathogenesis: Contagion in literature, arts, and media* (pp. 63–81). Routledge.

Craig, M. (2020, December 21). Time isn't supposed to last this long. *New York Times*. https://www.nytimes.com/2020/12/21/opinion/time-coronavirus.html

Dickey, C. (2021, December 6). The work of living goes on: Rereading *Mrs. Dalloway* during an endless pandemic. *Literary Hub*. https://lithub.com/the-work-of-living-goes-on-rereading-mrs-dalloway-during-an-endless-pandemic/

Douglass, P. (2013). Bergson, vitalism, and modernist literature. In P. Ardoin, S. E. Gontarski, & L. Mattison (Eds.), *Understanding Berson, understanding modernism* (pp. 107–127). Bloomsbury Publishing.

Ducharme, J. (2024, January 12). We're in a major COVID-19 surge. It's our new normal. *Time*. https://time.com/6554340/covid-19-surge-2024

Fernihough, A. (2007). Consciousness as a stream. In M. Shiach (Ed.), *The Cambridge companion to the modernist novel* (pp. 65–81). Cambridge University Press.

Fifield, P. (2020). *Modernism and physical illness: Sick books*. Oxford University Press.

Freeman, E. (2010). *Time binds: Queer temporalities, queer histories*. Duke University Press.

Honigsbaum, M. (2014). *A history of the Great Influenza pandemics: Death, panic, and hysteria, 1830–1920*. Bloomsbury Publishing.

Kindley, E. (2020, April 10). Why anxious readers under quarantine turn to 'Mrs. Dalloway.' *New Yorker*.. https://www.newyorker.com/books/page-turner/why-anxious-readers-under-quarantine-turn-to-virginia-woolfs-mrs-dalloway

Lundy, C. (2013). Bergson, history, and ontology. In J. Ó. Maoilearca & C. De Mille (Eds.), *Bergson and the art of immanence: Painting, photography, film* (pp. 17–31). Edinburgh University Press.

Moravec, M. (2020, December 2). A philosophical idea that can help us understand why time is moving slowly during the pandemic. *The Conversation*. https://theconversation.com/a-philosophical-idea-that-can-help-us-understand-why-time-is-moving-slowly-during-the-pandemic-151250

Outka, E. (2020). *Viral modernism: The influenza pandemic and interwar literature*. Columbia University Press.

Scott, D. (2006). The 'concept of time' and the 'being of the clock': Bergson, Einstein, Heidegger, and the interrogation of the temporality of modernism. *Continental Philosophy Review, 39*, 183–213. https://doi.org/10.1007/s11007-006-9023-4

Seshagiri, U. (2023). Family and place. In A. E. Fernald (Ed.), *The Oxford handbook of Virginia Woolf* (pp. 7–26). Oxford University Press.
Spencer, H. (1873). *The principles of psychology* (Vol. 2). Williams and Norgate.
Stephen, L. (1889, January). On some kinds of necessary truth (I). *Mind, 14*(53), 50–65. https://www.jstor.org/stable/2247346
Ter Shure, L. (2019). *Bergson and history: Transforming the modern regime of historicity*. State University of New York Press.
Venkatesan, S., & Joshi, I. A. (2022). 'The time is out of joint': Temporality, COVID-19, and graphic medicine. *Medical Humanities, 48*, e15. https://doi.org/10.1136/medhum-2021-012357
Whitworth, M. (2009). *Virginia Woolf*. Oxford University Press.
Wilson, J. (2024, March 12). Yes, time does feel different since the pandemic—And there's a reason why. *Huffington Post*. https://www.huffingtonpost.co.uk/entry/yes-time-does-feel-different-since-the-pandemic-and-theres-a-reason-why_uk_65f050e8e4b02ad7de1a53f3
Winkler, E. (2020, May 29). Through the smudged pane: Pandemic consciousness in *Mrs. Dalloway*. *Times Literary Supplement*, 6113, 16. https://www.the-tls.co.uk/articles/pandemic-consciousness-mrs-dalloway-essay-elizabeth-winkler/
Woolf, V. (1925/2000). *Mrs. Dalloway* (S. McNichol, Ed.). Penguin (Original work published 1925).

4

Temporality Must Be Cared For: Sensitive Trajectories of Time in Healthcare

Francisco Tirado, Jorge Castillo-Sepúlveda, Fernanda Bywaters-Collado, and Mariana Gálvez-Ramírez

La durée est hors de prix.
—Paul Valéry

The quote that opens this chapter is by the famous poet, writer, and philosopher Paul Valéry (1933), which—based on the Spanish interpretation of the French work—we translate as "duration is costly" (Valéry, 2004). This references the concept of "duration" (or "lived time") proposed by the French philosopher Henri Bergson (1913), which is

F. Tirado
Universitat Autònoma de Barcelona, Barcelona, Spain
e-mail: franciscojavier.tirado@uab.es

J. Castillo-Sepúlveda (✉) • F. Bywaters-Collado • M. Gálvez-Ramírez
Universidad de Santiago de Chile, Santiago, Chile
e-mail: jorge.castillo.s@usach.cl; fernanda.bywaters@usach.cl; mariana.galvez@usach.cl

K. Kenny et al. (eds.), *Timescapes of Health, Illness and Care*,
https://doi.org/10.1007/978-981-96-7055-0_4

distinguished from a spatialised construct of time that is measured, for example, by the clock. In the above quote, Valéry (1933) conveys that time is not something given and objective but a complex constructed dimension that requires effort and dedication. More briefly, it demands care.

Valéry's words allow us to contrast this definition of temporality with the definition commonly found in medicine. In the latter, time is considered from its "modern" concept, that is, as something exterior, linear, and sequential, which implies applying the same definition both to organisational activities and to the development of biological dynamics (Cloatre, 2019). However, for some decades, this way of thinking time in medicine has been indicated as ambiguous, and as an approach to time that was imposed to handle the uncertainty caused by changes and alterations in the mentioned biological structures (Roth, 1963). In the same way that transformations of cultural representations of time are intrinsic to socio-historical changes, as shown by sociology since the mid-twentieth century (Bourdieu, 1990; Gurvitch, 1964; Hassard, 1990), the link between time, efficiency, and action in health is also, at least, a sociocultural product. Therefore, some authors (e.g., Armstrong, 1985; Horobin & McIntosh, 1983) point out that our current understanding of time originates from the post-war period, when disease stopped being conceived as a fixed entity and started to be understood as a process. In a similar line, these post-war studies insisted on showing how socio-spatial arrangement practices that took place at healthcare centres directly determined the pace of organisational work (Zerubavel, 1979).

This chapter builds on previous critique of the conceptualisation of time as a unitary and homogeneous dimension, including how it is mobilised in medicine and health. As posited by Cloatre (2019): "Medicine is envisaged as a field in which time 'matters': knowledge practices are inherently shaped by particular, often divergent, senses of temporality; at the same time, they become conditioned by series of temporal assumptions predominant in the practice of medicine" (p. 130). Consequently, from approximations like the above, temporal processes and phenomena like duration, among others, whether of an action, a routine, or a biological process itself, cannot be understood as a homogenous and common whole, but as an emerging event based on the overlap between diverse practices that elaborate, situate, and configure in a given scenario.

Harrison et al. (2024) have previously indicated that sociological studies about temporality in medicine have had several trajectories. First, studies that are concerned with horology address the question: How do we measure time and how is time related to the practices of patient care? This is fundamental and, among other things, it allows us to understand how care time is organised beyond clinical contexts, such as through mundane domestic practices and personal care routines (Buse et al., 2018; Mol, 2008). Second, sociological studies have critiqued the conceptualisation of time as something linear and sequential. The speed of time and the scale we use when defining it in our studies becomes a critical topic in studies such as those by Rance et al. (2024) and Seear and Lenton (2021). Lastly, several works show that new sociotechnical arrangements in the organisation of healthcare reconfigure time for patients and health workers, producing new opportunities but also challenges for healthcare (Grønning et al., 2024; van Pijkeren et al., 2024). In this line, the contributions of cross-disciplinary sociological, anthropological, philosophical, and sociopsychological approaches to health (Scrimshaw et al., 2022) should be mentioned, which have integrated research repertories that extend the social and subjective nature of time to view it as a product of heterogeneous articulations that involve both humans and objects in the same plane. This approach has yielded works on health and time that can, to an extent, be associated with a heterochronic perspective that analyses the role of specific social and material techniques in the configuration of different temporalities in health. For example, in their study of "the medical record", Berg and Bowker (1997) argue that medical records and databases "mediate" the constitution of a body with a specific history and geography of disease, constructing an immovable medical past that is divorced from the day-to-day rhythms of patients' experiences, and inscribing and coordinating different temporalities (Craciun, 2017).

Regarding these conceptualisations of time in healthcare, it is interesting to recall that Latour (1993) introduces the metaphor of "sorting" to refer to a means of tracing the temporalities occasioned by the meetings of a wide range of elements and agencies, human and non-human, social and material, bringing a socio-material approach: from these, new temporalities emerge and act and have effects (Grabham, 2014). From this point of view, time (as a process) could be composed of different times, and by virtue of that trait alone it performs as another relational agent in the settings where it is practised. Temporalising is therefore a co-product of action, or an action itself, not a background for action. Hence, epistemologies and ontologies of health and illness depend on temporal schemata that entail experiences and practices of anticipation, preparedness, resilience, and response (Lynteris & Prince, 2016). In consequence, and as pointed out by Cloatre (2019): "The temporalities at play in medical practices, and in the law surrounding it, are never fixed or fully determined, but revisited as practices themselves come to be reshaped or experienced" (p. 130).

Following this literature, we attend to time as "a matter of concern" (Latour 2008). In other words, we engage with time as a matter of discussion and relevance for the analysis of situations related to health. To do this work, we present the concept of "sensitive trajectory", which is strongly inspired by Puig de la Bellacasa's (2017) "matter of care". Our use of the expression "sensitive trajectory" deepens the debate on time and health-related practices and discourses. In this chapter, we will define this concept, illustrating it with an empirical study conducted in Chile, and we will show how temporality can be viewed both as an effect of the everyday practices of maintenance of the sensitive trajectories that configure it and as the place where these trajectories subsequently emerge.

Sensitive Trajectories

The previous section delineates several consequences for the sociomaterial analysis of the relations of practices and discourses in healthcare and time. First, it is presumed that time does not precede the practices and discourses in which it is defined and analysed. Temporality appears as fragmented into several temporal lines embedded in the set of relationships between material elements and social practices established in a concrete and localised situation associated with healthcare. Instead of a uniquely technical or natural question, time in healthcare could be thought as the product of articulations between heterogeneous elements, that is, an alliance between linguistic components, technologies, biological processes, and social conventions, which participate in the elaboration of events (Serres & Latour, 1995).

Second, as noted by Moreira (2005, 2007), the problem that these multiple temporalities pose for the analyst is, precisely, the question of how they are articulated or scaled to be handled in a specific diagnostic and treatment. As this author argues, tensions between different schemes of medical temporality are engaged with each other in a multiplicity of ways; thus, stories are always incomplete accounts of a process and derive some of their value from their open-endedness. As we will show in our empirical analysis, medical practice faces the problem of combining, for example: the temporality derived from the patients and their daily routines, which must be aligned to the requirements of the temporalities of the health services; that of laboratory test takers and their conditions for organising demand; that of the duration of laboratory tests themselves; the temporality of nurses and the organisation of their work; or the temporality required by the computer programme that registers the arrival of people to specific department. These efforts are highly sensitive to the incorporation of the local variability of concrete material qualities and to the "human" conditions of those who interpret such norms and standards (Lynch, 2002).

Third, the socio-material and multiple nature ascribed to time (Grabham, 2016) poses the problem of traceability. This is relevant to the analyst because if time is composed of the association of entities embedded in concrete practices, the establishment of temporalities takes on various forms. Thus, we should understand how the traceability of these forms is configured or established in order to trace how they operate and through which agency configurations they become sensitive, whether by transforming or acquiring continuity, or creating slow-downs, accelerations or other specific temporality schemata (McNeilly, 2021).

To understand the action of time as another actor or agent in a set of practices and discourses in a health context, we intend to address two proposals in detail. Our first proposal involves differentiating between the notions of "temporality" and "time". In the literature discussed, authors often employ both terms as synonyms, and, alternatively, when they differentiate them, they fail to clarify what the difference consists of, which has resulted in ambiguities. On other occasions, it is unclear why individuals perceive temporality differently from how it is established by certain contextual conditions (we refer to the conditions that a physician can establish in their diagnosis, or a protocol used by nurses, for example). This ambiguity is well illustrated by Moreira (2007). When this author points out the need to articulate multiple temporal lines, we could legitimately ask if this refers to the articulation of different definitions of time offered by health system users or extracted from certain technologies, or if, on the contrary, it concerns the definition of a temporality as a relationship schema. For example, when a doctor interacts with a patient, the scheme proposed by Moreira does not make it clear whether the temporal lines that operate in this scene have to do with the temporal definition that each actor adds (the doctor has in his protocol a treatment time for a specific illness, the patient adapts the treatment to the temporal possibilities offered by his daily practices, etc.) or whether we are dealing with a final, local, and situated temporality that emerges as a combination of the previous ones.

To avoid such confusions, we will define temporality as the quality and condition of time. Put differently, temporality is a kind of schema that describes the relational effects of multiple entities. Its key feature is that it schematises a set of objectifiable bonds. Temporality is what Deleuze and Guattari (1987) expose as a diagram. It is a concept provided by the analyst and involves the creation of an abstract schema from a set of concrete relations between different elements or observable practices. It is the result of a specific analysis that is constituted as an explanatory condition of the elements included in such an analysis. The notion of time, however, is the objective measure, for example time controlled by a clock, of the performance of an action by a particular entity or associated with a practice. For instance, the temporality of a car is articulated by all the time action of its components and materials (wheels, steel, software, etc.). This temporality varies depending on the nature and organisation of the components of the car. Wheels that wear easily or combustion ratios and forces that demand or delegate greater traction will generate a temporality characterised by constant wheel problems, the need for frequent replacements, and so on. The sorting of the elements of the car makes it possible to measure the time it takes for it to start or to cover a distance; however, the temporality differs according to the relationships between the car's components (and their corresponding modes of interaction with the environment) and the movements themselves.

In the case of medicine, temporality can be extracted from the analysis of relations of a wide range of materials, including protocols, the (dis)continuity between tests and diagnosis, room infrastructures and links between technical elements, among others. Thus, a fast rate of implementation for a specific drug, for instance, has different temporalities as it can be enacted variously by different individuals as their organic relations with the medication and their daily routines vary from (as well as relate to) protocolised dosing and prescribing estimates (Mol, 1999); in turn, the deployment of all these combinations along with a clock or a calendar makes it possible to chronologically represent the time it has taken to implement the drug individually and collectively.

The above distinction seems relevant, as it allows us to generate the basis for the description and empirical analysis of the dynamics that emerge and that in turn configure temporalities, that is, specific temporal sortings, which differ from that of chronological time and the subjective conception or experience of time. To analyse these instances, we build on Timmermans's (1998) framework for attending to multiple trajectories of practice in medicine. The idea of trajectory shows how, in practice, modes of temporality are configured through the articulation of elements of a different nature, and indicates at which point these modes of temporality gain relevance or value (Timmermans, 1998). At this point, there become visible a set of varied and heterogeneous elements (e.g., social, technical, ideological, emotional, or material aspects) that play a role in the definition and constitution of a temporality. Furthermore, these various temporalities can clash with or contradict one another.

This brings us to our second proposal: the concept of the "sensitive trajectory". Here, we draw from Puig de la Bellacasa's (2017) concept of "care": care emphasises the reflexive and interdependent interaction in the shaping of realities during the process of paying attention and giving durability to things or issues. This means that care is not only a matter of attending to other humans but also a relational process that considers the concern for connections between humans and natural environments, processes, objects, and technological schemes. For Puig de la Bellacasa (2017), a “matter of care” consists of a process configured as vulnerable and that requires the articulation between humans and non-humans to attain its place in the world.

The relationship between the notions of trajectory and sensitivity alludes to the vulnerable and sometimes precarious condition and dynamics through which elements of diverse nature that compose temporalities in health are articulated in practice. With this, we consider a way to attend both to the relational and mundane character of the practices and objects that participate in this composition and to the sensitivity of these temporalities to the relations that configure them. As temporalities are elaborated by delicate articulations, for their permanence and duration, they must be cared for. This directs the analyst’s eyes to the small details and objects that strongly contribute to the establishment and duration of an assemblage but that are systematically forgotten (Michael, 2003). A good example is the effort that cleaning staff make every day using all the basic technology they manage in a laboratory. The concept also emphasises the importance of attending to emotionality and affectivity in our analysis. We will illustrate these assertions using examples taken from a long-term study of the Chilean healthcare system.

Caring Time in the Chilean Health System

This chapter is based on a long-term research project that began in 2014. To date, it has yielded a case study of the Chilean healthcare system consisting of two phases. During the first phase,[1] we focused on the practices and epistemic aspects involved in the design and management of population-level care policy. For the second,[2] initiated in 2018, we have focused on how epistemic, practical, and technological dynamics affect and participate in the configuration of the temporal dimension in political and clinical scenarios in the country. Both phases address the last

[1] Fondecyt de Iniciación en Investigación Project, N° 11140950, funded by CONICYT Chile.
[2] DICYT Regular Project, Code 032193CS, funded by University of Santiago de Chile; and Fondecyt Regular Project, N° 1241495, granted by ANID Chile.

major health reform in Chile and are related, as the question of the configuration of temporality emerges from the analysis of the practical aspects of this policy.

The reform is called Explicit Health Guarantees regime (*Garantías Explícitas en Salud*, or GES), and was initiated in 2004 with the main purpose of reorganising the care priorities of the two main health services in Chile: the public National Health Fund (*Fondo Nacional de Salud* or FONASA) and the private Social Security Health Institutions (*Instituciones de Salud Previsional* or ISAPRE), which serve 77.8% and 17.29% of the population, respectively (Sánchez, 2021).[3] For this purpose, GES regime establishes four legally enforceable guarantees related to *access* (meeting certain diagnostic criteria ensures incorporation into the scheme), *timeliness* (no more than a set period can elapse between each milestone of the treatment process), *financial protection* (a percentage of the total cost of treatment is covered), and *quality* (health providers are accredited only after a review process). These GES benefits are associated with a prioritised set of programs, diseases, or health conditions that are established taking into account a number of medical and financial analyses. These integrate "epidemiological studies that identify a list of health and treatment priorities based on the health status of the population, the effectiveness of each intervention, its contribution to quality of life or its prolongation, and, whenever possible, its cost-effectiveness" (Ferrer, 2004, p. 3).

As of this writing, the GES regime instituted in the public and private health systems has been used to prioritise 87 health problems within the national diagnostic caseload. This implies that for these diseases and biological conditions, relatively standardised technologies and services are made available, as well as deadlines for their implementation.[4] Thus, in order to implement the GES, regulatory and legal aspects must be

[3] These institutional transformations took place against a backdrop of reforms—encouraged by the World Bank (1993)—aimed at liberalising health, privatising services, promoting competitiveness, reducing state investment, and, above all, affecting the administration of care times for selected diseases.

[4] If a guarantee of timeliness is breached, a diagnosed person can sue his or her health provider before the Superintendence of Health, which will ensure that a second provider is assigned to provide the service.

articulated with the availability of human and technological medical equipment in clinical facilities, establishing subtle dynamics through which prioritisation can be made effective.

Our study stemmed from a very simple question: How could effective coordination be generated in a political healthcare project articulated upon the basis of an extremely wide range of material including political decisions, scientific criteria, technical protocols, users' opinions, and economic restrictions? To answer this question, we analysed several dimensions: (a) decision-making procedures, (b) the types of techno-scientific protocols used, (c) the role of medical experts, (d) the attention paid to users' opinion, (e) the definition and establishment of the so-called health space, and (f) the definition of time generated in each of the previous dimensions and how a single and general definition was articulated upon the basis of that variability.

In order to address the above, we developed focused ethnographies (Knoblauch, 2005) at the Ministry of Health, public hospitals, and private clinics. This approach involves making short visits to the centres in question and generating data through the making and recording of textual, visual and audible observations, in-depth interviews and the collection and analysis of available technical documents (Knoblauch, 2005; Trundle & Phillips, 2023). The main phases of information production in these spaces have taken place during 2014–2017, 2019, and from 2022 to the present. During this time span, we were able to access ministerial coordination meetings with experts and methodological advisors, as well as standards update sessions at the Ministry of Health, transit and waiting spaces, and care scenarios and clinical case analysis sessions in a public hospital and a private clinic. Interviews were conducted by members of the research team in different facilities (ministry, hospitals, and the university), gathering so far 16 experts in in health economics, politics design, and clinical guidelines design; 55 healthcare professionals specialised in different diseases, 4 patient associations, and 12 individual patients have taken part in the research.

For the analysis of the information, we adopted what Tavory and Timmermans (2014) call abductive analysis. This involves identifying elements in the phenomenon or process under study, describing them and then looking for theoretical references that allow us to reflect on these elements. From there, it is necessary to return to these elements by formulating new hypotheses that contribute to their understanding. Unlike the inductive approach and the deductive approach, the abductive method focuses on generating plausible new ideas from the observed material.

This study was performed in line with the principles of the Declaration of Helsinki. Approval was granted by the Ethics Committee of University of Santiago de Chile and the care organisations that have been part of the studies. Informed consent to participate and to publish was obtained from individual participants, ensuring their voluntary, consented to, and anonymised involvement. Further details about the study and methods have been published elsewhere (Castillo-Sepúlveda et al., 2022, 2023; Castillo-Sepúlveda (in press).

Sensitive Trajectories in the Chilean Health System

The following field note was written by one of the study authors while doing fieldwork in a hospital:

> Just before reaching the counter, I register a conversation between a woman in her mid-sixties and the nurse coordinating the medical appointments in the Endocrinology ward. The woman states that, approximately one year earlier, she had received a doctor's order to have four tests done. Today, she had returned with the results. After the nurse's question, the woman states that she cannot remember the name of the doctor who had treated her and given her the order. At that point, the nurse asks her to see her National ID card. The woman finally notes that she had had a second meeting with the doctor, during which she had showed him two of the tests, but he had stated that he would need all the results to diagnose her. After looking for some documents in a filing cabinet, entering information into her computer, and quickly glancing at the screen, the nurse tells the woman to have a seat in the waiting room. (Field note, March 17, 2017)

This fragment reveals two noteworthy aspects that are repeatedly found in our work. First, it reveals the social (patient, nurse), material (national ID card, computer, database), and epistemic entities (legitimate knowledge in this setting) that must be coordinated in a simple interaction aimed solely at determining the patient's situation and resuming her treatment. Professionals' biological rhythms, machines, and test validity must be connected in a way that allows the patient's case to be interpreted as a single temporal flow. It is only through the alignment of subtle elements such as an identity card and a registration in the database, and the social interplay among them, that biological conditions, test times, multiple appointments, and the personal circumstances of the woman can be configured as a single trajectory. Second, it highlights the sensitive nature of the various elements that take part in the configuration of this temporal trajectory: all the individual elements establish a difference in the possibility of configuring the temporal continuity of the patient's treatment. Put differently, the trajectory of the disorder and the temporality that it configures are sensitive to the participation of the entities that compose and configure them. The continuity of the medical process is not granted directly but must instead be produced or developed.

Therefore, the existence and possibility of supporting a single medical temporality—that is, a single scheme signalling the deployment of individual experiences over time—in healthcare settings is associated with the synchronisation of different temporality trajectories that coexist with one another. In other words, it is necessary to make an extra and explicit effort to obtain a central and coherent chronology. In this regard, Timmermans (1998) has pointed out that "these mutual tunings form the main dynamic of trajectories: they are shaped by others and shape others in turn; they define and are defined by, they align and are aligned vis-a-vis other trajectories" (p. 433). Nevertheless, our fragment goes somewhat further, showing that emergent moment when time is cared for and emerges as a problem to be solved. This is what we refer to as sensitive trajectories.

However, our study revealed a second issue. The effort above has certain particularities. Its existence depends on the activities of certain actors, who play a key role in ensuring that different flows can be aligned with one another. Without their participation, the consideration of a single time would be hard to achieve (von Arx, 2023). This situation is illustrated by the following fragment of an interview with a doctor responsible for a health centre:

> Not all healthcare programs or strategies stem from the maturation of something. Sometimes they are generated by somebody's will, and here the personal factor appears again. So, for example, if I know someone who's on the autistic spectrum, and I'm in a place where decisions are made, I'm going to propose a strategy, because we realize that it's a shortcoming, a gap, and so it depends on the position I have to drive this initiative, that will determine how much traction it's gonna get and how many other people I can convince. If I'm in a strategic position, I can talk to an authority and say, "Look, autism is important, I need help to treat people for free, we need to treat autism free of charge". "Okay, let's estimate how many people have autism in the country", "How many children aged 0 to 2 are there?" (Tamara, personal communication, September 1, 2022)

This fragment shows how the composition of a temporality—in this case, of prioritisation or acceleration for the attention of a diagnosis—would be expressed by the strategic exercise of association exercised by an agent. In situations like the above, it was possible to detect how certain agents, human beings in this case, play a key role in the sensitive trajectory. These actors were able to impose their projects over other choices, drive other practices in the same direction, or even redefine and change their format. We have explicitly noted that they were human agents, because the situation may also have involved non-humans; for instance, a cancer treatment imposes a sensitive trajectory that has nothing to do with the biological evolution determined by the pathology and which is articulated by the need to use certain chemical substances before their effectiveness expires or by the opportunities to distribute or administer these elements in a specific clinical centre (Callon & Law, 1982). This can also be seen in the following extract from an interview with the Head of the Emergency Service of a private clinic, in which it can be seen how the incorporation of more simple diagnostic technology, but strategically placed in a location close to the clinical care space, configures a different temporality to that of its remote location:

> [For the last year, in the emergency room] we have been using Point of Care tests. We call them SPOC [Single Point of Contact] tests, which require a sample that can even be a capillary one, for example a finger prick, and with a fast machine it gives you a general test result that allows you to make decisions. With this, they don't have to travel to the lab for viral tests (...) [with this] we go from a test that takes between 45 and an hour, to 10 or 15 minutes. With the result the doctor makes a very good decision for serious patients. (Andrés, head of the Emergency Service at Private Clinic, individual interview, September 5, 2024)

Alternatively, these processes may be steered by the presence or absence of information, "evidence", or data in health policy decision-making. This is illustrated in the following field note, which describes a situation in an expert meeting to update a GES clinical practice guide, specifically, to modify the temporality and regularity of depression care:

> One of the attendees asks whether there is any information about depression treatment waiting lists. Another attendee notes that database records are only generated for treatment provided by specialist physicians, not psychologists, and that, therefore, the databases contain no records or information about this (…) In consequence, it is impossible to determine the actual costs involved, as the information from other countries that is indeed available can only be used to make an estimate. Although the participants use these statistics to try to ascertain the size of the target population and the number of sessions needed, they ignore the total number of sessions that their planned measures will require. (Field note, October 25, 2016)

As the above fragment shows, a trajectory that orients the temporality of healthcare processes is configured both by the care that humans express and by the conditions for the establishment of agency that non-humans provide. Interestingly, these problems tended to resolve when temporary trajectories were established. In other words, the problem reflected by the sensitive trajectory operated as a black hole that absorbed the other problems. This led us to believe that sensitive trajectories could be understood as a mechanism necessary for the creation of meaningful entireties that facilitate single and coordinated action.

How Do Trajectories Work?

In the GES regime, diseases that are added to the listing are associated with complex infrastructures that make it possible to control the relative temporality of their processes. Trajectories do more than indicate a problem with temporality: they establish that it is necessary or logical to introduce some type of anticipation. In these situations, an unavoidable temporality is established (based on certain elements such as political involvement or the characteristics of a pathology) and then imposed over every other aspect of a given healthcare-related practice. In the following fragments, we see how a sense of inevitability is introduced as an argument to impose this temporality:

> It's like the message we have to convey, we couldn't put seventy-nine diseases on the list, it looked inadequate [since 80 looks better], because there's an underlying political motivation. So, the Minister of Health called me and said: "I need to inform you that we can't include glaucoma, we're over budget". And I tried to sway him a little... "But, Minister, you know it's important...". And he said: "I'm not asking you", he said, "I'm telling you, because otherwise the President won't give us the budget for GES". Such a terrible thing to say... (Fernanda, individual interview, April 9, 2015)

> Oh, no, but before the glaucoma thing! The boss told us she had a new vision, but the process was coming to an end at the time, so she didn't do much (...) So she informed us that it wasn't going to, due to budget issues, I don't remember which pathology, but it wasn't going to be included, and one pathology would have to be split in two, mitral and aortic regurgitation, well. And actually, we had to divide it into subcategories. So that's what happened. (Fernanda, personal communication, April 9, 2015)

In the examples above, the logic of evidence is not enough to define this prioritised care process in the care system. This logic also incorporates unexpected events, which are incorporated into the relational play of previous elements and introduce a variation on the relationship between speed and pathology. This prioritisation is a sensitive process that attends to the infrastructural, social, political, and ethical conditions of the settings where prioritisation is exerted. In other words, this trajectory organises how temporalities become accelerated or acquire a distinctive rhythm in relation with various epistemic, ethical and political concerns.

In other cases, we have identified sensitive trajectories that express the need for total *synchrony* in the health system. For example:

> You know the Ministry of Health has several divisions (…) We managed the healthcare networks and are always going to meetings with them during the day because our challenge here is to articulate this, work together, because it would be pointless to work in isolation, primary care in its own lane, specialists in another, in the end we're not looking at the whole person. The person moves through the system, actually, they don't just stay in primary care. So, on a normal day, we have meetings with them, meetings with inter-sectoral counterparts [other institutions involved in social care], we need to strengthen this and repeat these meetings, and make sure they have concrete products. (María José, personal communication, September 21, 2022)

> Timing is important when you're giving an answer. Some things require immediate answers, because after a while the window of opportunity to do something has already passed (…) [To do that,] the network should activate itself, and you only need to monitor how it operates (…) there are periodic meetings with people. When things happen, local agents should activate automatically and we, at the central level, what we do is check that it actually, the things that have to be done are actually being done, and check if they need further support or if they can handle things at the local level (…) we have periodic meetings precisely to make sure they activate automatically and then check that things have actually happened. (Samantha, personal communication, January 11, 2022)

These examples highlight a need for a single articulation of different temporalities. In some cases, problems stem from a temporality that demands that certain events occur simultaneously, as observed in Samantha's case. Both extracts illustrate the careful work required to configure a common synchronous temporality that allows both regular and unexpected events to be dealt with, as well as for the care networks to operate in a timely manner. Without this care, the network would probably not operate in terms of expectations or achieve its intended health, political, or intervention outcomes.

In the excerpts above, sensitive trajectories perform with a common synchronous temporality, which enables a large set of resources to be mobilised in a specific moment enacted by a collective that the trajectories define. In turn, it is also enacted as a collective temporality, that is, defined as the effect of a coordinated and organised activity at a single time. But this collectively enacted time is not given. Here, sensitive trajectories materialise through practices of caring for and monitoring relationships over time to ensure that many temporalities can be reconfigured in synchrony when required. This temporality does not emerge as a "natural", fully formed, or spontaneous effect; rather, it is produced by progressive and simultaneous care aimed at preserving, protecting, and monitoring connections. In these cases, synchronicity is woven by the activity of agents who care for their event.

Where the above examples enact synchrony as the primary problem to be cared for, we also identified cases where temporality became constituted as a problem of *continuity*:

> You hold these meetings, mainly with people from other teams, you prepare minutes, send them by e-mail, leave a paper trail of what goes on, so that if anyone leaves the process, whoever replaces them can stay on the path that we had previously defined. (Samantha, personal communication, January 11, 2022)

> If I leave, that program will still be there [in the specification sheet for the relevant social scheme]. All the objectives are there, all the coverage details are there. I make sure to leave all the formulas, how I calculated everything, because when people leave, you say, "Hey, why did you calculate it like this? Why do we want to get that result? Is this objective badly described or did they describe it this way for a reason?". How can we reconstruct history when it's so dependent on people? And the only way to do it is to be rigorous, we must do it in a way that is understandable when it's presented like this, in a specification sheet. (Tamara, personal communication, September 1, 2022)

These fragments reveal concerns over whether social and healthcare schemes will continue to operate if changes in decision-making occur when those responsible for them switch positions in their organisation or when new protocols are introduced. Tamara, for example, indicates that if she abandons the project in which she is involved, it will continue there, in the corresponding institution, compiled in a series of documents and schemes. Tamara represents a temporality, and another time; when new relationship networks are incorporated, they will contribute this element that will need to conjugate with other contributions from other agents, and combine into a timeline, that is, in the definition of a time that is operational and that stands out over all these temporalities.

In these examples, the fluidity and continuity of the temporality of processes and programmes is cared for through concrete activities and their conversion into durable materialities that can be easily articulated into habitual routines and practices. In all cases, a sensitive trajectory is prefigured that problematises the issue of continuity—the establishment of a single or a fixed temporality that does not harm the system or the patients. All this is linked to the problem of how to generate continuity and the registering processes that make it possible to reconstitute it if necessary. Again, this flow is not the product of a natural phenomenon, but a cared-for process that stems from practices and the articulation of specific objects used to monitor the ways in which relationships have been composed, thus facilitating their reconfiguration.

Discussion and Conclusions

The trajectories we have explored throughout this chapter describe different situations and articulations of human and non-human elements; however, they share some relevant features. The sensitive trajectory signals the moment when time is cared for, is problematised, and becomes a matter of care. This step towards the resolution of the complexity problem does not emerge from nowhere; it comes from, and simultaneously updates, a scheme of relationships among heterogeneous elements that we have termed *temporality*. The coherency produced through this scheme enables the multiple actors implicated in our study, as well ourselves as analysts, to discuss something we call *time*.

These trajectories are deemed to be sensitive for two reasons. First, they clearly show the precariousness of the articulation of temporality by revealing that this is composed of diverse and heterogeneous elements. Second, they stress the fact that temporality coexists with other schemes that constitute other similar or neighbouring practices. Nevertheless, in the trajectories examined, we detected the prevalence of certain actors and characteristics that are shared with other trajectories. These two elements, a prominent actor and the existence of common terms, make it possible to understand how some temporalities predominate over others or how general syntheses are attained and situations where various temporality schemes coexist are homogenised.

This characteristic is in line with works that put forward the question of how from a network of diverse elements there emerges some sort of cohesion or meaningful entirety (Moreira, 2005). Our study has shown that in such relationship networks, there is no naive symmetry. On the contrary, there are always agents of elements that for diverse contextual reasons have some pre-eminence that grants them the possibility of imposing themselves or stand out in the relationship with other entities.

The traits of sensitive trajectories enrich the studies conducted thus far on similar topics. For instance, in their editorial on matters of time in health and illness, Harrison et al. (2024) point out the problems of ambiguity and uncertainty that regularly emerge in the sociological literature in this field. These sociological studies highlight that health interventions often reorganise how illness is experienced over long periods of time, and the complexity of the organising limits of the clock when health, illness, and care are investigated at larger scales. Sensitive trajectories, as we have mentioned, offer approaches to articulating how this ambiguity and uncertainty is closed in each particular context.

Other scholars in this field show how difficult it is to integrate into a meaningful totality practices and discourses that often operate in different directions (e.g., Moreira, 2005, 2007; Mol, 2002; Mol & Law, 1994). Moreover, they cleverly show how the medical professional faces the challenge of such coordination and how the analyst, in turn, has to explain such actions. Once again, the trajectories of sensitivity, based on their differentiation between temporality and time, their insistence on the existence of dominant actors in the schemes of temporality, or the existence of practices that impose themselves on others by appealing to common terms, shed light on (a) how to understand the creation of totalities with meaning and (b) how the analyst, based on the notion of temporality that functions as a diagram of intelligibility, explains and understands the creation of this articulation.

If we consider medicine to be a field in which time "matters" (Cloatre, 2019), the concept of the sensitive trajectory is concerned with *how* and *why* time matters. A sensitive trajectory operates as the basic infrastructure that gives meaning to that individual experience and connects it with similar experiences. The various sensitive trajectories that can be established as certain practices represent, above all, a problematisation of temporal experience. In other words, they constitute that experience as a problem that has certain effects, over which an action must be exerted, and which grounds one's operation. Echoing the words of Puig de la Bellacasa (2017), we can say that they turn that experience into a matter of care because they turn time into a problem that must be addressed, analysed, and understood in its evolution. Temporality, in this sense, can be viewed both as an effect of the everyday practices of maintenance of the sensitive trajectories that configure it, and as the place where these trajectories subsequently emerge. They signal a moment when change may occur, that is, the irruption of an event that can have certain effects on a concrete practice. Likewise, they indicate that experience associated with the temporal domain is more important than it has usually been said to be in healthcare. Such experience tends to be treated as a merely technical problem, involving activity management, the rational usage of human resources, or the establishment of protocols of varying effectiveness; alternatively, it can be viewed as a biological problem, that is, as something related to the natural course of a process.

The examples that we have included in our case study have involved the articulation of differentiated temporal regimes, inducing acceleration vectors for those health problems that satisfy a series of evidence requirements, based on a complex and dynamic epistemic network used to prioritise certain bodies and the medical and economic activities and technologies associated with timely care (Castillo-Sepúlveda, 2019;

Castillo-Sepúlveda et al., 2017, 2022). Our analysis attends to time as an emergent process based on relations between epistemic, ethical, political, material, and even spatial processes, which enact it differently in each health entanglement. In applying our concept of sensitive trajectories, we show that temporality, and the time that can be derived from it, is relevant enough to affect the definition of a pathology, the implementation of a treatment process, or even the composition of a whole public healthcare service. In addition, these trajectories show that tension and dissent—that is, difference—are the norm and not the exception, even in a sphere as delicate as that of healthcare. This differentiation concerns local and wholly situational practices and problems. Thus, these trajectories insist that something apparently as objective and abstract as "time" is yet another matter open to discussion.

Competing Interests This study was funded by DICYT, Project Code 032193CS, granted by University of Santiago de Chile, and Fondecyt Regular Project N° 1241495, granted by ANID Chile.

References

Armstrong, D. (1985). Space and time in British general practice. *Social Science and Medicine, 20*(7), 659–666. https://doi.org/10.1016/0277-9536(85)90054-1

Berg, M., & Bowker, G. (1997). The multiple bodies of the medical record: Toward a sociology of an artifact. *The Sociological Quarterly, 38*(3), 513–537. http://doi.wiley.com/10.1111/j.1533-8525.1997.tb00490.x

Bergson, H. (1913). *Time and free will. An essay on the immediate data of consciousness.* George Allen & Company, Ltd.

Bourdieu, P. (1990). Time perspectives of the Kabyle. In J. Hassard (Ed.), *The sociology of time* (pp. 219–237). Palgrave Macmillan.

Buse, C., Martin, D., & Nettleton, S. (2018). Conceptualising 'materialities of care': Making visible mundane material culture in health and social care contexts. *Sociology of Health & Illness, 40*(2), 243–255. https://doi.org/10.1111/1467-9566.12663

Callon, M., & Law, J. (1982). On interests and their transformation: Enrolment and counter-enrolment. *Social Studies of Science, 12*(4), 615–625. https://doi.org/10.1177/030631282012004003

Castillo-Sepúlveda, J. (2019). Gubernamentalidad y somatocracia en el Régimen de Garantías Explícitas en Salud en Chile. *Revista de Estudios Atacameños, 62*, 247–275. https://doi.org/10.22199/issn.0718-1043-2019-0009

Castillo-Sepúlveda, J. (in press). Opening the black box of time in health: Analysis of temporal sorting through objects in Chile. *Saúde e Sociedade.*

Castillo-Sepúlveda, J., Bywaters-Collado, F., & Gálvez-Ramírez, M. (2022). On the production of certainty in public health: Biopolitics and speculative objects. *Saúde e Sociedade, 31*(1), e200891. https://doi.org/10.1590/S0104-12902022200891

Castillo-Sepúlveda, J., Espejo, M., Tapia, J., Catalán, M., Toro, J., & Gálvez, M. (2017). Tecnologías, episteme y subjetivación en un régimen de garantías en salud. *Psicoperspectivas, 16*(3), 6–16. https://doi.org/10.5027/psicoperspectivas-vol17-issue3-fulltext-1069

Castillo-Sepulveda, J., Tirado, F., & Galvez, A. (2023). Biopolitics and speculative objects in Chilean health projects. *Social Studies of Science, 53*(2), 194–212. https://doi.org/10.1177/03063127221136804

Cloatre, E. (2019). Traditional medicines, law and the (dis)ordering of temporalities. In S. Beynon-Jones & E. Grabham (Eds.), *Law and time* (pp. 128–144). Routledge.

Craciun, M. (2017). Time, knowledge, and power in psychotherapy: A comparison of psychodynamic and cognitive behavioral practices. *Qualitative Sociology, 40*(2), 165–190. https://doi.org/10.1007/s11133-017-9355-x

Deleuze, G., & Guattari, F. (1987). *A thousand plateaus. Capitalism and schizophrenia.* University of Minnesota Press.

Ferrer, M. (2004). Plan AUGE y Reforma a la Salud: ¿Vía a la equidad en salud? *Agenda Pública, 3*(4), 1–13.

Grabham, E. (2014). Legal form and temporal rationalities in UK work-life balance law. *Australian Feminist Studies, 29*(79), 67–84. https://doi.org/10.1080/08164649.2014.901280

Grabham, E. (2016). *Brewing legal times. Things, form, and the enactment of law.* University of Toronto Press.

Grønning, A., Simonsen, L. M., Lüchau, E. C., Assing Hvidt, E., & Klausen, M. (2024). My time, your time, our time. Older patients' and GPs' time sensibilities around email consultations. *Health Sociology Review, 33*(1). https://doi.org/10.1080/14461242.2024.2316742

Gurvitch, G. (1964). *The spectrum of social time.* D. Reidel.

Harrison, M., Smith, A. K. J., & Adams, S. (2024). Matters of time in health and illness. *Health Sociology Review, 33*(1), 1–9. https://doi.org/10.1080/14461242.2024.2319943

Hassard, J. (1990). *The sociology of time*. Palgrave Macmillan.

Horobin, G., & McIntosh, J. (1983). Time, risk and routine in general practice. *Sociology of Health and Illness, 5*(3), 312–331. https://doi.org/10.1111/1467-9566.ep10491839

Knoblauch, H. (2005). Focused ethnography. *Forum Qualitative Sozialforschung Forum Qualitative Social Research, 6*(3), 1–14.

Latour, B. (1993). *We have never been Modern*. Harvard University Press.

Latour, B. (2008). What is the style of matters of concern? In N. Gaskill & A. J. Nocek (Eds.), *The Lure of Whitehead* (pp. 92–126). University of Minnesota Press.

Lynch, M. (2002). Protocols, practices, and the reproduction of technique in molecular biology. *The British Journal of Sociology, 53*(2), 203–220. http://doi.wiley.com/10.1080/00071310220133304

Lynteris, C., & Prince, R. J. (2016). Anthropology and medical photography: Ethnographic, critical and comparative perspectives. *Visual Anthropology, 29*(2), 101–117. https://doi.org/10.1080/08949468.2016.1131104

McNeilly, K. (2021). How time matters in the UN human rights council's universal periodic review: Humans, objects, and time creation. *SSRN Electronic Journal*. https://doi.org/10.2139/ssrn.3813061

Michael, M. (2003). Between the mundane and the exotic: Time for a different sociotechnical stuff. *Time & Society, 12*(1), 127–143. https://doi.org/10.1177/0961463X03012001372

Mol, A. (1999). Ontological politics. A word and some questions. In *Actor network theory and after* (pp. 74–89). Blackwell.

Mol, A. (2002). *The body multiple: Ontology in medical practice*. Duke University Press Books.

Mol, A. (2008). *The logic of care. Health and the problem of patient choice*. Routledge.

Mol, A., & Law, J. (1994). Regions, networks and fluids: Anaemia and social topology. *Social Studies of Science, 24*(4), 641–671. https://doi.org/10.1177/030631279402400402

Moreira, T. (2005). Diversity in clinical guidelines: The role of repertoires of evaluation. *Social Studies of Science, 60*(9), 1975–1985. https://doi.org/10.1016/j.socscimed.2004.08.062

Moreira, T. (2007). How to investigate the temporalities of health. *Forum Qualitative Sozialforschung, 8*(1), Article 13.

Puig de la Bellacasa, M. (2017). *Matters of care. Speculative ethics in more than human worlds*. University of Minnesota Press.

Rance, J., Grebely, J., & Treloar, C. (2024). The time of cure: Hepatitis C treatment and the matter of reinfection among people who inject drugs. *Health Sociology Review, 33*(1). https://doi.org/10.1080/14461242.2024.2315031

Roth, J. (1963). *Timetables: Structuring the passage of time in hospital treatment and other careers*. Bobbs-Merrill.

Sánchez, M. (2021). *Análisis Estadístico del Sistema Isapre con Perspectiva de Género. Año 2020*. Superintendencia de Salud.

Scrimshaw, S. C., Lane, S. D., Rubinstein, R. A., & Fisher, J. (2022). *The SAGE handbook of social studies in health and medicine* (2nd ed.). SAGE Publications.

Seear, K., & Lenton, E. (2021). Becoming posthuman: Hepatitis C, the race to elimination and the politics of remaking the subject. *Health Sociology Review, 30*(3), 229–243. https://doi.org/10.1080/14461242.2021.1971102

Serres, M., & Latour, B. (1995). *Michel Serres with Bruno Latour. Conversations on Science, Culture, and Time* (R. Lapidus, Trans.). University of Michigan Press.

Tavory, I., & Timmermans, S. (2014). *Abductive analysis. Theorizing qualitative research*. The University of Chicago Press.

Timmermans, S. (1998). Mutual tuning of multiple trajectories. *Symbolic Interaction, 21*(4), 425–440. https://doi.org/10.1525/si.1998.21.4.425

Trundle, C., & Phillips, T. (2023). Defining focused ethnography: Disciplinary boundary-work and the imagined divisions between 'focused' and 'traditional' ethnography in health research—A critical review. *Social Science & Medicine, 332*. https://doi.org/10.1016/j.socscimed.2023.116108

Valéry, P. (1933). *L'idée fixe*. Editions Gallimard.

Valéry, P. (2004). *La idea fija*. A. Machado Libros.

van Pijkeren, N., Schuurmans, J., Wallenburg, I., & Bal, R. (2024). 'The night is for sleeping': How nurses care for conflicting temporal orders in older person care. *Health Sociology Review, 33*(1). https://doi.org/10.1080/14461242.2024.2316737

von Arx, M. (2023). The illusion of immediacy: On the need for human synchronization in data-intensive medicine. *Frontiers in Sociology, 8*, 1120946. https://doi.org/10.3389/fsoc.2023.1120946

World Bank. (1993). *World development report 1993. Investing in health*. World Bank.

Zerubavel, E. (1979). *Patterns of time in hospital Life. A sociological perspective*. University of Chicago Press.

Part II

Institutionalised Temporalities

5

A Rhythm of Unpredictability: Conceptualizing Temporalities in the Emergency Department

Andreas Wagenknecht, Johannes Deutschbein, Anna Schneider, Daniela Krüger, Martin Möckel, and Liane Schenk

The emergency department (ED) is generally regarded as one of the most time-sensitive settings in the healthcare system. In the public imagination, the ED appears as a hectic place. Severe acute and life-threatening emergencies require immediate, rapid response. Media representations of EDs work with fast cuts, short scenes, and flickering lighting effects, showing the fast-moving personnel providing care for severely injured patients for whose survival every minute and every second counts. This 'classic narrative' of work in EDs has not only informed the public

---

A. Wagenknecht (✉) • J. Deutschbein • L. Schenk
Institute of Medical Sociology and Rehabilitation Science, Charité - Universitätsmedizin Berlin, Berlin, Germany
e-mail: andreas.wagenknecht@charite.de; johannes.deutschbein@charite.de; liane.schenk@charite.de

A. Schneider
Ankerland Trauma-Therapiezentrum gGmbH, Hamburg, Germany
e-mail: anna.schneider@ankerland.de

K. Kenny et al. (eds.), *Timescapes of Health, Illness and Care*,
https://doi.org/10.1007/978-981-96-7055-0_5

imagination for decades but also informed the scientific reasoning of different disciplines, distorting the analysis of time and temporalities in the ED.

Quantitative health services research includes time as a variable for quality and performance measurement (McClelland et al., 2012; Otto et al., 2022), and studies from the field of psychology assess time allocation, changes in activities, and interruptions during work in the ED (Schneider et al., 2021a; Weigl et al., 2021). Waiting times, their management, and their consequences (e.g., treatment satisfaction) have been issues in health services research focusing on patients and nurses (Burström et al., 2013; Innes et al., 2018; Nyce et al., 2021; Pitrou et al., 2009; Thompson et al., 1996). Medical sociologists have also explored patients' experience of temporality as well as the regulation of time in the ED. Their research has provided insight into trajectories and the experience of long waiting times in the ED that conflict with perceived urgency (Hillman, 2014; Schwartz, 1975), the role of conflicts and struggles in the definition of urgency (Krüger, 2023), and how these aspects relate to triage processes (Ellebrecht, 2020; Wamsiedel, 2022).

The latter has been of special interest as it can be considered as a first step within the treatment trajectory that determines waiting times. Triage is a procedure implemented to save lives as EDs face an inadvertent public service dilemma (Lipsky, 2010): the number and needs of clients usually exceed the resources available to frontline staff to see every client immediately or with equal attention. Consequently, triage staff prioritize patients based on their level of urgency (Möckel et al., 2020). Triage and its potential biases through typification and moral evaluations have

D. Krüger
Emergency Medicine Care Research / Emergency and Acute Medicine, Charité - Universitätsmedizin Berlin, Berlin, Germany
e-mail: daniela.krueger2@charite.de

M. Möckel
Division of Emergency Medicine Campus Mitte and Virchow, Charité - Universitätsmedizin Berlin, Berlin, Germany
e-mail: martin.moeckel@charite.de

garnered much sociological interest as it affects service distribution and risks reproducing stigma and disadvantage (Fry, 2012; Johannessen, 2017; Vassy, 2001; Wamsiedel, 2020). The emphasis on triage processes has focused on the agency and capacities of triage personnel to regulate the ED workflow. This places triage staff at the forefront of the patient's temporal experience. While ED staff have a degree of control over, for example, waiting times, there are other departments and processes—often referred to as 'contextual factors'—that also influence the patient's experience. Following triage, patients may receive diverse examinations, consultations, and treatments that are beyond the control of the triage and ED staff. Even though the time following triage and initial treatment dominates an ED stay quantitatively, there is limited knowledge regarding the patterns that define the time patients spend in an ED from initial care to discharge.

Research focused on the triage processes may inadvertently perpetuate the 'classical narrative' of emergency medicine and its focus on rapidly saving lives within EDs. While time-critical urgent care remains a central part of the ED's mandate and portfolio, numerous studies demonstrate that ED personnel treat a more diverse range of health (and social) complaints, including providing treatment that vary from critical, lifesaving care to minor symptoms (Ruegenberg et al., 2023; Schneider et al., 2021b). Accordingly, cases differ in their temporal unfolding. In less urgent cases, which represent the majority of ED cases, ED care after triage is less structured and predetermined. Cases can have heterogeneous and complex timelines. This means that the understanding of the particular temporality in the ED requires a broader perspective. Our contribution in this chapter, therefore, firstly, aims to develop a conceptual heuristic to study temporalities within the ED; and secondly, it uses empirical data to study the temporal structure of ED stays.

This chapter delineates the temporal rhythms of the ED by exploring the conceptual tools provided by sociology and develops a heuristic for studying *time* in the ED. The chapter highlights the benefit of a temporal perspective to care provision in the ED and the patient experience, putting emphasis on the 'time-in-between' triage and admission to the hospital ward or discharge. This 'time-in-between' is experienced as unpredictable by patients—and appears to be 'out of hands' of providers.

The Temporal Rhythm of the ED

Our main approach for comprehending the significance of time in the ED revolves around *rhythm* and a *practice theory* approach. We will explain both and the analysis they allow, suggesting them as analytical heuristics. The ideas presented in this section enable us to understand the specificity of temporal processes in the ED from a patient's perspective.

Practice theory scholars have continued to stress the conceptual relationship between social practice and temporality. Following general considerations on the significance of temporality for the understanding of social practices (Schatzki, 2006, 2010; Reckwitz, 2002), scholars developed a deeper understanding of this issue. This encompasses that time involves more than just the past, present, and future, but aspects such as duration, synchronicity, and various 'temporality functions' that influence the shape of social life (Moran, 2015); how networked social practices produce temporal rhythms (Shove & Pantzar, 2010); the role of socially different experiences of the everyday organization of social practices and their temporal demands (Southerton, 2006; Atkinson, 2019); or, as particularly relevant to our study, the dialogue of practice theory and rhythm analysis to understand institutionalization processes (Blue, 2019).

Social practices possess a distinct temporal order, and, conversely, the temporality of a phenomenon is intertwined with the execution of social practices. As Bourdieu (1990, p. 81) states: "practice unfolds in time [...]. Its temporal structure, that is, its rhythm, its tempo, and above all its directionality, is constitutive of its meaning". Temporalities become taken for granted and persist through their practical enactment, as long as their logic is not questioned (Atkinson, 2019). Temporal regularity functions as a social norm and obligation, as well as a device for orientation (Bourdieu, 1990; Zerubavel, 1985). Individuals derive their temporal orientation and form judgments about what is acceptable in terms of temporality, such as acceptable waiting times in a healthcare setting.

Rhythms have been discussed in the context of practice theory research since Henri Lefebvre's work (Lefebvre, 2004; Blue, 2019), and recently, it is being applied to healthcare topics (Ihlebæk, 2021; Meadows et al.,

2017; O'Connor & Fotakopoulou, 2023; Osborne et al., 2023). Meadows et al. (2017), for example, showed how sleep rhythms contribute to recovery from substance abuse. These interdisciplinary and multimethod studies show the complex intersection of institutional rhythms of healthcare organizations and quasi-natural, individual, and physical rhythms of patients. These studies in rhythm analyses illustrate the significance of the stability made possible by rhythms, the embeddedness of rhythms in networks of heterogeneous rhythms (e.g., 'medical time', 'patient time', and 'hospital time'; see Ihlebæk, 2021), as well as attempts at stabilization and synchronization by the actors involved and the implications of moments of disruption.

In line with Shove and Pantzar (2010) and Blue (2019), we see a key role of rhythms in temporally linking various social activities and the production of socio-temporal orders. They affect and shape individual behavior and connect social practices by forming time-based relationships, for example the coordinated efforts of hospital departments or the operating theater in patient care. In contrast to this temporal cohesion, rhythms can also create conflicts that may occur when a dominant rhythm is altered or challenged (Atkinson, 2019), for example while ED medical personnel may follow a certain treatment order based on standardized procedures, patients may demand earlier consultation or treatment according to their perceived urgency or order of appearance.

Therefore, we argue that emergency medicine consist of a multitude of routinized social practices interwoven by their temporal rhythms. The ED consists of a "multiplicity of times" (Moran, 2015, p. 292) and differing but related rhythms. Specific time-sensitive pathways, which regulate the interaction of professions and interdisciplinary collaboration, intervene with a seemingly spontaneous chain of events.

The experience of time (or rhythm) is different for social actors, and access to the means of shaping temporal rhythms is associated with social inequality. Bourdieu (1986, 1990) argues that habitus and capital place social actors differently in a social structure, thereby positioning them accordingly as well as unequally to the means and opportunities to influence a field's temporal organization (Atkinson, 2019; Suderland, 2020). The power over schedules as a means to control the course and timing of relevant events and the possibilities of negotiating sequences are unequally distributed depending on the social position of actors. In this context, the concept of 'imposed timings' is of particular relevance. It refers to situations in which actors are "laying out timelines" (Atkinson, 2019, p. 961) for others, influencing their opportunities and experiences. In the ED, there are unequal conditions for managing conflicting temporalities, for example the occurrence of treatment-relevant events (from which patients can read the progress of their treatment) and the control over the treatment chronology (over which overview and power lies on the healthcare provider side).

Methods and Data

The empirical data used in this analysis are part of the mixed-methods research project EMAAge II, which is part of the research network EMANet (Schmiedhofer et al., 2018). The project investigates various facets of ED care for older patients (Deutschbein et al., 2024). To achieve a deeper understanding of older patients' ED stays, encompassing the trajectories of their treatment, their physical and mental conditions during the stay, specific problems and needs, and how they cope with the challenging situation, we conducted ethnographic observations. Observations were designed as overt and passive bedside company, if possible from the beginning of ED admission until discharge. A semi-structured observation protocol was used to capture all events in chronological order, including timestamps for each event. The observations strictly focused on patients; activities of ED personnel were only captured with regard to the observed patients. The primary aim of observations was to systematically collect data that come close to representing ED stays as experienced by these patients. Staff-related activities and processes that happen primarily in the background remained indiscernible for observers, as for the patients. Our analysis, therefore, cannot go into the temporal processes, mechanisms, and resources that affect the staff's experience or the ED as an organization. Given that this study focused on older patients' experiences of the ED, our sample and analysis is not representative of the wider possible cases in the ED.

The sample included patients aged 60 years and older who were conscious and able to verbally consent. The sample consisted of 72 cases, mostly low-acuity visits. The average age of patients was 79.9 years, with a median of 7.9. There were equal proportions of men and women. The sampling strategy aimed to reach a wide range of variation in patient characteristics. Observations were conducted on weekdays between March and December 2021 by nine observers in six different EDs in the central district Mitte of Berlin, Germany, which included hospitals of different sizes and structures. Prior to fieldwork, all observers were introduced to the observing technique, its rationale, potential pitfalls, and general considerations regarding the ED setting, and the observed population by the lead investigator (JD). In addition, regular meetings were held to reflect on the experiences and challenges of the observers in the field. Field notes were drafted into protocols immediately after the observation.

For analysis, all protocols were coded using an inductive and adaptable coding system. The coding process was accompanied by regular team meetings of the authors, other involved observers, and qualitative health researchers to discuss questions regarding the identification and content scope of identified codes. In this process, differences in the interpretation of specific descriptions in protocols were discussed to reach a shared understanding of potential meanings. Additionally, the intra-case level was addressed by a case summary for each observation. Quantitative temporal analysis of ED cases was mapped by extracting all relevant time data in a table. For each case, the timestamps of arrival, discharge, procedures, and all medical and nursing events were entered. We operationalized events as moments when actions were performed related to the patient's treatment and care. This included medical and nursing procedures, as well as communication between patients and staff.

Dimensions of Temporality and the Rhythm of ED Care

Our analysis identified that each presentation to the ED exhibits a certain rhythmic pattern. Various temporal aspects (see Fig. 5.1) characterize ED presentation cases and their rhythmic unfolding. The terms used in this section are in line with practice theory and rhythm analysis as outlined above, serving to make analytical sense of case trajectories, their temporal dimensions, and the ED rhythm as experienced by patients. These terms are 'events,' 'duration,' 'sequentiality,' 'idle', and 'body time', as well as 'schedules'. We suppose that these terms together characterize temporal rhythms.

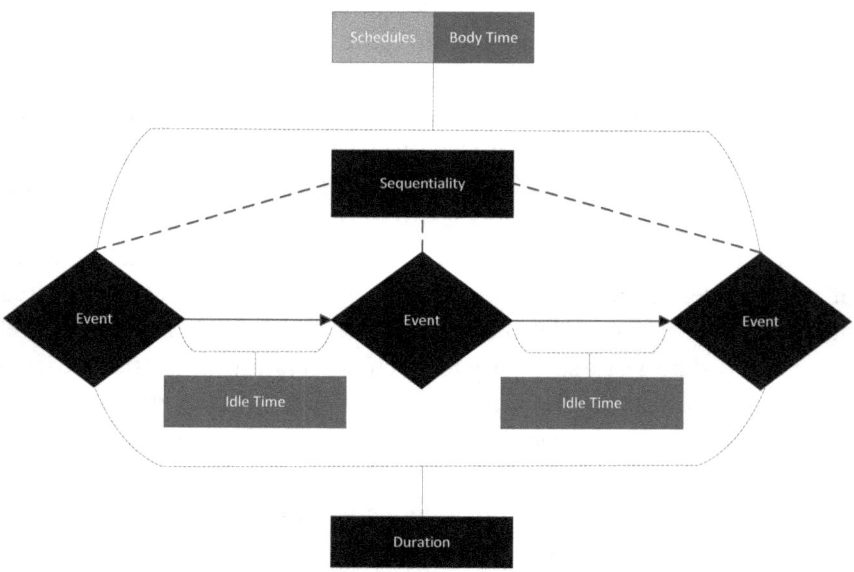

Fig. 5.1 Schematic overview of temporal concepts

Duration

A central issue concerning time in medical practice is how long things take. Duration can be understood as the amount of time devoted to specific activities, specified as an "uninterrupted succession and integrated change of affairs" (Schatzki, 2006, p. 164f). Additionally, duration can refer to the amount of time between two distinct events. Such idle time appears to be of particular importance for ED stays and will be discussed in a following section.

A first temporal aspect of a medical case is its overall length. Generally, ED cases can range from 25 minutes for serious injuries requiring immediate surgery or the treatment of a stroke following strict clinical protocols, to several hours. In our sample, the mean duration of observed stays was 4 hours and 38 minutes, with a large standard deviation of 2 hours and 8 minutes.[1] Half of the cases lasted approximately 3 hours or less, including around 10% of very short cases lasting less than two hours. The other half ranged between 3.5 and 11 hours, with less than 20% of the sample spending more than 6 hours in the ED.[2]

For example, an 80-year-old male ED patient (case #44) was treated as an inpatient for prostate cancer in another hospital, and then was sent to a study hospital for a computer tomography (CT). After the CT scan, the patient experienced acute back pain and nausea:

> 10:59 Patient comes around the corner with two nurses, they say they were at the CT and then the patient felt bad, nausea and back pain, they actually wanted to drive him back to the other hospital where he is currently hospitalized but he will now stay here (...)

[1] The mean duration of stay in our sample is underestimated since not every case could be observed until discharge. For these censured cases, there was usually data available on the time of discharge in the hospital information system. Based on this additional information, the longest case had a duration of more than 15 hours and the mean duration of stay for the sample was 5 hours and 20 minutes with a standard deviation of approximately 3 hours. However, data on time stamps in hospital information systems need to be interpreted cautiously since they can be biased by different factors, for example documentation practices of health professionals.

[2] There were mostly no single and objective medical reasons that explained variations and especially the very long stays. The temporal unfolding of a case often seemed to depend on available resources (e.g., ED staffing), organizational issues (e.g., general patient load in the ED at the time of the patients' stay), and external factors (e.g., the timely availability of hospital beds).

> 13:09 Nurse enters the room, patient seems very pleased, nurse has a cup in his hand and an infusion, he tells the patient that his potassium is too low, so he gets potassium in water and the infusion, the nurse also says transport has already been ordered (…)
>
> 19:00: Patient asks me (the observer) if I've been here the whole time, I say "yes, mostly", patient says he can't comprehend the length of time, he thinks he's going to "hand in his dinner pail"

The patient waited for about six hours for the return transport. The reasons for this waiting time remain unclear, and, in the meantime, the patient's condition worsened.

In contrast, a 76-year-old female patient (case #29) with suspected uncontrolled diabetes underwent blood sampling, a physical examination, medical history assessment, and infusion completed within the first half-hour. Afterwards, she 'only' waited for the infusion to run through and for the return of lab results. Finally, it was determined that no acute treatment in the ED was necessary, and she was admitted as an inpatient after an hour and three quarters.

A second aspect of duration pertains to the *length of procedures*: Depending on the specific procedure, they can be very short (e.g., a quick visual monitoring encounter of a patient's vital signs) or last for more than 20 minutes (e.g., an anamnesis, radiology exam). Additionally, it is common for procedures to be interrupted, which diffused and extended their total duration. For instance, the anamnesis of a 70-year-old male ED patient (case #7) with an abscess took about 33 minutes: It was conducted by two physicians who alternated during the anamnesis, with one leaving to take care of other tasks. Time gaps occurred, and nursing care as well as documentation were performed in between. It was also observed several times that blood collection took a relatively long time and sometimes had to be repeated. Here is an example from an 80-year-old patient with reduced general condition due to refusal of food and fluids (case #36):

> Doctor now approaches the patient's stretcher with a blood collection tray and announces to the patient that he "has to take the arm again, but this time it won't take so long"; patient yawns but does not visibly react to what is said, his eyes keep closing.

The patient's experience of exhaustion due to the repeated lengthy procedure of blood sampling of approximately 10 minutes appeared to be of relevance in this situation.

In general, the duration of the stay as a whole, and specific procedures in particular, is a regular topic of staff-patient interactions. In such conversations, different temporal rhythms within a hospital and the respective ward become a topic of discussion (Ihlebæk, 2021). Generally, communication about the duration of interim periods, or any temporal specifications, serve as a resource for temporal orientation for patients (Zerubavel, 1985). Most striking, however, was the widespread lack of discussion of time in our sample. In at least half of the cases, the length of stay in the ED, when to expect the next step of treatment, how long certain procedures will take, or when discharge will occur were not discussed at all. Around half of the observed patients inquired at least once about the length of their stay; however, explicit complaints about waiting times were rare. Following are two possible explanations: (a) Cases were processed quickly, that is, diagnostic and treatment events followed each other in short intervals, making discussions about duration seem irrelevant to those involved. It can therefore be assumed that in terms of time, the treatment was adequate for the parties involved. (b) A large part of the patients silently endured longer waiting times. Due to the limitations of the observation method, we can only speculate about the reasons.[3]

If temporality was communicated by healthcare personnel, it primarily occured in the form of vague formulations and phrases that avoided concrete specifications of temporal frames or exact time specifications in minutes or hours. We identified the following variations:

- Phrases such as 'soon', 'in a moment', 'shortly', 'really not much longer', and 'later' were used when an event had been completed and the period until the next event needed temporal qualification. In most cases, these imprecise statements corresponded to about ten minutes until the announced event, but we also observed patients waiting for an hour for a doctor who claimed to "come back in a moment".

[3] Also, in some cases, patients are in such a severe state of health that they are hardly able to express their needs, including the need for temporal orientation.

- 'if… then' or 'first…then': if event A (e.g., the blood/urine sample is examined or the infusion runs through), then event B (e.g., further diagnostics/consultations/discharge) will follow. This way, a certain causality of events that occupy the respective actor backstage is determined and communicated—but without temporal qualification.

- Concrete time specifications by ED personnel were rather rare but nevertheless occurred, mostly in connection with certain procedures: for example, checking/observing cardiac values in the next two hours, waiting for blood testing results in about 30 minutes, or stating that an infusion will run through for another 30 to 40 minutes. As the stay progressed, case processing became less standardized and communication about expectable events and progression became less frequent.

Another aspect was communication with patients' relatives, who usually waited outside the ED. Occasionally, patients tried to communicate exact times to their relatives by 'translating' statements of ED staff, without having concrete information on the duration of the stay, as exemplified in the following excerpt (case #39):

> 16:03 Patient makes a voice message to assumedly his wife. He tells her that the electrocardiogram (ECG) is normal, that he thinks the pain is due to heavy lifting and that he is just waiting for the x-ray and labs.
>
> 16:10 He makes another voice message and says "we're halfway through now".
>
> 16:15 He makes another voice message in which he says: "we're just waiting for the lab results".
>
> 17:28 The doctor explains to the patient that they are just waiting for the lab results. After the doctor has left, the patient makes a voice message and says: "The doctor said I'm almost done".

To summarize, what was most striking concerning duration was that not only the total duration but also, to a certain extent, the durations could neither be estimated nor anticipated by both ED staff and patients. This impacted patient-staff-interaction. The conversational technique of 'vaguely approximating' and 'not being able to specify' prevailed as the most common form of communication. This 'blurred' but relevant information is needed for both parties to estimate durations relevant to the patients' ED stay. Due to the lack of designation of specific time measurement marks (minutes, hours), which are usually used in everyday communication to express the duration of certain activities, the respective communication between staff and patients fulfills the function of temporal orientation only to a limited extent.[4]

Events

Events are a limited condensation of time, in which social elements (bodies, things, humans, etc.) interact (Hillebrandt, 2023). Events are not without preconditions and consequences but are connected with other events, forming some sort of series or sequence (for sequentiality, see next section). A distinction can be made between events that always occur at the same time due to a predetermined structure (e.g., institutional or organizational), events that occur with a certain regularity, and events that occur fully unexpectedly and unpredictably. Social actors also have different capabilities to generate or participate in events, according to their agency, capital, position, and power in the field (Suderland, 2020).

We observed that most cases consisted of an average of ten events. In about 40% of cases, more than 9 events occurred (with a few cases having over 20 events), 20% involved 6 to 8 events, and 13% had less than 5 events to completion. For example, a 79-year-old female patient (case #57) presenting with a nosebleed underwent treatment starting with body temperature and blood sample collection, followed by medical history, a brief physical examination, and immediate sclerotherapy of a vein in the nose. After some time, the doctor checked the wound, and, shortly after, the patient received her doctor's letter and could leave the ED. The immediate link between diagnostics and treatment resulted in few events and a very short overall length of stay. On the other end of the spectrum,

[4] This is not to argue that the way staff communicates is wrong or problematic. It follows its own logic, and the vagueness of the communication makes sense for the staff and the organizational processes. Staff themselves sometimes do not have more precise information and do not want to incite unrealistic expectations.

the treatment of an 83-year-old male patient (case #1), who independently stopped taking his dehydration drugs and experienced shortness of breath, involved more than 20 events. Due to the suspicion of water in the lungs, additional diagnostic measures were conducted alongside standard procedures. Extensive nursing activities followed, particularly concerning the patient's incontinence.

Patient actions were only one factor influencing the total number of events. Other, more significant factors included the necessity of diagnostic procedures, diagnostic uncertainties, complications, or the availability of ED and other hospital personnel. Therefore, events were usually initiated by ED staff. If initiated by patients, events typically involved expressing needs. Patients' ability to express their needs often increased the number of events but was not automatically linked to it. Individual needs included assistance with toileting, thirst, hunger, feeling cold, or changing their position on the stretcher. Receiving help with these needs, which initiated additional events for ED personnel, could require several attempts from patients, and the satisfaction of expressed needs could take some time, depending on the availability of suitable ED staff. Two examples:

> Patient (case #72) sits up and calls into the corridor: "Sister Maria!" A nurse enters the room, and the patient complains that he's been waiting so long without receiving any food or drink.
>
> The patient (case #63) opens his eyes and looks around. He then rings the bell and gazes at the door. A nurse enters, and the patient, visibly annoyed, asks what is going on and what should happen next. The nurse responds that he has to wait until the doctor decides what to do, and this might take a little while. The patient quietly and sarcastically remarks, "a 'little while', that's good."

So, can events and their consequences be reasonably anticipated? Following the conclusions on duration, we would deduce that the implementation and execution of a treatment-relevant events by ED staff are characterized by a low level of anticipation, as is the total number of events. Initial procedures such as blood sampling, temperature taking, and history taking have a relevantly high degree of probability. However, beyond and after that, it is not easily predictable for the patient what will happen next. This is a typical feature of acute and emergency presentations, as the underlying cause of the presentation is mostly unclear at the beginning, and the case unfolds over an unforeseen period.

Idle Times

A general temporal pattern is the alternation between periods of activity and periods of inactivity (Zerubavel, 1987). In our case, this refers to the (idle) time between two medical or nursing events. The ratio of events and idle time was one of the most important aspects shaping the rhythm of an ED stay, particularly from the patient's perspective. Much sociological research has explored the social significance of idle or waiting time, considering 'letting someone wait' as an indication of social insignificance or low priority (Schwartz, 1975; Sellerberg, 2008; Auyero, 2011; Hansen, 2020). Studies beyond clinical settings have revealed the strategic role of imposing waiting time as part of institutional power dynamics in organizations. Studies focusing on patients have demonstrated how waiting can create a hostile atmosphere within nurse-patient interactions and worsen the patient's treatment experience (Akerström, 1997; Nyce et al., 2021).

Patients in our sample experienced significant amounts of idle time. Idle time was defined as a period of at least approximately 15 minutes between the end of one event and the beginning of another. The ratio of eventful to idle time varied: some cases had almost no idle time or significantly shorter idle time compared to eventful time; others had a balance between eventful and idle time, while some had longer idle time than eventful time. In our sample, idle time between two events lasted up to 90 minutes or more in extreme cases. Overall, across all observed cases, the proportion of idle time was 57%. Idle periods typically lasted much longer than the events themselves, with the cumulative idle time duration often far exceeding that of events. For instance, a 78-year-old female patient (case #46) with visual disturbances after a shingles infection (varicella-zoster virus) waited more than two hours between anamnesis and physical examination (lasting from 9:15 to 9:30) and a neurological consultation (lasting from 11:50 to 12:00).

Longer stays tend to correlate with longer idle periods, reflecting the complexity of cases. The longest idle periods were typically observed in the latter third of a stay, although lengthy periods could also occur shortly after admission or following diagnostic procedures. For instance, an 84-year-old male patient (case #17) having problems with breathing, a low oxygen saturation, and a weak pulse was admitted to the hospital for further observation. Diagnostic procedures, with idle times of 50 and 30 minutes between them, yielded no clear findings. Subsequently, at 15:54, a decision was made to have the patient picked up by the transport service, which finally occurred at 17:29.

From the patient perspective, the cause of idle times often remains unclear. Several factors influence this ratio, including the medical characteristics of cases and organizational processes. While some empty periods, such as waiting for laboratory results, could be anticipated in certain cases, their duration remained unpredictable. In many instances, the occurrence and duration of idle time were unpredictable, significantly affecting patients' time orientation.

Sequentiality

Sequentiality refers to the order in which events occur. It is a general feature of social interaction, processes, and experience that constitutes their coherence (Schatzki, 2006; Rawls, 2005; Hillebrandt, 2023). Each event conditions the next, creating meaning through their connection. In an ED, events follow a typical sequence: arrival, triage, stabilization, diagnosis, treatment, and discharge. However, this sequence may not always be clear or explained to patients, leading to unpredictability. For example, blood samples and medical history may be repeated, and causally linked events may vary in temporal distance, therefore diffusing their relation.

However, this is merely superficial. Complexity arises when examining the temporal structure, particularly the sequential arrangement of events and idle time. In our sample, cohesive event sequences typically occurred at the start of ED stays during the diagnostic phase. As the duration of the stay increased, events became sporadic and disjointed. Evenly distributed event sequences throughout the stay were rare in our sample of older adults with low acuity visits. We identified four ideal-typical structures:

- A prolonged idle period at the outset of treatment, suggesting a delayed start. An example is an 82-year-old female patient (case #13) with suspected thrombosis in her left leg. After initial care, she waits an hour and a half for a doctor to take her medical history and perform diagnostics. An hour later, she's informed she doesn't have thrombosis.
- A second structure involves a longer idle period in the middle of the case. After initial intensive measures, there is a gap until events resume. An example would be an 81-year-old female patient (case #11) with suspected internal bleeding, who receives intensive treatment for three hours (including repeated insertion of venous catheters and X-rays), then experiences a lull from 14:30 to 16:00. "*At 16:10: Physician A1 arrives and asks the patient how she is, the patient says in a tearful voice that she no longer knows how to lie down, 'everything hurts*". The last medical and nursing activities take place until 17:30, then the patient is discharged.

- Thirdly, some cases show multiple empty periods toward the end. Initially coherent treatment events are followed by increasing idle time until discharge. Example: The 83-old male patient (case #1) mentioned earlier experiences a coherent hour and a half of treatment, followed by idle periods of 38 minutes, 1 hour, and finally 2.5 hours.

- Lastly, certain cases are characterized by idle time throughout, resulting in a prolonged overall duration.

Only a portion of the cases in our sample could be distinctly categorized into these structures. Many exhibit mixed forms or lack recognizable patterns. Additionally, these structures were discerned only in hindsight through methodological and interpretative efforts. Nevertheless, the sequential oscillation between events and idle times gave the impression of a disordered sequentiality.

Schedules and Body Time

Schedules, a component of social time and rhythms (Zerubavel, 1976), prestructure the occurrence of events and actions in a collective manner. They dictate the sequence, timing, and duration of events, exerting significant influence. Particularly in healthcare settings, schedules are crucial for maintaining temporal order, enhancing predictability and optimizing resource utilization. In the ED, schedules must adapt to the dynamic environment and diverse medical disease patterns.

As outlined earlier, different rhythms can intersect, impacting patients and their bodily rhythms known as body time (Cohen, 2011; Holmes, 2018). In the ED, bodily phenomena are inevitable, such as basic needs like eating and drinking, but also blood extraction, and pain management. Such physical processes generate specific events (Schillmeier, 2014) that are relevant for processes in the ED. If schedules refer to bodily phenomena, it involves considerations of duration, pace, and efforts to expedite bodily processes. But, schedules and the human body may also sometimes clash, as "bodies and their temporality are, however, frustratingly unpredictable" (Cohen, 2011, p. 193).

We describe this aspect with reference to urination. Typically, ED staff responded promptly, within minutes, to a patient's request to urinate, facilitating actions such as monitoring cable adjustments, toilet escort, or providing urinals/bedpans. For instance, the 83-year-old male patient (case #1), presenting with shortness of breath, repeatedly seeks diaper changes due to incontinence, a process taking up to 20 minutes. After an hour in the ED, a nurse and the patient agree to a toileting schedule: "*he should go to the toilet every 2 hours as a safety precaution*" to manage enuresis, minimizing diaper changes. However, later, the patient's requests for assistance are dismissed, with the diaper being suggested instead, countering his urge to urinate. Conversely, in another case, acceleration of urination is attempted. A 90-year-old female patient (case #42), admitted for vomiting and severe pain, is informed of receiving an infusion to "*speed up the urge to urinate*", aiming to obtain a urine sample promptly and overcome the patient's physiological resistance as a temporal obstacle and serving the organizational need for timely diagnosis and treatment.

The examples illustrate how the patient's body becomes a treatment element, factored into staff calculations as a temporal consideration or obstacle. Efforts are made to regulate urine flow to fit time constraints by administering substances affecting its speed. Toilet use, crucial for older patients, is initiated by the patient as a social event, with the time until assistance being critical. Here, individual body rhythms intersect with organizational ones, influencing each other. Synchronizing medical procedures with quasi-autonomous embodied temporalities necessitates coordination to reduce unpredictability.

Conclusion: A Rhythm of Unpredictability

Our contribution demonstrates the value of examining ED processes through a temporal lens and focusing patients. We analyzed the rhythm of ED care utilizing concepts from practice theory and rhythm analysis. Conceptually, we argue for using rhythms and related terms (duration, events, idle time, sequentiality, schedules, body time) to understand time experiences and regulation capacities in the ED. This approach additionally emphasizes the 'time-in-between' triage and ED discharge, and complements previous studies on ED triage (Fry, 2012; Johannessen, 2017; Vassy, 2001; Wamsiedel, 2020).

To conclude, our analysis reveals the ED rhythm's predominant temporal characteristic: unpredictability. Our contribution is part of the multifaceted medical sociological research on the topic of uncertainty and unpredictability (Calnan, 1984; Peter & Funcke, 2003; Mackintosh & Armstrong, 2020; Lian et al., 2021; Robinson, 2004; Serra, 2016). Research into the phenomenon of uncertainty, based on the principles of the sociology of knowledge, examines the influence as well as techniques and technologies of dealing with uncertainty, focusing on medical practices and decision-making, diagnostics and prognostics, staff-patient-relationship, patient experiences, and communication of uncertainty. A few studies specifically address the connection between temporality and uncertainty (Timmermans & Stivers, 2018; Hautamäki, 2018). Our specific contribution sheds light on how one form of temporal uncertainty is dominant in a particular healthcare institution due to typical practices, routines, and rhythms: unpredictability.

While ED personnel and the organization may perceive an overarching rhythm, patients often find the logic and reasons behind their stay's rhythm obscure. The incomprehensible schedule imposed by the ED disrupts some patients' sense of time, resembling a 'time-anomic' situation lacking "any definite norm that regulates their duration" (Zerubavel, 1976, p. 88f) and other temporal dimensions. A sense of unpredictability dominates and contradicts the notion of a practical sense of time. Such a sense typically arises from actors' habitus, manifesting itself in the form of anticipation. The "practical (…) sense of the forthcoming" (Atkinson, 2019, p. 954; Bourdieu, 2000) is enabling effective action within collectives. ED patients not only experience an imposed rhythm but also appear to lack a sense of anticipation. The ED schedule remains largely obscure and difficult to grasp, leaving patients at the mercy of others who regulate their treatment. With limited knowledge or experience of the ED's temporal structure and their individual case, patients feel incapable of action. Other studies have shown how predictability of events as well as long waiting times influence the relationship of healthcare workers and patients and lower patient satisfaction (Akerström, 1997; Ihlebæk, 2021; Nyce et al., 2021). Our study adds to this by focusing on the patient's perspective and the aforementioned conceptual assumptions. We showed that it is neither waiting alone nor only certain phases of treatment that are formative for the experience of time in the ED. The specific constellation of duration, events, idle times, and sequences create an absence of expectability and anticipation, what we call a rhythm of the unpredictable.

We suggested that much of ED care and its pace appear to be 'out of the hands' of ED staff as well. The flexibility of ED schedules may be exacerbated by the organizational dependence of EDs on the schedules of other entities (Ihlebæk, 2021). EDs are typically interconnected with the schedules of laboratories, medical consultation services, hospital wards, external hospitals, or patient transport providers. Consequently, the rhythm of an ED stay is nontransparent on two levels: patients are unable to comprehend the ED's schedule that determines their stay, and ED personnel often cannot influence or predict the capacities of organizations they depend on. Although synchronicity is sought, the rhythm of the ED and the patient's rhythm tend to be less synchronous or difficult to synchronize at least.

Due to the limitations of our data, we could not fully ascertain the extent to which the aforementioned temporal dimensions of the ED stay act as stressors and thus influence the physical and emotional state of the patients. The lack of information and ability to anticipate the duration of the stay and 'when it will continue' diffused temporal orientation, which may also have serious medical consequences (e.g., delirium). Nonetheless, we occasionally observed how the duration of stay had a negative impact on patients. A dynamic of exhaustion could be observed, with patients visibly weakened physically, some becoming apathetic, nervous, frustrated, or repeatedly falling asleep. It can also be noted that temporal orientation and sovereignty pose a particular challenge for older people, who are typically brought to the ED for nursing reasons or minor medical issues, comprising the population of our study. Time-related aspects and associated challenges are likely to become more acute with the increasing vulnerability of this patient population. Finally, we would like to mention that communication strategies addressing temporal aspects, as well as strategies for dealing with idle time, are further topics promising interesting sociological insights. Further research on the impact of temporal anomic situations is likely to be relevant as it can also contribute to improvement initiatives in healthcare institutions and patient satisfaction.

Acknowledgments The authors would like to thank the participating hospitals in the EMANet research network, all study participants, as well as all EMANet researchers and study personnel responsible for study planning, patient recruitment, and data management.

Competing Interests The authors have no conflicts of interest to declare that are relevant to the content of this chapter.

References

Akerström, M. (1997). Waiting—A source of hostile interaction in an emergency clinic. Qualitative Health Research, 7(4), 504–520. https://doi.org/10.1177/104973239700700405

Atkinson, W. (2019). Time for Bourdieu: Insights and oversights. *Time & Society, 28*(3), 951–970. https://doi.org/10.1177/0961463X17752280

Auyero, J. (2011). Patients of the state: An ethnographic account of poor people's waiting. *Latin American Research Review, 46*(1), 5–29. https://doi.org/10.1353/lar.2011.0014

Blue, S. (2019). Institutional rhythms: Combining practice theory and rhythmanalysis to conceptualise processes of institutionalisation. *Time & Society, 28*(3), 922–950. https://doi.org/10.1177/0961463X17702165

Bourdieu, P. (1986). The forms of capital. In J. G. Richardson (Ed.), *Handbook of theory and research for the sociology of education* (pp. 241–258). Greenwood Press.

Bourdieu, P. (1990). *The logic of practice.* Stanford University Press. https://doi.org/10.1515/9781503621749

Bourdieu, P. (2000). *Pascalian meditations.* Polity Press.

Burström, L., Starrin, B., Engström, M.-L., & Thulesius, H. (2013). Waiting management at the emergency department—A grounded theory study. *BMC Health Service Research, 13*, 95. https://doi.org/10.1186/1472-6963-13-95

Calnan, M. (1984). Clinical uncertainty: Is it a problem in the doctor-patient relationship? *Sociology of Health and Illness, 6*(1), 74–85.

Cohen, R. L. (2011). Time, space and touch at work: Body work and labour process (re)organisation. *Sociology of Health & Illness, 33*(2), 189–205. https://doi.org/10.1111/j.1467-9566.2010.01306.x

Deutschbein, J., Wagenknecht, A., Gilles, G., Möckel, M., & Schenk, L. (2024). 'The stay here is, of course, not appropriate for an old person': The perspective of healthcare providers on older patients in the emergency department. *BMC Geriatrics, 24*, 890. https://doi.org/10.1186/s12877-024-05429-9

Ellebrecht, N. (2020). *Organisierte Rettung Studien zur Soziologie des Notfalls.* Springer VS. https://doi.org/10.1007/978-3-658-30162-0

Fry, M. (2012). An ethnography: Understanding emergency nursing practice belief systems. *International Emergency Nursing, 20*(3), 120–125. https://doi.org/10.1016/j.ienj.2011.09.002

Hansen, L. S. (2020). 'It's not even the leaders out here who have any say at all in how long they're gonna have to wait': A study of waiting time, power, and acceptance. *Time & Society, 29*(4), 1128–1149. https://doi.org/10.1177/0961463X20950983

Hautamäki, L. (2018). Uncertainty work and temporality in psychiatry: How clinicians and patients experience and manage risk in practice? *Health, Risk & Society, 20*(1–2), 43–62. https://doi.org/10.1080/13698575.2018.1442918

Hillebrandt, F. (2023). *Ereignistheorie für eine Soziologie der Praxis. Das love and peace Festival auf Fehmarn und die Formation der Pop-Musik*. Springer VS. https://doi.org/10.1007/978-3-658-39022-8

Hillman, A. (2014). 'Why Must I Wait?' The performance of legitimacy in a hospital emergency department. *Sociology of Health & Illness, 36*(4), 485–499. https://doi.org/10.1111/1467-9566.12072

Holmes, H. (2018). Self-time: The importance of temporal experience within practice. *Time & Society, 27*(2), 176–194. https://doi.org/10.1177/0961463X15596461

Ihlebæk, H. M. (2021). Time to care—An ethnographic study of how temporal structuring affects caring relationships in clinical nursing. *Social Science & Medicine, 287*, 114349. https://doi.org/10.1016/j.socscimed.2021.114349

Innes, K., Elliott, D., Plummer, V., & Jackson, D. (2018). Emergency department waiting room nurses in practice: An observational study. *Journal of Clinical Nursing, 27*(7–8), e1402–e1411. https://doi.org/10.1111/jocn.14240

Johannessen, L. E. F. (2017). Beyond guidelines: Discretionary practice in face-to-face triage nursing. *Sociology of Health & Illness, 39*(7), 1180–1194. https://doi.org/10.1111/1467-9566.12578

Krüger, D. (2023). 'It Has Become Normal to Call 112'—Classificatory struggles over the increased use of emergency care in urgencity. [Doctoral Dissertation, Humboldt-Universität zu Berlin].

Lefebvre, H. (2004). *Rhythmanalysis: Space, time and everyday life*. Continuum.

Lian, O. S., Nettleton, S., Wifstad, A., & Dowrick, C. (2021). Negotiating uncertainty in clinical encounters: A narrative exploration of naturally occurring primary care consultations. *Social Science & Medicine, 291*, 114467. https://doi.org/10.1016/j.socscimed.2021.114467

Lipsky, M. (2010). *Street-level bureaucracy: Dilemmas of the individual in public services*. Russell Sage.

Mackintosh, N., & Armstrong, N. (2020). Understanding and managing uncertainty in health care: Revisiting and advancing sociological contributions. *Sociology of Health & Illness, 42*(S1), 1–20. https://doi.org/10.1111/1467-9566.13160

McClelland, M. S., Jones, K., Siegel, B., & Pines, J. M. (2012). A field test of time-based emergency department quality measures. *Annals of Emergency Medicine, 59*(1), 1–10.e2. https://doi.org/10.1016/j.annemergmed.2011.06.013

Meadows, R., Nettleton, S., & Neale, J. (2017). Sleep waves and recovery from drug and alcohol dependence: Towards a rhythm analysis of sleep in residential treatment. *Social Science & Medicine, 184*, 124–133. https://doi.org/10.1016/j.socscimed.2017.05.016

Möckel, M., Reiter, S., Lindner, T., & Slagman, A. (2020). 'Triagierung'—Ersteinschätzung von Patienten in der zentralen Notaufnahme: Eine Übersicht mit systematischem Review ['Triage'-primary assessment of patients in the emergency department: An overview with a systematic review]. *Medizinische Klinik—Intensivmedizin und Notfallmedizin, 115*(8), 668–681. https://doi.org/10.1007/s00063-019-0589-0

Moran, C. (2015). Time as a social practice. *Time & Society, 24(3)*, 283–303. https://doi.org/10.1177/0961463X13478051

Nyce, A., Gandhi, S., Freeze, B., Bosire, J., Ricca, T., Kupersmith, E., et al. (2021). Association of emergency department waiting times with patient experience in admitted and discharged patients. *Journal of Patient Experience, 8*, 23743735211011404. https://doi.org/10.1177/23743735211011404

O'Connor, J., & Fotakopoulou, O. (2023). Using rhythmanalysis to explore the synchronicities and disruptions in children's everyday lives in England and Greece during the 2020 lockdown. *Methodological Innovations, 16*(1), 27–37. https://doi.org/10.1177/20597991221144571

Osborne, T., Lowe, T. A., & Meijering, L. (2023). Care and rhythmanalysis: Using metastability to understand the routines of dementia care. *Social Science & Medicine, 331*, 116099. https://doi.org/10.1016/j.socscimed.2023.116099

Otto, R., Blaschke, S., Schirrmeister, W., Drynda, S., Walcher, F., & Greiner, F. (2022). Length of stay as quality indicator in emergency departments: Analysis of determinants in the German Emergency Department Data Registry (AKTIN registry). *Internal and Emergency Medicine, 17*, 1199–1209. https://doi.org/10.1007/s11739-021-02919-1

Peter, C., & Funcke, D. (Eds.). (2003). *Wissen an der Grenze. Zum Umgang mit Ungewissheit und Unsicherheit in der modernen Medizin*. Campus Verlag.

Pitrou, I., Lecourt, A. C., Bailly, L., Brousse, B., Dauchet, L., & Ladner, J. (2009). Waiting time and assessment of patient satisfaction in a large reference emergency department: A prospective cohort study, France. *European Journal of Emergency Medicine, 16*(4), 177–182. https://doi.org/10.1097/MEJ.0b013e32831016a6

Rawls, A. W. (2005). Garfinkel's conception of time. *Time & Society, 14*(2–3), 163–190. https://doi.org/10.1177/0961463X05055132

Reckwitz, A. (2002). Toward a theory of social practices: A development in culturalist theorizing. *European Journal of Social Theory, 5*(2), 243–263. https://doi.org/10.1177/13684310222225432

Robinson, S. (2004). Uncertainty. In J. Gabe, M. Bury, & M. A. Elston (Eds.), *Key concepts in medical sociology* (pp. 101–107). SAGE.

Ruegenberg, A., Schmiedhofer, M., Kreutzberg, A., Henscke, C., Möckel, M., & Slagman, A. (2023). Blackbox: Psychosoziale Fälle in der Notaufnahme. *Medizinische Klinik—Intensivmedizin und Notfallmedizin, 119*, 10–17. https://doi.org/10.1007/s00063-022-00981-x

Schatzki, T. R. (2006). The time of activity. *Continental Philosophy Review, 39*, 155–182. https://doi.org/10.1007/s11007-006-9026-1

Schatzki, T. R. (2010). *The timespace of human activity: On performance, society and history as indeterminate teleological events*. Lexington Books.

Schillmeier, M. (2014). *Eventful bodies. The cosmopolitics of illness*. Ashgate.

Schmiedhofer, M., Inhoff, T., Krobisch, V., Schenk, L., Rose, M., Holzinger, F., et al. (2018). EMANet: A regional network for health services research in emergency and acute medicine. *Zeitschrift für Evidenz, Fortbildung und Qualität im Gesundheitswesen, 135–136*, 81–88. https://doi.org/10.1016/j.zefq.2018.07.009

Schneider, A., Riedlinger, D., Pigorsch, M., Holzinger, F., Deutschbein, J., Keil, T., et al. (2021a). Self-reported health and life satisfaction in older emergency department patients: Sociodemographic, disease-related and care-specific associated factors. *BMC Public Health, 21*(1), 1440. https://doi.org/10.1186/s12889-021-11439-8

Schneider, A., Williams, D. J., Kalynych, C., Wehler, M., & Weigl, M. (2021b). Physicians' and nurses' work time allocation and workflow interruptions in emergency departments: A comparative time-motion study across two countries. *Emergency Medicine Journal, 38*(4), 263–268. https://doi.org/10.1136/emermed-2019-208508

Schwartz, B. (1975). *Queuing and waiting: Studies on the social organization of access and delay*. University of Chicago Press.

Sellerberg, A.-M. (2008). Waiting and rejection: An organizational perspective 'Cooling out' rejected applicants. *Time & Society, 17*(2/3), 349–362. https://doi.org/10.1177/0961463X08093428

Serra, H. (2016). Gamble on the uncertain. Negotiating medical decision-making. *Qualitative Sociology Review, 12*(4), 44–59. https://doi.org/10.18778/1733-8077.12.4.03

Shove, E., & Pantzar, M. (2010). Temporal rhythms as outcomes of social practices. *Ethnologia Europaea, 40*(1), 19–29. https://doi.org/10.16995/ee.1061

Southerton, D. (2006). Analysing the temporal organization of daily life. Social constraints, practices and their allocation. *Sociology, 40*(3), 435–454. https://doi.org/10.1177/0038038506063668

Suderland, M. (2020). Grundlage einer soziologischen Theorie der Zeitlichkeit? Bourdieus theoretische Denkwerkzeuge als Erkenntnispotenzial für qualitativ-empirische Forschung. *Forum Qualitative Sozialforschung / Forum: Qualitative Social Research, 21*(2). Art. 13, https://doi.org/10.17169/fqs-21.2.3472

Thompson, D. A., Yarnold, P. R., Williams, D. R., & Adams, S. L. (1996). Effects of actual waiting time, perceived waiting time, information delivery, and expressive quality on patient satisfaction in the emergency department. *Annals of Emergency Medicine, 28*, 657–665.

Timmermans, S., & Stivers, T. (2018). Clinical forecasting: Towards a sociology of prognosis. *Social Science & Medicine, 218*, 13–20. https://doi.org/10.1016/j.socscimed.2018.09.031

Vassy, C. (2001). Categorisation and micro-rationing: Access to care in a French Emergency Department. *Sociology of Health and Illness, 23*(5), 615–632. https://doi.org/10.1111/1467-9566.00268

Wamsiedel, M. (2020). Credibility work and moral evaluation at the ED. *Social Science & Medicine, 248*, 112845. https://doi.org/10.1016/j.socscimed.2020.112845

Wamsiedel, M. (2022). Temporal typifications as an organizational resource: Experiential knowledge and patient processing at the emergency department. *Time & Society, 31*(2), 157–176. https://doi.org/10.1177/0961463X211031881

Weigl, M., Händl, T., Wehler, M., & Schneider, A. (2021). Beobachtungsstudie ärztlicher und pflegerischer Aktivitäten in der Notaufnahme. *Medizinische Klinik—Intensivmedizin und Notfallmedizin, 116*(3), 229–237. https://doi.org/10.1007/s00063-020-00657-4

Zerubavel, E. (1976). Timetables and scheduling: On the social organization of time. *Sociological Inquiry, 46*(2), 87–94. https://doi.org/10.1111/j.1475-682X.1976.tb00753.x

Zerubavel, E. (1985). *Hidden rhythms: Schedules and calendars in social life*. University of California Press.

Zerubavel, E. (1987). The language of time: Towards a semiotics of temporality. *The Sociological Quarterly, 28*(3), 343–356.

6

Finding Yourself Waiting: The Spatio-Temporal Semiotics of the GP Waiting Room

Michael J. Flexer

Queue-Jumping: Some Last Thoughts First

> First last moment. Grant only enough remain to devour all. Moment by glutton moment. (Beckett, 1981, p. 59)

When initially researching and drafting this chapter in early 2020, the objective was, through a semiotic critique of the temporalities produced by the waiting room, and placed onto the patients navigating and being constructed by it, only to be a call to arms to rethink waiting for GP services. Events have overrun this ambition. In a matter of days in late March 2020, the accumulated traditions of waiting for GP services were swept aside. There is no need to call for change. Change has been forced. As the turmoil and destruction of the pandemic receded, so did practices of care and of the management of care, similarly return. Like so much

M. J. Flexer (✉)
University of Exeter, Exeter, UK
e-mail: m.flexer@exeter.ac.uk

K. Kenny et al. (eds.), *Timescapes of Health, Illness and Care*,
https://doi.org/10.1007/978-981-96-7055-0_6

that came back, these revenants were familiar but different. They are lessened, hollowed by their time in the grave, and their return articulates their absence; '[t]here is something disappeared, departed in the apparition itself as reapparition of the departed' (Derrida, 1994, p. 50). At the current time of writing, in mid-2024, the machinery of waiting—and the services for which we waited—are doubly haunted, by an ill-retrieved past and a lost future.

In October 2020, the author had to collect paperwork for a referral from his GP practice in Walthamstow, London. Although his GP consultation had been conducted entirely over the phone, supported by emailed self-taken digital photographs in lieu of a physical examination, it was still necessary to present at the practice. No GPs were working out of the practice building anymore and no patients were allowed to enter. Only the management and administrative staff, mostly fielding incoming calls from patients hoping for telephone appointments, populated the building. Buzzing at the front door of the practice, patients were either sent home to make an appointment by telephone or redirected to a side street and a ground-floor window, only ajar, situated near the practice's bins, to collect or drop off paperwork. On this occasion, a small queue formed, and the author was requested to wait, socially distanced, whilst the administrative staff contacted the GP—working from home outside London—to arrange the paperwork to be collected. It felt not much different from waiting in the waiting room: the sense of neglect, of being refused or being a problem, of being on the periphery, of being a foreign interloper, or, worse, of being a foreign object out of place and ripe for expulsion were all present. In fact, these feelings were perhaps less anxiety producing, less angering, than in the waiting room, because at least the waiters were now situated appropriately: shut off, to one side, down with the rubbish, out in the street, barred from the practice.

This chapter's proposed critical analysis of the spatio-temporal semiotics of the waiting room would, prior to COVID-19, have been activism. Within the conjuncture of the pandemic, it became merely archaeology. In semiotic terms as used by Uspenskij, there was a shift in the temporal model for situating the GP waiting room, as the COVID-19 pandemic ushered in a 'new era': 'the cosmological model of time perception may be foregrounded or symbolically resurrected, in the perception of historical events which inaugurate a *new era* that is assumed to be significant for all mankind or for the fate of a given people' (Uspenskij, 2017, p. 236). Whereas in the historical model there is a subjectivity, linearity and future-orientation to time, based on at least supposed chains of causal relations, in the cosmological model, as described by Uspenskij, there is an objectivity, concentricity and past orientation to time, based on symbolic relations. As such, it is not that the present was caused by the past or goes on to cause the future (as a future present) but, instead, the present manifests the past and portents the future. Cosmologically, that pandemic 'present' manifested the myths of the Black Death or the Spanish Flu and equally portended oncoming catastrophes, not merely the epidemiological catastrophe of COVID-19, itself now rendered 'past,' and its concurrent economic and political crises, but those greater catastrophes of antimicrobial resistance and climate change, still gathering on the horizon.

In cosmological time, the GP waiting room as archaeological relic exists as the consequence of a past and as a haunting foundational myth of a future era only just arriving. Originally, this chapter was to claim that waiting rooms represented the last public space, and a form that was thriving—in terms of frequency and of attendance, if not sociability or conviviality—compared to youth centres, libraries, community cafes and other vanishing commons. Of course, a pandemic wiped away this time-space, and this chapter, which might have been a bill of health, or, at worst, a diagnosis, is now partially a post-mortem. As the 'first last moment' of life in Beckett's *Ill Seen Ill Said* is both minute and yet able to gluttonously gobble up all the moments preceding it, and all the world around it, so the small quiet death of the GP waiting room is in microcosm the end of an era in healthcare provision, a synecdochic sign of a closed, sold or abandoned commons, and symbolically the birth of a new world.

A Short Note on Methodology and Context

This chapter is based on fieldwork conducted in late 2019 at four different GP practices in the UK: one in Hackney, London; one in Alum Rock, Birmingham; one in a small village in Devon; one in a coastal town in north Wales. It is worth briefly characterising these four practices and their local areas. Practice one is a large multi-clinician practice, with 14 doctors and a considerable practice staff. Hackney itself is a highly diverse inner-city London borough, where one in four people speak a first language other than English, and according to the 2011 census, around one-third of residents identify as White British, with one-quarter identifying as Black or Black British. As with many parts of London, the borough is home to both some of the poorest and the wealthiest people in the UK. Practice two has two GPs, only one of whom is full time. Alum Rock is more homogeneous in both ethnicity and income: over three-quarters of the population identified on the 2011 census as Asian or British Asian; residents have lower-paid jobs, fewer educational qualifications, are less likely to own property and more likely to be unemployed than the average person in England. Practice three has four GPs working three or four days a week. The village in Devon has 1500 residents, and three pubs. Almost everyone who lives there identifies as White British, the benefit claimant count is significantly below the national average and the population is disproportionately elderly and wealthy. Practice four is a four-partner practice, with two salaried GPs. The coastal town in Wales has a population of around 500, and the residents are educated to a higher level, in higher-paying jobs, less ethnically diverse and significantly more likely to speak Welsh than the average Welsh person.

The fieldwork comprised discussions with administrative and clinical staff, as well as extended periods of time exploring waiting spaces. Specifically, the researcher conducted a series of consultation meetings with staff—some of these were one-to-one or two-to-one discussions with GPs and practice managers and assistant practice managers; others were group consultation discussions. These were freeform consultation discussions aimed more at framing the research interests, rather than answering research questions, as initially the intention was to develop, in collaboration with the clinical and clerical staff of all practices specific workshop programmes for patients and staff, using storytelling and other methodologies. Unfortunately, COVID overran these plans. An initial wave of site visits was completed by the researcher, which entailed extensive photographing of the built environments and observation of how people—patients, staff and others—moved through, and constructed, the time-space of the waiting room. Notes were made on the design and actual use of the spaces, including signage, reading material, televisions and additional information, and the uses made of the spaces for waiting and other activities. The researcher did walk-thrus of the spaces, observing and recording the interaction points with the architecture, the staff, the furniture and the clinic as mediated through third-party objects (e.g. touchscreen self-check-ins). Levels of light, noise, heat and smell were also considered. The observational and analytical approach was semiotic throughout, and the visits comprised a semiotic 'audit' of the clinics as spatio-temporal sites of waiting. For other limited applications of a material-semiotic and/or general social semiotic approach to clinical spaces, see McPhail et al. (2022), Veinot and Pierce (2019) and Caronia and Mortari (2015).

Motivating this research were comments from practice managers and clinicians at three of four practices to the effect that there was something amiss about the waiting rooms and waiting 'experience' (as one practice manager termed it).[1] It is worth noting that there was commonly expressed satisfaction by staff with the waiting room at practice three in rural Devon. At the other three practices, though, staff had a sense or intuition that everything was not quite as it should be. They noticed as well that instructions and signs were not followed, that waiters behaved out of step with guidance offered, that they queued when they should not, and did not queue when they should, and that despite the absolute superfluity of health information available, waiters engaged very little with any of it all. Could a semiotic account of the waiting room, and the ways in which time was spent within it, offer insights into some of these problems?

This chapter is also based on stories told in online story-sharing sessions from January through to July 2021. This was a period that began in the UK with the reimposition of a near-full lockdown on 4 January and ended with the cessation of all COVID restrictions (beyond isolation rules and mask mandates) on 19 July. The author worked with a national provider of specialist housing and care for those in later life, which was

[1] The elucidation and exploration of the experiences of waiting for healthcare are at the heart of the Waiting Times project. See Baraitser and Brook (2020), Baraitser et al. (2024) and Salisbury et al. (2023).

participating in a pilot scheme to provide residents with online classes, well-being support and social events through their televisions. This particular service was designed for older people with either no or limited computer or online device access. Over the course of research, the author ran four story-sharing workshops weekly. (They also played a lot of bingo.) Through these sessions, an alternative time-space of caring was created, not *after* a time-space of waiting—as with the clinical encounter as sequel to the waiting room wait—but from within it. Within this practice of care, accounts of the time-spaces of waiting—both new and old—emerged, and some are included here as vignettes, placed (waiting?) in silent dialogue with the close semiotic reading of GP waiting spaces. Methodologically, the approach was similar to that employed by the researcher and their colleague Kelechi Anucha in another series of storytelling workshops conducted at a day hospice in Devon in 2018–2019, (Anucha et al., 2021) and built on the engaged research practices developed at the University of Exeter's Wellcome Centre for Cultures and Environments of Health (Hinchliffe et al., 2018). Stories from these workshops are included as vignettes at the end of each section of this chapter and offer a part-ironic, part-critical, part-sympathetic reflection on (and of) the particular quality or function of waiting rooms, as semiotic and relational machine, being outlined in that section. These human stories are offered without comment or analysis or exegesis, in contrast to the rigorous deconstruction of the effects and affects of the waiting room machine; the power relations embedded in the time-space of the clinic are rightly subjected to a dynamic and perhaps accusatory interrogation; the stories are left to speak for themselves and stand with all their human dignity.

Knowing Your (Non)place: The Spatio-Temporal Powerplay of Neglect

> The cabin. Its situation. Careful. On. At the inexistent centre of a formless place. Rather more circular than otherwise finally. Flat to be sure. To cross it in a straight line takes her from five to ten minutes. Depending on her speed and radius taken. (Beckett, 1981, p. 8)

What kind of time-space, what kind of place, was the waiting room? Before the advent of COVID-19, and the sudden shutting of GP surgeries to waiting patients, the GP waiting room had for years enjoyed a contradictory status as simultaneously a site of care and of neglect: a site of care, as this is where you came to be seen, and a site of neglect, as here in the waiting room was most certainly where you were not seen, a place where you became temporarily (and temporally) invisible and suspended. It was a space of neglected objects, a depository for flotsam and jetsam, years-old magazines, broken children's toys, masses of dumped unread flyers and cacophonous posters, blank TV screens, forgotten umbrellas, chairs positioned awkwardly in eccentric nooks and round blind corners. Each object holding, compacted within it, a similarly neglected moment, a museum of materialised lost times. Later, in the pandemic, shuttered up and taped off, the waiting room itself was a neglected object; since then, it has failed to return in quite the same deep, complex materiality.

It is unclear if the waiting room really is a place at all. It is perhaps a pose, an attitude, or a temporal decentring, which is why, on at least one level, the waiting room could be so familiarly recovered, re-engineered, in a street by the side of a practice. A productive problem emerges trying to categorise the GP waiting room using Marc Augé's typology of places and non-places. For Augé, anthropological place is centred, spatially and temporally, on a monument that is an organic expression of a cultural history. Conversely, the non-places he describes are peripheral and time does not constructively and creatively accumulate here, according to historical progress; rather, it is fleetingly spent, it dissipates in the present; instead of vertical accretion and stratification, there is a horizontal dispersion to vanishing horizons: '[w]hat reigns there is actuality, the urgency of the present moment. Since non-places are there to be passed through, they are measured in units of time' (Augé, 1995, pp. 83–84).

The GP waiting room though is an untypical non-place, which is no doubt why it does not feature in Augé's text next to out-of-town supermarkets, motorways, airport departure lounges and cash machines. It is a temporal place of transit, but without departure, destination or itinerary: there is only suspended arrival. Similarly, it is architecturally, socially and temporally central—being often the largest and centrally structuring space, being where most people within the practice are at any moment in time, being the place where most of the time is spent—and yet it is simultaneously peripheral, extraneous and desocialised, where people exist in a de-agentive, non-social form. Partly, this speaks to something Augé misses in his critique of non-places: their democratic nature. Granted, an individual might have more or less money to withdraw from their cash machine, or might be able to accelerate more or less on a motorway, or even have access to an expensive first-class airport lounge. Regardless, everyone gets on the same plane, and lands at the same time. The supermarket cashier works in the same space that the customer waits or pays, and, crucially, their tempo is in harmony, if not in unison, with those waiting. In a traffic jam, there is no first place. For all their problems and petty tyrannies, these non-places cannot ration time.

Conversely, the GP practice is anti-democratic, in spatio-temporal terms. It is imperial and autocratic, and is organised hierarchically according to strict asymmetric power relations. Its analogue is not the motorway hotel but the Forbidden City. There, large open spaces were not the locus of centralised authority. Although spatially dominant, they were subordinate, in terms of power and time, and they were where bureaucrats and the military waited. Indeed, the largest space, Tiananmen Square, was located outside the city walls entirely. Power resided within the smaller enclosed spaces, behind and beyond. It is no coincidence that it was deep within the city walls where the *rigui* (日晷) set the time for Imperial China, as an extension of the emperor's power: it is a power over the material content of the empire and also over the temporal form. The place of time is true centre, regardless that Beijing was never the physical centre of China, any more than Greenwich is the centre of the world, and where time is set, there can be no waiting, as it is always the right time. The emperor, like the clinician, never waits. As a common rule, and specifically in practices one and two, the clinicians do not enter the waiting room. Patients, waiters, are called forth. In practice one, the patient has to be admitted through magnetically locked doors. The parallels with the sequence of gates within the Forbidden City signifying the progress towards the seat of power are striking.

Consider the position, spatial and temporal, of reception desk in this cosmology of power. In the ground-floor waiting room of practice one and in practice two, the desk sits directly opposing waiters. Their seats angle expectantly towards this, as if towards a stage (see Image 6.1). This

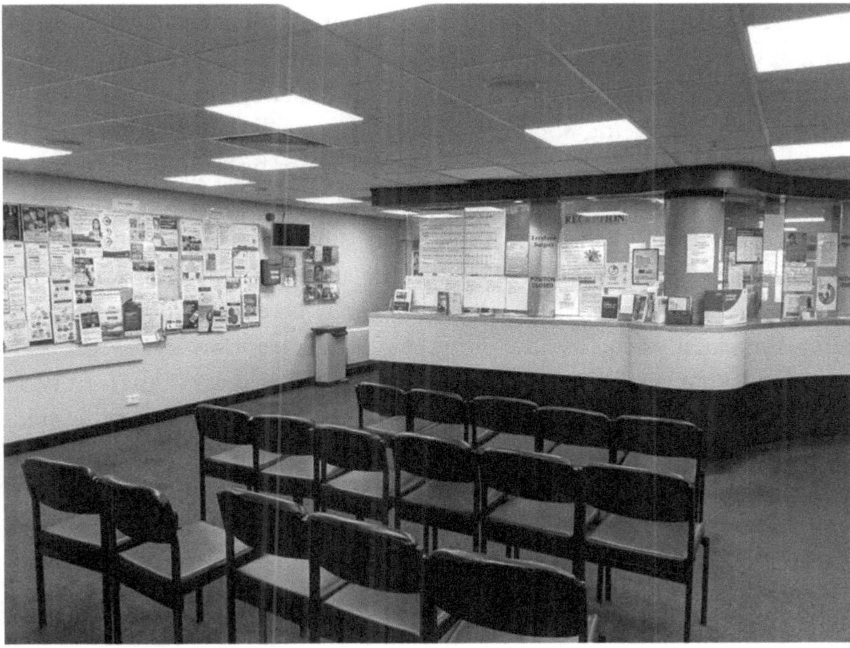

Image 6.1 The reception desk as the centre of power

creates the anticipation of spectacle: waiters are orientated towards the action. But the action of the desk is absolutely not for the consumption of the waiters. Within the power arrangements of the practice, the desk is a boundary, portioning off not only two distinct spaces—one of the public, of waiting, of subordination; one of the institution, of working, of authority—but also two distinct temporalities. Indeed, these temporalities, and the tensions between them, contribute generously to the frustrations of waiting in the GP waiting room. For just out of reach for waiters (but not out sight), there is a tempo of energy, or agency, of time used and time recognised, or even time reimbursed (the best recognition of all). Who would put people working freely in the same spatio-temporal network as people suspended, delayed and abstracted from their day? It is the aesthetic disjunction of the zoo but the energies and interests of agentive party (here, the administrative staff) are pointedly not directed to the pacified and contained beasts (the waiters). It is a perverse arrangement. When approached afresh, separated from the traditions of waiting for doctors, the design choice seems as cruel as putting holidaymakers in gardens overlooked by prison cells. The reception is a staged performance of time. That is what time looks like: activity, agency, interaction, maybe power. And it is being spent at a frenetic pace. For the waiter to step towards it is to feel the heat of it, and yet it cannot be approached, almost as an opposite magnetic pole. The actors know their parts well. They cannot be distracted. And they know their authority, and know who is authorised and who is not to enter the performing space and time. Temporally and spatially, this arrangement is eccentric, in the sense of being abnormally centred. The boundary of the reception is the temporal-spatial axis that displaces and decentres the waiting mass (a mass of both time and flesh) and therefore maintains the power hierarchy of the practice as a whole.

In this sense, the reception desk is the boundary, and an eccentric axis, separating clinical knowledge and truth from a non-meaning time-space that is necessarily ignorant. Here is a simple semiotic explanation for why no one reads the information sheets in the waiting room—there is a spatio-temporal hierarchy of medical meaning. Meaning can only be constructed beyond the boundary and so, conversely, whatever is within the waiting space is without medical knowledge.

In terms of the authority to communicate and construct signs of medical meaning, the waiting space is definitionally a diminished space and moment—despite the fact that architecturally, or literally, these waiting spaces are the largest and often physically central in the surgery, yet they are experientially peripheral, and this is because of their temporal-power situation rather than their spatio-structural one. The whole temporal arrangement is that meaning is *only* sanctified or validated within the consultation, so what use are the attempts to construct meaning through leaflets or posters?

For the waiter, this experience of the waiting room, regardless of architectural insistence, is of being in a non-time, non-place, non-centre. The 'inexistent centre of a formless place' is endured by the ageing solitary female figure in Beckett's *Ill Seen Ill Said*. What gives that space any sort of definition is the duration of transgressing it. But just as the figure herself requires to be seen—by a circle of 12 other figures, by the eye of the narrative perspective—so does the eccentricity of the arrangements of the waiting room, and its relations to the reception desk and the consulting rooms, demand the spectatorial presence of waiters to operate. Lotman gives this account of the relationship between the theatricality and geography of Petersberg, and how both operate in tandem as semiotic processes that explain the generation of that city's mythology: '[t]he need for an audience has a semiotic parallel in eccentric positioning in geography. Petersberg does not have its own point of view on itself—it has always to posit a spectator' (Lotman, 1990, p.198). Similarly, general practice lacks a point of view on itself. There is little or no medicine performed out of sight: few procedures performed and few medications administered. The invisible and concealed pharmacological or physiological mechanistic procedures that are the assumed gold standard for scientific evidence-based medicine's point of view on itself take place elsewhere and elsewhen. General practice is an open performance of medicine *qua* performance and cannot be done on a patient who is either absent or anaesthetised out of consciousness. Part of the performance is the rationing of time; the wait is the semiotic exchange of prestige, and the temporal divestment of the waiter is coin to the GP's coffer. As nothing is *done* but only performed in the medical encounter, the wait is what gives this its weight. The delay is what allows for a feeling of arrival. This is then an integral element of the affective journey of the waiter and the vitalising of the theatrics of the consultation. Waiting is not a structural failure; it is the structure itself, as Jerry Seinfeld observes:

> The waiting room. I hate when they make you wait in the room. Because it says waiting room. There's no chance of not waiting. Because they call it the waiting room. They're going to use it. They've got it. It's all set up for you to wait. ('*The Ex-Girlfriend*' *Seinfeld*, 1991)

Vignette: The Magical Performance of Medicine in the General Practice Clinical Encounter

The following story was told by a former reception manager of practice three, as part of sequence of open-ended interviews about their several decades of experience working at the practice:

> There was this lady who had obviously got some issue going on and she would go and see and one of our GPs, Marcus, and be in there for 40 minutes and then she'd come out all teary and book an appointment for the next week and the next week go in for another forty minutes. She didn't ask for a long appointment, but I started giving her one automatically because I knew that she would make him run late.
>
> Then, one morning, he was ill, with something. He couldn't come in for some reason or other. She'd booked her normal weekly session with him. Marcus was ill and we couldn't get hold of her. So we thought, 'Well, what are going to do about Mrs so-and-so. She's coming to see Marcus. She's not going to be able to see him. She's going to have to see the other GP, Arthur. She won't like him.' We were dreading her coming and she came, and I explained what had happened. Arthur said, 'oh, I'll see her.' Not a problem. She went in. She went in on time. She had 10 minutes. She came out smiling and she walked out of the door and she didn't book another appointment and we all said, 'what have you done to her?' And he just shrugged his shoulders and said, 'I just told her she was better.'
>
> I mean, this had been going on for weeks [...] Marcus had obviously given her the time that she needed but was unable himself to finish it somehow or other, so maybe there was a need in him.
>
> That was what really struck home about this waiting thing. It is being held that is important to people and feeling that they're not being forgotten about.

Derangement or Plurality of Sense: Literary Language vs Metalanguage

> The coffer. Empty after long nocturnal search. Nothing. Save in the end in a cranny of dust a scrap of paper. Jagged along one edge as if torn from a diary. On its yellowed face in barely legible ink two letters followed by a number. Tu 17. Or Th. Tu or Th 17. Otherwise blank. Otherwise empty.
>
> —Beckett (1981, p. 38)

In *Ill Seen Ill Said*, a time that was once an historic time—some particular Tuesday or Thursday on some particular 17th of some particular month—is reduced to an indeterminate and oscillating fragment, violently extracted from a perhaps coherent and complete (at least chronologically) narrative. Two different languages have been thrown into fierce and comic juxtaposition. There is the metalanguage of the diary, how time would like to talk about itself: ordered, balanced, defined and progressing clearly and regularly, to completion. Then there is the literary language of the torn scrap: partial, displaced, ambiguous, recursive and lingering without resolution.

A similar distinction can be discerned in the waiting room, between a metalanguage and a language. And it is worth stressing here that these languages do not have to be purely verbal, but may contain verbal languages. Lotman uses this binarism to consider the dual registers of the city: it has a metalanguage that speaks of its spatio-temporal order, its zoning, its routes and locations, and a literary language which is the heterogeneous clatter of its multiple perspectives, its polyphonous exchanges, its encounters, surprises, blockages and ruptures. In the metalanguage, the institutional voice of the practice, there is a complete and clear narrative. (One practice manager deliberately uses the corporate customer service terminology of the 'journey' to describe this.) This entails an arranged attendance, temporally situated by the practice within a matrix of other attendances corresponding to a matrix of available units from the production side (the clinicians' apportionable time slots), or an unarranged attendance that is more loosely temporally situated within a period for 'walk-in' consultations. This contingency—if allowed for by the practice—will still be ordered according to a temporal supply-side calculation (and will be undergirded by dedicated additional funding). The service user's wait will be in designated, purpose-designed spaces, populated with targeted information (some commercial) and entertainment. Their wait in this space will be calculated according to a measured average for the practice: there will be targets and monitoring, and these data will generate an *Ideal* (rather than actual) sense of the time spent. From waiting, they will progress to consultation. From there, either onwards to secondary care or to a pharmacy or to home. In this metalanguage, there are delineated times and spaces, and spatio-temporal algorithmic routes linking these into what might be a narrative.

And, of course, this relates to a lived dialogic movement through a GP service in the same way the sterile clarity of Google Maps directions relate

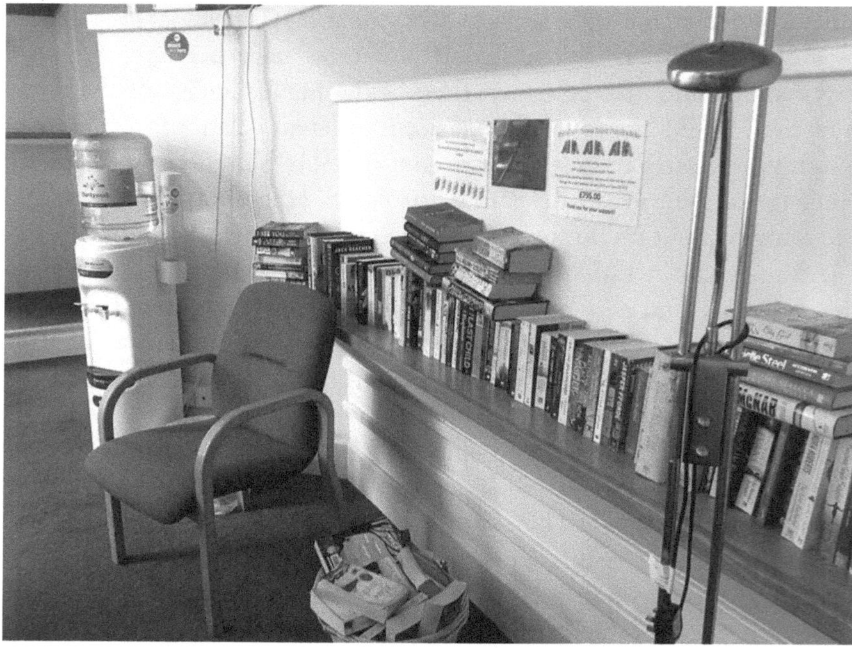

Image 6.2 The bookcase augurs poorly for how long one might be waiting

to the roar and clutter of a walk through a city. 'Take a seat, you won't be waiting long,' may be the official voice; the never-ending story bookcase urges a different temporality (Image 6.2).

The metalanguage of the spatio-temporal algorithmic journey constructs discrete meaningful syntagmatic chains. The narrative and determining power of these chains is remarkable. Should a service user not attend between making the appointment and its allotted time, a narrative journey is still constructed by the metalanguage of the NHS: appointment arranged; non-attendance; the automatic generation and dispatch of a did-not-attend (DNA) letter; an nth instance of non-attendance automatically triggering a request that the patient deregister at the practice. Whilst this narrative is being built up, the actual service-user may have died or been abducted or suffered a profound psychotic incident and be experiencing a wholly temporally coterminous narrative of a very different structure and in a very different language from that auto-constructing within the practice bureaucracy.

But obviously, two kinds of rupture occur between the metalanguage of the practice and the literary language of the individual subject and their experience. The first is the simple deviation, where the lived narrative is irreconcilably different in its construction, in its tempos and events, from that constructed by the practice. The above is an example of this. But there can be subtle and nuanced divergences where, importantly, the patient might not be aware that a radically different narrative is being constructed about them. Again, the simplest example is the patient whose presence has somehow not been registered. They may be living a narrative of extended waiting, whilst in the practice's metalanguage, the patient has completed a standard narrative arc of non-attendance as described. The temporal divergence is remarkable here. The metalanguage short-circuits lived time. Within a reasonably short duration after the appointment time, a prefabricated narrative is written onto the patient, and whilst this narrative itself extends—through the letter to be sent, through further reprimanding action to be taken—perhaps outwards by many days, this period of 'many days,' although a real time in the objective world, is only a feature of diegetic time from the perspective of the practice, and the narrative is already complete (as written). Conversely, though the patient continues to wait and is arrested in terms of syntagmatic progression, and has a narrative that cannot progress to any meaning beyond a spiralling out into empty duration, into an experience of timelessness and abandonment, yet this exponentially increasing time actually has a real-world fixed endpoint beyond which it cannot go, that is, no matter how ignored or forgotten they are, at some point the practice will close and they will be seen to be there, if only in the act of being asked to leave.

The importance of this divergence—when illustrated by these extreme limit cases—is that essentially the bureaucratic time of the metalanguage narratives of the practice is inherently fictitious and a fantasy, whilst simultaneously exhibiting the qualities of historical time, as being future-orientated and causal. So, a spontaneously emerging, self-organising narrative of causality reaching out into an imagined future can outpace actual events and superimpose itself on them as a 'that which will happen as already happened'—a fate *accompli*. Paradoxically, the thick durational experience of the patient, sinking beneath an ever-rising waterline of time, has them living a period tending towards the infinite through the suspension of the next syntagmatic element, as a broken off sentence vanishes into an ellipsis. This is cosmological time, where they are a consequence, and they experience an abandonment that is imaginatively open-ended. If the two syntagms were plotted on a graph, the first would have to be a sequence of disconnected points, and the other would be a line exponentially rising upwards.

The second kind of rupture occurs because the real, lived syntagmatic-meaning constructions of the people passing through the waiting time-space are both subject to and generative of semiotic static and interference. The simplest example of this is perhaps in the proliferation of information sheets. In three of the practices, and most notably in practice one, these were duplicated across a variety of languages: Turkish, Kurdish, Vietnamese and Urdu are all immediately obvious. And, naturally, they are directed to a broad range of ailments or interests but without structural differentiation: cancer, diabetes, dementia, mental distress, pregnancy, heart disease, giving up smoking, applying for benefits, parent and baby support groups, Zumba, drug addiction recovery, deafness, all coexist and shout each other down. The rationale from the metalanguage perspective of the practice is that individuals will select their relevant material, through a movement along the paradigmatic axis of meaning between alternatives, but this is based on a fundamental misapprehension of how meaning is semiotically constructed. A bundle of disparate posters, as in Image 6.3, are not experienced separately but compositely. There are not individual, differentiated clear lines of syntagmatic meaning for each patient navigating through this time-space. Instead, there is a tangle of incoherent meanings. The signs construct and situate their interpretants so that a wall positing that you might be in the early stages of type 2 diabetes, or looking to foster a child or, in a particularly thoughtless juxtaposition, the victim of or witness to abuse communicates very simply: 'this practice does not know who you are.' The attempted denotation of care ('this is for you') actually connotes neglect ('who are you?') and a neglect that is reciprocated by waiters shunning the material.

When menopause awareness hides the early signs of prostate cancer, or admonishments for being feckless in antibiotic usage drags the eye away

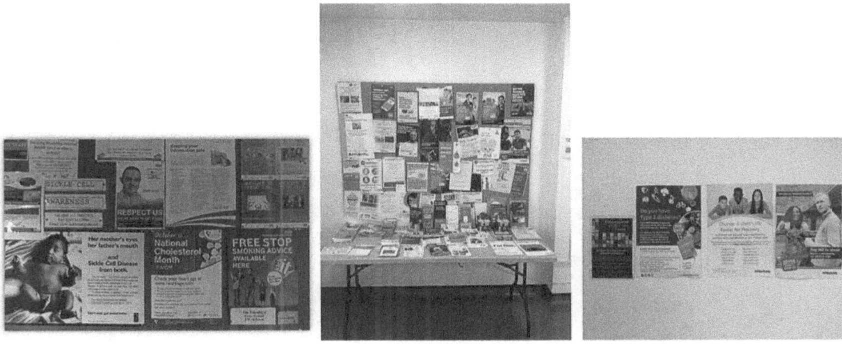

Images 6.3–6.5 The discordant clamour of disparate posters

from carer support, the semiotic excess is that the addresser—constructed in the mind of the waiter as some supposed monolithic entity 'the NHS,' represented symbolically in the person of the GP or time-space of the practice—does not, for all its protestations, really care. In truth, these patchwork welters of quasi-clinical white noise are an honest anatomy of the piecemeal services and competing interests that jostle in the tremulous, barely held rattle bag that is the NHS (Bramwell et al., 2023) One practice manager could not account for who might have any responsibility for what was on the walls of their own practice, recognising few of the posters. At another practice, one clinician remarked wryly, 'it remains a mystery where the leaflets come from.' What is not a mystery is where the leaflets go. Nowhere, except eventually swept away by more leaflets. This discordant clamour (Image 6.4) dissolves the patient in an interpretant space that cannot contain the contradictory lives, identities, and narratives: Are you worried about data protection or sickle cell anaemia? There is something blithe and dismissive about the sidesteps from shingles to hearing aids (Image 6.5). Who wants to be presented with a smorgasbord of fantasy pathologies and invited to tuck in?

The sense of neglect, the sense of derangement or the derangement of sense is more than a merely aesthetic response to the hysteria of the waiting room, and its jumble of offered temporalities and narratives, though it is certainly that as well. In *The Logic of Sense* (1969), Deleuze describes 'sense' as a fourth plane of meaning generation in the proposition,

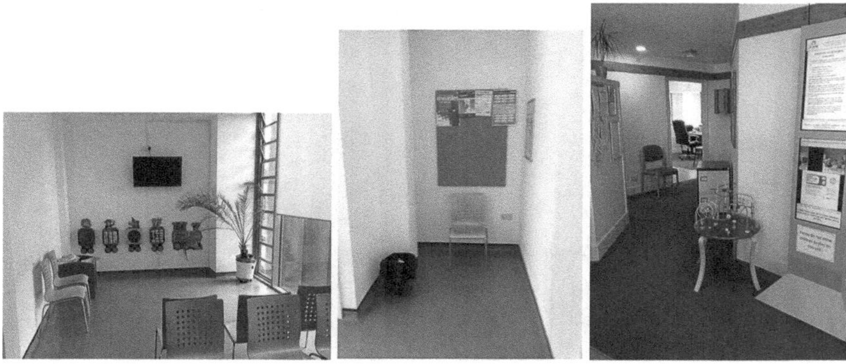

Images 6.6–6.8 The physical arrangement of deranged senses

complementing the three internal components of denotation (a form of direct reference), manifestation (which might be termed 'dietic contextual relationality') and signification (which might be understood as connotation or universalised meaning). In contrast to these generative manoeuvres, not only inherent to the proposition but also evidently extending out into the world through the semiotic exchanges, sense is a surface effect: 'sense, *the expressed of the proposition* [...] an incorporeal, complex, and irreducible entity, at the surface of things, a pure event which inheres or subsists in the proposition' (Deleuze, 2004, p. 22). As such, it might be thought of as either meaning as aesthetic or an aesthetics of meaning. Sense's meaning is not referential, relational or universal, but tonal or sculptural. When we are confronted with arrangements as in Images 6.6, 6.7 and 6.8, it might be possible to articulate the derangement of sense they produce, but those articulations will miss some of the irreducible, complex essence of what has been mis-meant.

Vignette: Lost in the Post

This story was told by a participant in one of the series of online story-sharing workshops in 2020–2021:

> I had quite a bad fall recently and went to A&E. They did the job beautifully. I then waited four and a half hours to come home. I went to downstairs dispatch, upstairs dispatch, downstairs dispatch, upstairs dispatch, upstairs ... And it went on like that until finally they let me sit in upstairs dispatch for four and a half hours. They are busy, I know, but apparently, they'd lost me. I was a parcel and they weren't sure of the address. It's quite funny in a way.
>
> After an hour, I said to somebody, 'I'm not very obvious here, should I be somewhere where I can be seen?' He said, 'no, stay there.' Then, after another hour, he said. 'what are you still doing here?'

Save Your Time: The Inequitable Fungibilities of Time in the Waiting Room

> Close-up of a dial. Nothing else. White disc divided in minutes. Unless it be in seconds. Sixty black dots. No figure. One hand only. Finest of fine black darts. It advances by fits and starts. No ticks. Leaps from dot to dot with so lightening a leap that but for its new position it had not stirred. Whole nights may pass as may but a fraction of a second or any intermediate lapse of time soever before it flings itself from one degree to the next. None in any moment overleaping in all fairness be it said. (Beckett, 1981, p. 46)

These lightening leaps of time might echo the unconnected dots of the algorithmic syntagms of the practice's metalanguage. However, there is an economy of time in the waiting room which, whilst as highly fungible as the divisions of the figureless, one-hand dial, are not traded 'in all fairness' but replicate the power asymmetries already identified at play.

Image 6.9 represents a temporal currency, a sign of time, exchanged within the time-space of the waiting room. There is simply no way that these mountains of paper are retained and maintained to entertain waiters. Rather, they form a clear monument to the institution's power to compel waiting. More charitably, they also signify a public space. As the magazines are outside ownership—and the pile can no doubt be added to and subtracted from by patients with relative freedom—they simultaneously represent and enact a form of sociality, indeed the form of sociality

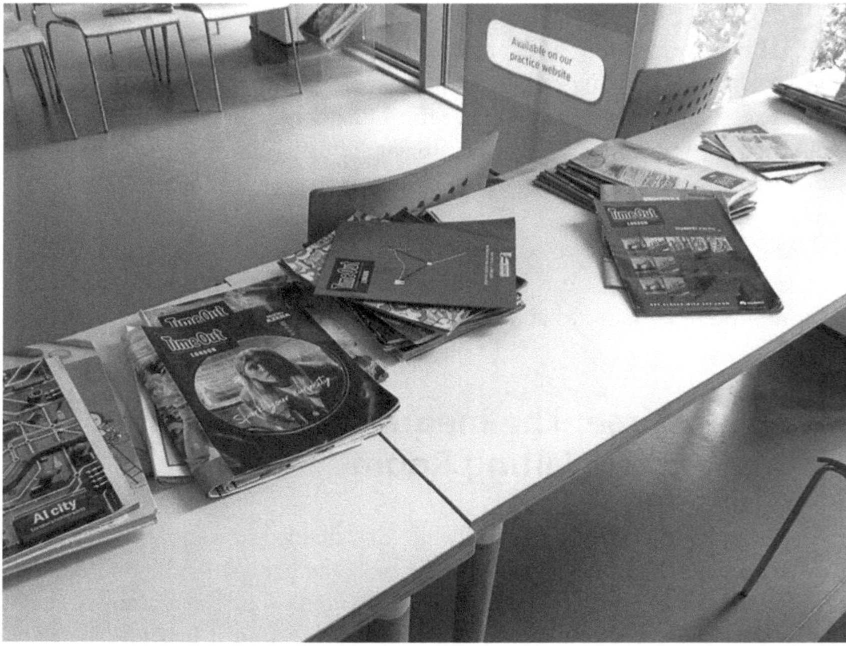

Image 6.9 A temporal currency

at the conceptual heart of the NHS. In conjunction with the leaflets already described, they comprise a polyphonic chorus of detritus, a tyranny of objects that insubstantialise—physically and temporally—the waiter and within which they then disintegrate as a product of their uncanny effect. Schweizer describes this as an oscillating process—the waiter is depersonalised in the inchoate semiotic noise and then repersonalised in particularity: ‘Like the objects the waiter sees and does not see, he appears to himself once present once absent from his scene of waiting, once in exaggerated particularity, once re-absorbed into the flux of the whole’ (Schweizer, 2008, p. 31).

Each object is an instance of compacted temporality and, as a semiotic sign, serves to construct an interpretant (which can be the individual waiter) as interpellated subjectivity that renders that sign intelligible. Yet what kind of interpretant is interpellated by an object-sign like a stack of *TimeOut* magazines, spiralling back over many months? *TimeOut* is a culture magazine and its content is almost entirely composed of two, very time-contingent, informational texts: listings and reviews. Published weekly on Tuesdays, it is a rapidly informationally redundant text. Given the weighting of nightlife events, within a few days of being printed around half the listings have transmuted from informational data to historical anecdote. Piled up haphazardly in the waiting room, the copies of *TimeOut* are a rebuke: a chronicle of adventures either distantly or never experienced by the waiter. They are dead time physicalised as waste; ephemeral or missed events materialised into unmissable bulk.

Further, *TimeOut* is given away for free, on Tuesday mornings at London underground stations. Their only value, to any reader, is that they might divert them in their current journey, either literally or at least in fantasy, or offer them the opportunity of planning some future action. In that context, perhaps, their meaning is approximately: 'your time is an asset, and we freely tell you how and where you might spend it profitably (to you, for pleasure; to our advertisers, as ticket revenue; and then back to us, through their advertising spend).' That it is given to people when they speed to work on mass transit is not because that is an ideal moment to access a large number of people, but rather it is because these are people at a moment of need. They are in the very process of handing over their time as labour, despondent and alienated, and so very susceptible to the compensatory inducements of cultural capital. 'You race to work. You expend your time for others. Take the money you earn to buy some of this "time out" time for yourself as reward.' So, for obvious reasons, *TimeOut* is not distributed as people exit football matches or wait outside West End theatres.

There is lots that is already objectionable about this as it is. But when this semiotic discourse is displaced, in time and space, from the rush hour tube to the inert waiting room, then its meaning-making processes repeat as a grotesque parody. So, for the waiter, as interpretant, they offer the following meaning: 'your time is so valueless, not only can you not spend it now as you might like, but here is a lifetime of ways you could have spent it earlier.'[2] Cosmologically, the temporal economy of the waiting room uses the present as a consequence to symbolically foreclose the past, as portent of a future that repeats this foundational myth of the wastage of time.

Yet while your time is wasted, you are simultaneously exhorted, with the raised voice of the exclamation mark, to 'save time.' But although you are to do the saving, you are not the one who will be banking that time. All time saved accrues to the practice. All time wasted was the time of the waiter. Even if you seem to waste the time of the clinician, it remains, in this exchange economy, *your* time with them that is wasted. Fundamentally, responsibility and resources for managing time are not aligned.

Vignette: *Il n'y a pas de hors-attendant*[3]

This story was told by a participant in one of the series of online story-sharing workshops in 2020–2021:

> Well, I've found it's frustrating to get an appointment. If you wanted to speak to a doctor in my surgery, they always say to you, 'No, you have to first get a …' Well, you have to tell them what's the matter and then otherwise you just have to speak to a nurse. And you know, personally, I like to go to church in the morning and if I have to wait to speak to a nurse, that means that I have to sit in from 8.30 until he can ring you, you see? In the meantime, I could have gone to church and come home, because sometimes, he doesn't call you until 10.30 or 11 o'clock. It means my morning is just wasted.

---

[2] The author would also like to include here the observation of the peer-reviewer of this chapter, who astutely noted that this particular choice of journal imagines a reader (and a waiter) who is able-bodied, privileged and essentially healthy; in other words, exhibiting all the qualities that might constitute a 'full person' from both a socio-economic and medico-economic point of view. The mission of the clinic might even be understood as the restoration of that full personhood, which includes within in it economic and cultural vitality as natural extensions of physical vitality. Those waiting are not just interrupted in their physical health, but in their economic and cultural health too. These magazines then become yet another way in which the ill or disabled are further abnormalised through the practices of the clinic. With all credit here to the peer-reviewer.

[3] 'There is no outside-of-waiting.'

I said to them, 'Can't you ask him to ring me at 10.30 or 11' and they say, 'no, I'm sorry, they will call you from now until that time.' I find that very frustrating because I like to go to church. I like to start my day that way and then I've wasted my whole morning not to get a call until probably 10.30, maybe even 11 o'clock. So, the same thing is, I had an issue with a doctor, and he said to me, 'Why didn't you discuss with me.' And I said to him, 'Well, when you ring the receptionist, she will say, you cannot speak to the doctor, first you have to speak to the nurse.' You know, things like this. Before, it was lovely, you could just make an appointment and you saw the doctor. You got things sorted out. I know it's difficult now but I find all the wait distressing.

You Are (Not) Here (Now): Residues and Deixis

The oval handle is wrought to a semblance of scales. The shank a little bent leads up to the hook the eye so far still dry. A lifetime of hooking has lessened its curvature. To the point at certain moments of seeming unfit for service. Child's play with a pliers to restore it. Was there once a time she did? Careful. Once once in a way. Till she could no more. (Beckett, 1981, p. 18)

What is left over now, from which to fashion some conclusions?

There is an ethical and practical requirement to be seen, to be placed in deictic relations that establish the subject as an object in the world for others. As the waiting room is a time and space where one waits to be seen, definitionally (if over simplistically) it is a space in which they are not seen or pre-seen, waiting to have their subjectivity reactivated through being seen.

Attendance, and the experience of not being seen, disrupts (or at very least pauses or estranges) a person's deictic orientation in the world, the set of shared material and identifying coordinates necessary for the mutual recognition between subjects constitutive of social, intersubjective existence. To not be acknowledged as present, to have one's presence erased through waiting, is the stuff of deictic crisis. Such crisis—and the disintegration it threatens—can be a source of genuinely creative destruction. Architecture theorist Peter Bishop identifies the horizontal temporal expansive opportunities of the waiting room as a liminal space:

> Waiting rooms [...] whether formally designated as such or as ephemeral micro-spaces, become liminal, in-between, and initiatory places and waiting becomes an initiatory event – not in terms of a 'horizontal' linear movement from past to future, ut as an entrance into imaginative and experiential depth. (Bishop, 2013, pp. 135–49)

In waiting rooms, as sites of deictic disintegration as described in this analysis, the collective is fractured into individual temporal narratives of waiting; there is no waiting *with* but rather a waiting *against*, an asymmetric race, where temporal distances to be crossed vary and even oscillate. Yet in this fracturing, there is the time-space for an initiatory event. Our initial hypothesis had been that we would ignite these events through a physical intervention, and the insertion of the researcher, as story-sharer, into the time-space of the waiting room, and this was our intent in the first months of 2020. Instead, we—indeed we all—experienced a collective derangement of time and space; the pandemic brought a sick spatio-temporality, which erupted out from and overlaid itself onto all moments and places. The lucky majority of us not sick, or not profoundly sick, with COVID-19, were infected instead with COVID-19 spatio-temporality. We collectively convalesced from an illness we hadn't had.

Yet, if our enforced confinement took us out of the world, and the waiting room, as our universal lying-in, it become how we rebirthed our world. Forced into improvised modes of connection and of unprecedented novel spatio-temporal forms and arrangements, new opportunities arose. This waiting, without possibility of being seen, offered an absolute, systemic, global rupturing, in place of the isolated and quotidian fractures identified as possible sites for initiatory events. So here, we found, or made, such interstitial events through the story-sharing workshops, where lonely, isolated, unseen moments of waiting were transformed into collective and affirming narratives for sharing and exchange. The telling—the careful to and from between tellers and listeners—constituted itself an act of mutual collective care, drawing together these atomised moments into a dynamic intermolecular flow.

At the very least, these constituted the very things impossible to leave in clinical waiting spaces. Enduring marks and traces of our specificity, of our once-presence. Something that says, in the style of the archetypal scribbled exclamatory graffito: yes, once we were here!

> Last example the flagstone before her door that by dint by dint her little weight has grooved. Tears. (Beckett, 1981, pp. 17–18)

Vignette: No Time Is the Right Time

This story was told by a participant in an online story-sharing workshop series for British Caribbean women over retirement age, most of whom had worked in healthcare and/or the NHS:

> If I go early in the morning [to the pharmacy], I still have to wait for it to unlock. If I go in the afternoon, it's the same problem. She'll just say to me ... I think the reason why I know that they have to wait for it is one, I went and everybody is coming and getting and served and I'm still sitting down there like an idiot and nobody is ... and I got really angry and I said, hang on, I've got other things to do in my house. Not to sit down here like a statue. I've been here over 20mins now. And the guy, one of the guys came out, right, because he knows me so well, he says, I'm sorry but the safe is on a time lock and we can't just open it when we want. We have to wait until the time that it's set to open so that we can go in there. And I thought, okay. So now when I go in, I don't moan.

Acknowledgements For the support and wisdom and generosity of my colleagues on the Waiting Times project and my collaborators in our online storytelling sessions—you kept me sane, or sane-adjacent.

Competing Interests This research was funded in whole, or in part by the Wellcome Trust [Grant number 205400/A/16/Z]. For the purpose of open access, the author has applied a CC BY public copyright licence to any Author Accepted Manuscript version arising from this submission

References

Anucha, K., Baraitser, L., Davies, S., Flexer, M. J., & Robinson, D. (2021). Investigating waiting: Interdisciplinary thoughts on researching elongated temporalities in healthcare settings. In B. C. Clift, J. Gore, S. Gustafsson, S. Bekker, I. C. Batlle, & J. Hatchard (Eds.), *Temporality in qualitative inquiry: Theories, methods and practices* (pp. 39–56). Routledge.

Augé, M. (1995). *Non-places: An introduction to supermodernity* (J. Howe, Trans.). Verso.

Baraitser, L., & Brook, W. (2020). Watchful waiting: Temporalities of crisis and care in the UK National Health Service. In V. Browne, J. Danely, T. Managhan, & D. Rosenow (Eds.), *Vulnerability and the politics of care*. Oxford University Press.

Baraitser, L., Anucha, K., Catty, J., Davies, S., Osserman, J., Salisbury, L., Flexer, M., & Moore, M. (2024). (Un)timely care: findings from the Waiting Times project [version 1; peer review: 1 approved, 1 approved with reservations]. *Wellcome Open Research,* 9490. https://doi.org/10.12688/wellcomeopenres.22556.1

Beckett, S. (1981). *Ill seen ill said* (Samuel Beckett, Trans.). John Calder.

Bishop, P. (2013). Surveying 'the waiting room'. *Architectural Theory Review, 18*(2), 135–149. https://doi.org/10.1080/13264826.2013.814558

Bramwell, D., Checkland, K., Shields, J., & Allen, P. (2023). 2010–2015: The health and social care act, NHS fragmentation. In *Community nursing services in England: An historical policy analysis* (pp. 75–82). Springer International Publishing.

Caronia, L., & Mortari, L. (2015). The agency of things: How spaces and artefacts organize the moral order of an intensive care unit. *Social Semiotics, 24*(4), 401–422.

Deleuze, G. (2004). *The logic of sense* (C. V Boundas, Ed.; M. Lester & C. Stivale, Trans.). Continuum.

Derrida, J. (1994). *Specters of Marx* (P. Kamuf, Trans.). Routledge.

Hinchliffe, S., Jackson, M. A., Wyatt, K., Barlow, A. E., Barreto, M., Clare, L., Depledge, M. H., Durie, R., Fleming, L. E., Groom, N., Morrissey, K., Salisbury, L., & Thomas, F. (2018). Healthy Publics: Enabling cultures and environments for health. *Palgrave Communications, 4*(57), 1–10. https://doi.org/10.1057/s41599-018-0113-9

Lotman, Y. M. (1990). *Universe of the mind: A semiotic theory of culture* (Ann Shukman, Trans.). I.B. Tauris.

McPhail, d., Lorway, R., & Chevrier, C. (2022). Safe spaces that matter: Material semiotics, affective bodies and queer readings of clinical spaces in Winnipeg, Canada. *SSM - Qualitative Research in Health, 2*. https://doi.org/10.1016/j.ssmqr.2022.100126

Salisbury, L., Baraitser, L., Catty, J., Anucha, K., Davies, S., Flexer, M., Moore, M., & Osserman, J. (2023). A waiting crisis? *The Lancet, 401*, 428–429.

Schweizer, H. (2008). *On waiting*. Routledge.

"The Ex-Girlfriend" Seinfeld. (1991, January 23). [Broadcast]. NBC.

Uspenskij, B. (2017). Semiotics and culture: The perception of time as a semiotic problem. *Sign Systems Studies, 45*(3–4), 230–248. https://doi.org/10.12697/SSS.2017.45.3-4.02

Veinot, T., & Pierce, C. (2019). Materiality in information environments: Objects, spaces, and bodies in three outpatient hemodialysis facilities. *Journal of the Association for Information Science and Technology, 70*(12), 1324–1133.

7

'Sorry If I Was a Bit Whistle Stop!': Boundary Work and Whistle Stop Teaching in X-Ray Image Interpretation with Medical Students

Peter Winter

In the United Kingdom, the demand for medical imaging is rising at a faster rate than that of most other National Health Service (NHS) services, reaching a point where radiology services "cannot cope" (Maskell, 2022, p. 1). The increasing workload for radiology services, combined with the high demand for complex imaging modalities such as computed tomography (CT) and magnetic resonance imaging (MRI) and a national shortage of both radiologists and radiographers, has significantly reduced the time available for teaching radiology to medical students (Royal College of Radiologists, 2020). This increased demand for radiology services has placed pressure on the dual role of radiologists as both clinicians and educators, thus threatening the teaching time available for radiologists and not adequately preparing medical students for postgraduate practice as junior doctors (Lewis et al., 2016; Blazar et al., 2020; Ayesa

P. Winter (✉)
School of Sociology, Politics and International Studies (SPAIS), University of Bristol, Bristol, UK
e-mail: Peter.winter@bristol.ac.uk

K. Kenny et al. (eds.), *Timescapes of Health, Illness and Care*,
https://doi.org/10.1007/978-981-96-7055-0_7

et al., 2021). In response, radiologists have been compelled to reorganise their priorities and methods of teaching, and to reconstitute their epistemic territory of teaching interactions to manage this dual responsibility effectively (Huang et al. 2009; Vavasseur et al. 2020).

This chapter explores how the temporal demands of increased information and the complexities of interpreting newer imaging technologies create new temporal pressures on radiologists, particularly in the context of teaching radiology to medical students. Drawing on my video ethnographic field research in an NHS teaching hospital's radiology department, I examine the practices and strategies through which these time constraints and teaching obligations are organised and managed.

Building on Thomas Gieryn's (1999) concept of boundary work, I argue that teaching time and professional expertise in radiology are managed through anticipatory practices. These practices focus on what is common or 'obvious' to streamlining the learning process. 'Whistle stop' teaching practices, which prioritise chest x-ray image interpretation and emphasise common abnormalities and spot diagnoses, serve as a proactive and reactive strategy to manage the temporal pressures faced by radiologists. These practices allow radiologists to cope with their dual responsibilities by quickly imparting essential skills, although often at the expense of more in-depth, comprehensive knowledge.

The implications of these temporal practices are significant. While they provide an immediate solution to balancing clinical and educational duties, they risk compromising the depth of radiology education that medical students receive. This chapter argues that while whistle stop teaching practices are a necessary adaptation to current pressures, they underscore the need for a re-evaluation of how teaching and clinical duties can be balanced to ensure the development of well-rounded medical professionals capable of handling the challenges of modern radiology.

Time, Radiology Teaching, and Radiological Expertise in the Making

Much literature has been published on the role of time in medical work, providing valuable insights into how medical work is intricately organised and structured in relation to time, influencing both the delivery and experience of healthcare (e.g., Atkinson, 1981; Frankenberg, 1992; Berg, 1996; Harrison et al., 2024). The analysis of time in medical work has seen a resurgence in recent years, driven by new expectations and burdens emerging from health crises. For example, in a recent special issue on "Matters of Time in Health and Illness," Harrison et al. (2024) highlight how the clock measures and orders various aspects of healthcare, such as appointment scheduling and treatment durations. The rigid structure of clock time often conflicts with the fluid, processual nature of care, which can unfold in unbounded and relational ways (Davies, 1994; Twigg, 2000). This conflict was notably exacerbated during the COVID-19 pandemic, necessitating a reorganisation of care practices through multitasking and peer collaboration (Harrison et al., 2023). Furthermore, chronic illness and disability disrupt linear temporalities, emphasising the need for flexible and patient-centred time management in medical settings (Samuels, 2017).

These insights underscore the complexity of temporal structuring in medical work and its significant impact on both healthcare providers and patients (Harrison et al., 2024). However, much of this work pays little attention to how medical fields, such as radiology, organise teaching time and materials, including the content of their performances and recipients' responses, which centre around the logic of clinical reasoning. There is also a predominance of quantitative approaches in the study of time in medical education, which emphasise the evaluation of teaching at the expense of deeper qualitative analyses (Chew et al., 2021). This chapter addresses this gap by analysing the relationship between temporality and clinical reasoning, focusing on how this is deployed in the teaching of radiology.

Drawing from Gieryn's (1983, 1999) concept of 'boundary work,' this chapter examines how teaching practices both organise time and shape radiological expertise in relation to specific knowledge and clinical domains. Existing scholarship in fields such as science and technology studies (STS) and medical anthropology (e.g., Saunders, 2008; Winter, 2019) has investigated how radiology teaching organises its objects of scrutiny, yet these fall short of exploring how teaching itself is organised through practices of boundary work. Gieryn uses the term 'boundary work' to describe the efforts made by scientific communities to establish, maintain, and defend the borders of what is considered legitimate science and what is not. According to Gieryn, the boundary between science and non-science is a matter of power and authority, rather than a set of essential characteristics or methods. Boundary work is performed through discursive practices, which reshape and organise stimuli as objects of knowledge that animate the discourse of a profession. Boundaries thus operate as "interpretive walls [that] protect [scientists'] professional authority" from outside powers that may "compromise the material and symbolic resources of science inside" (Gieryn, 1999, p. 17).

The concept of boundary work has been extensively explored in STS and related fields to understand how medical technologies and practices authorise and legitimise specific forms of expertise and evidence, thereby shaping professional boundaries and authority within healthcare (Moreira et al., 2006; Burri, 2008; Reed et al., 2016; Lindberg et al., 2017). While Gieryn's concept of boundary work is not explicitly framed as a time management strategy, its application in various fields often involves managing and optimising time and resources through the strategic organisation of tasks and responsibilities. Of particular relevance to this chapter is Burri's (2008) application of the concept, which highlights the ways medical experts, notably radiologists, do boundary work through interactions to enhance their reputation and safeguard their professional identity, which had become threatened with the advent of MRI. Radiologists were forced to renegotiate responsibilities and professional competences and to reconstitute their epistemic authority and identity due to the transformations in radiology brought about by the introduction of new visualisation technologies. This focus on the ways in which staff are organised around new technologies to (re)gain professional authority, underscores the limited direct application of this concept specifically as a strategy to manage time, attention, and labour in conditions of professional overload or contestation.

This chapter traces some of the rising workload in radiology caused by radiologists meeting clinical demands at high standards and points out the epistemic challenges they face when teaching medical students and adjusting radiological skills. Drawing on video footage of radiologists, it shows how boundary work, aimed at organising facts and the practice of seeing, has organised both the teaching practices of radiology education and the focus of student attention on compulsory images to help manage radiological workload in the department. It highlights the intersection of temporality and clinical reasoning, showing how time management not only influences the pacing and depth of learning but also serves as a form of boundary work that delineates professional expertise and authority. By situating radiology teaching within the framework of boundary work, it offers a nuanced understanding of how temporal practices shape and are shaped by the professional identities and epistemic practices of radiologists.

The Temporal Demands of Increased Information and New Uncertainties in Radiology

Radiology is pivotal in patient diagnosis and management, but advancements in imaging technology have paradoxically introduced new uncertainties. Over the last 30 years, there has been a global surge in medical imaging services, particularly in CT and MRI. Radiologists now analyse hundreds of images for every patient daily due to the proliferation of cross-sectional imaging examinations (Kwee & Kwee, 2021). In the United Kingdom, CT scans doubled from 250,000 per month to 500,000 per month, and MRI scans rose from 170,000 to 320,000 per month between 2012 and 2019, leading to what the Royal College of Radiologists (2020) described as a "workforce in crisis."

Newer visualisation technologies such as MRI are often positioned as more objective compared to 'low-tech' procedures, which are labelled as subjective (see Burri 2008; Joyce 2008). This distinction is also applied to CT, which, since its introduction, has been considered a significant upgrade over traditional x-rays, providing highly detailed cross-sectional images (Barley, 1990). However, this perceived objectivity and detail come with increased complexity and the potential for uncertain findings. Radiologists often resolve these uncertainties by proposing further imaging (Maskell, 2022). Moreover, the shortage of radiologists and the demands of interpreting these complex images have led to a rise in unreported images,[1] increasing the risk of missed or delayed diagnoses (Royal College of Radiologists, 2020). The Care Quality Commission (CQC) reported in 2018 that the growing number of unreported images has contributed to multiple investigations and legal actions against healthcare providers, highlighting significant concerns about patient safety and the reliability of radiological services (Care Quality Commission, 2018).

The temporal demands of dealing with these new uncertainties have fundamentally altered the radiological profession. Radiologists' time is increasingly consumed by the need to interpret complex CT and MRI scans, reducing the time available for clinical, administrative, educational, and technological duties. This shift has been compounded by societal demands for precise anatomical depictions and the critical role imaging plays in patient management today (Maskell, 2022).

Despite the pressures, the evolving role of radiographers has provided some relief. Historically, radiographers produced images and conducted initial assessments, while radiologists and junior doctors engaged in interpretive work. However, the growing demand for imaging technologies has allowed radiographers to expand their roles to include reporting CT, MRI, and x-ray images, moving towards a diagnostic profession (Royal College of Radiologists, 2020; Price & Le Masurier, 2007; Snaith et al., 2015).

Clearly, advancements in imaging technology have increased the volume and detail of medical images. However, they have also introduced new uncertainties, requiring additional interpretive efforts and further straining time as a resource in an already-overburdened radiology workforce. This paradox, where greater information creates new uncertainties and "complexity in reading" (Saunders, 2008, p. 75), has significantly contributed to the reorganisation of radiological work and expertise, revealing how time is distributed between new and old imaging technologies. This tension calls for further investigation not only with a view that new uncertainties carry their own temporal demands but also because of

[1] Unreported images refer to medical scans that have not been reviewed and interpreted by radiologists, which can result in critical diagnostic information being overlooked. This situation has led to increased scrutiny from independent regulators and a rise in medical malpractice lawsuits due to missed or delayed diagnoses.

their effect on teaching and training. This chapter attempts to identify the different ways that radiologists organise their teaching to medical students in response to the temporal priorities of MRI and CT technologies.

Teaching, Chest X-Rays, and Time Practices

This chapter is based on a six-month video ethnography of an NHS teaching hospital's radiology department between 2015 and 2016, referred to here as Bridgestock Hospital (a pseudonym). It is part of a multi-sited video ethnography focusing on radiologists and radiographers teaching x-ray image interpretation to undergraduate medical and radiography students in various 'academic' settings such as classrooms, seminar rooms, meeting rooms, offices, and lecture theatres (Winter, 2019, 2022). The focus of this chapter is on radiologists teaching chest x-ray image interpretation to third-, fourth-, and fifth-year medical students in Bridgestock Radiology Meeting Room (BRMR).

Located away from patients, BRMR was situated within a network of corridors leading to departmental offices used by radiologists and radiology administrators. While BRMR is mainly used by radiologists as a space to discuss follow-up investigations, audits, discrepancies, and management, the room also doubles up as a space for Specialist Training (ST) in radiology, for both radiologists and medical students, on their rotation[2] in the radiology department. ST radiologists opt to undertake undergraduate teaching duties and are administered BRMR as the locus of formal teaching. They participate in a complex system that combines clinical work and formal rotation teaching (Winter, 2019).

Video ethnography is a qualitative research method that involves the use of video recordings to capture naturally occurring interactions and events in their real-life context. The method provides a rich, multimodal dataset that includes not only verbal communication but also non-verbal cues such as body language, gestures, spatial arrangements, and interactions with objects, which are often lost in purely textual data (Heath

[2] In this rotation, 15 medical students are divided into five groups of three, rotating every two weeks.

et al., 2010). The decision to conduct a video ethnography and use video data to explore teaching interactions is grounded in the theory developed to understand the training of 'professional vision' (Goodwin, 1994). According to Goodwin (1994), 'professional vision' provides a framework for understanding how professionals are trained to interpret and act upon visual information in ways that are specific to their field. This involves the practices of highlighting important features, coding information in systematic ways, and creating visual representations, all of which emerge through the interplay with a domain of scrutiny (e.g., x-ray images made available by the radiologist). Video data can be, as Goodwin (2000, p. 6) suggests, an appropriate method to "maintain as much information as possible about the setting, bodily displays and spatial organisation of all relevant participants, their talk, and how events change through time."

I proposed video ethnography as my primary source for data collection because I was interested in providing a detailed description of the spatial-material features of the learning environment and the nuances of talk and body in learning to see as a competent practitioner (Winter, 2019). Excerpts from video footage are transcribed according to the complex character of 'professional vision' (Goodwin, 1994). Each excerpt illustrates how the participants (both professionals and students) talk, gesture, and interactionally engage their bodies as they attend to images, materials, and each other (Alač, 2011) within the specifics of the three modes of practice used to accomplish professional vision: coding, highlighting, and graphic representation.

Transcription focused on situating these practices with respect to their textual landmark and where they appeared in the transcription. This operation was generated using a combination of text and italics to mark how the text should be read. For example, when a participant uses a body part (e.g., hand) to make image content perceptually salient against an ambiguous background (the highlighting practice), the extract is represented by means of italicised text in square brackets included in the talk; for example, 'It's really important to try and look behind the diaphragm and actually how superior it goes' [*Highlighting 1: On the posterior anterior (PA) chest x-ray (CXR) the radiologist hovers the mouse cursor over the highest point of the right lower lobe (RLL)*]. In my analysis, I label two types of highlighting practice (Highlighting 1 and Highlighting 2), which both chime with Ivarsson's (2017) and Gegenfurtner et al.'s (2019) analysis of highlighting gesture in radiological practice. Highlighting 1 refers to highlighting that selects, elaborates, and makes salient features "of the world within sight" (i.e., that are present). Highlighting 2 evokes "phenomena that are not present and depict imaginary and abstract worlds" (Ivarsson, 2017, p. 15). Including these bracketed descriptions helps clarify the participants' actions and enhances the reader's understanding of the teaching interactions being described.

All participants consented to being video recorded, and the names used in this chapter are pseudonyms. The x-ray images that have been video recorded are used as teaching resources and have been anonymised by the radiologists by removing any individual identifiers, such as the patient's name, date of birth, or treating hospital.

The next section tracks three discursive contexts of boundary work as a way of organising teaching time in x-ray image interpretation to medical students: the teaching of chest x-rays as a priority; the structured and expectant interpretation of chest x-rays; and spot diagnosis and 'obvious' appearances for speeding up the learning process. Doing so also reveals boundary work as a knowledge-making practice that is performed in relation with the organising of time, emphasising boundary work as a pedagogical practice in shaping medical education.

Top Priority: Teaching Chest X-Rays as a Practice of Frontline Intervention

In Bridgestock Hospital's radiology department (BHRD), radiologists teach medical students to interpret x-ray images—but not to interpret all kinds of x-ray images concerning different body parts. The sense here is that radiologists, responding to demand, prioritise CT and MRI and that there is a need to find ways of managing demand for other imaging examinations such as chest x-ray. Below, for example, is Dr Maxwell—a consultant radiologist from BHRD—introducing a group of medical students to a chest x-ray image interpretation seminar and giving them a gentle warning that as junior doctors they will be "first in line" to interpret chest x-rays, mainly "on the ward" or "in A&E" whereby they interact with patients of varying chest/lung concerns.

> I've just got to kind of prepare you in terms of really spotting an abnormal finding early on, because you guys as presumably as junior doctors might be the first and only people to look at the film for quite a while until the radiologist gets round to reporting it, because they'll be busy with the acute CTs, the acute intervention, you know, vascular intervention, that kind of thing, and get round to the plain films maybe a bit later on, and you've got the patient in front of you; if you've got an acutely deteriorating patient in front of you and someone says 'oh, here's the chest x-ray!' you know, it's nice for you to know what to spot and what not to spot. (Dr Maxwell, BHRD radiologist)

Dr Maxwell sees junior doctors as contributors to the radiological workforce in the hospital. The assignment of chest x-rays—frequently talked about as the most requested x-ray image in BHRD—reflects a division of labour in which junior doctors are allocated to a particular x-ray image; the role of the junior doctor, in turn, extends to what is commonly described by radiologists as the "first and only people to look at the film for quite a while until the radiologist gets round to reporting it." Here, radiologists perform boundary work by strategically assigning medical students (imagined as junior doctors) to interpret x-ray images rather than MRI or more complex imaging, thereby preserving their control over more advanced imaging techniques (Burri, 2008). This helps reinforce the perception that advanced imaging technologies like MRI and CT require the specialised expertise of a fully trained radiologist ("they'll [the radiologist] be busy with the acute CTs, the acute intervention, you know, vascular intervention, that kind of thing"). This contrasts with older imaging technologies like x-rays, which are seen as more routine, less specialised, and less prestigious compared to newer and more sophisticated technologies such as MRIs (Barley, 1990; Burri, 2008; Joyce, 2008). This places junior doctors at the bottom of the interpretive hierarchy and radiology's division of labour.

While limiting medical students to x-ray image interpretation may preserve the hierarchical professional expertise of the radiologist, it also enhances training and skill development. Medical students can develop their foundational skills with x-ray images, which are generally less complex. This gradual learning curve ensures that medical students gain competence in basic imaging before advancing to more sophisticated technologies. Moreover, Dr Maxwell's warning serves as a timely reminder that abnormalities must not be missed. The next section explores in more detail the concerns of radiologists about missing or not seeing abnormalities and how a structured approach not only prevents these issues from arising but also provides temporal affordances, helping to manage time effectively.

Reviewing Areas and Anticipating Abnormalities

Radiologists emphasise the importance of a systematic approach to medical image interpretation through a 'structured review.' This approach involves a consistent, organised method for examining medical images, ensuring no critical areas are overlooked (Sandell, 2010; Winter and Linehan, 2014; Van der Gijp et al., 2014; Kok et al., 2016; Winter, 2019). By following a consistent method, radiologists can quickly identify and analyse key areas, reducing interpretation time and improving diagnostic accuracy (Higashi et al., 2012). Radiologists in BHRD frequently encouraged medical students to adopt a structured approach to interpretation practices. This involves developing a routine that helps them become aware of what they might miss or forget, allowing them to navigate the image with focused urgency and speed up the review of specific areas of the chest.

This structured approach to image interpretation defines the boundaries of the review, standardising certain areas as points of focus for anticipating abnormalities. When a radiologist introduces a structured review, it is typically done at the beginning of the session using a normal chest x-ray and diagrams of the normal chest. Teaching radiologists usually guide the review steps by 'highlighting' areas where abnormalities are likely to occur, even if the current image is normal (Goodwin, 1994). These 'norms of abnormal expectation' mean that certain areas are routinely emphasised because they are common sites for potential abnormalities (Saunders, 2008; Ivarsson, 2017; Winter, 2019). In these instances, drawing attention to specific areas of the body also functions as a temporal practice of boundary work by prioritising life-threatening abnormalities (such as lung tumours) that require immediate attention:

> It's really important to try and look behind the diaphragm and actually how superior it goes [*Highlighting 1: On the posterior anterior (PA) diagram of the chest the radiologist hovers the mouse cursor over the highest point of the right lower lobe (RLL)*] so sometimes you can see a mass here [*Highlighting 2: cursor hovers across the PA diagram of the chest between the right upper lobe (RUL) and right middle lobe (RML) to indicate expectant abnormality* (Fig. 7.1)] and you don't know if it's in the middle lobe [*Highlighting 2: cursor hovers of RML to indicate expectant abnormality*], the upper lobe [*Highlighting 2: cursor hovers over expectant abnormality on PA in RUL*], or the lower lobe [*Highlighting 2: cursor hovers over expectant abnormality on PA in lower lobe*] because it can be any where around here [*Highlighting 2: on lateral CXR cursor hovers over midpoint of RUL/RML/RLL*]. (Dr Delichon, BHRD radiologist)

Each review is informed by abnormal expectation. In the case of the diaphragm, Dr Delichon explains that because the diaphragm sits in front of the lung lobes (right upper lobe, right middle lobe, and right lower lobe) the lung lobes are partially obscured. This means that a 'mass' can hide 'behind the diaphragm.' Dr Delichon's demonstration draws attention to common abnormalities that junior doctors are likely to encounter, thus enabling medical students to scrutinise areas in which these abnormalities might dwell.

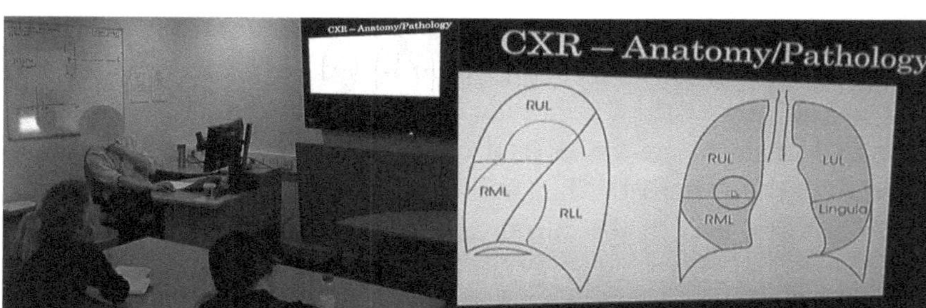

Fig. 7.1 Diagram of lateral (LA) and posteroanterior (PA) CXR anatomy

Yet the practice of the structured review can also be seen as an important time-saving device that enables greater efficiency, as well as affording a degree of legal protection. Indeed, Dr Maxwell (BHRD radiologist) encapsulates this point eloquently when he informs a group of medical students that a structured approach will protect them against "a conspiracy of little things that kind of lead people up the garden path." This advice illustrates some of the boundary-making practices through which radiologists navigate the messiness and ambiguity of the chest x-ray and thus save time—a practice that is tinged with the ever-present fear of litigation and malpractice (Joyce, 2008; Burri, 2013; Winter, 2019).

Practices of boundary work become even more visible in the use of case presentations in teaching. As we have seen, x-ray image interpretation is introduced to radiology students through the reading of a normal chest x-ray image and diagram. Radiologists then shift their focus to case presentations where the legibility of abnormalities is crucial. These presentations often feature images (or sometimes a series of images) selected for their "ontological ambiguity" (Måseide, 2007, p. 203). Such images are treated with suspicion, considered potentially misleading, and used to introduce uncertainty and error (Winter, 2019). Saunders (2008) refers to these case presentations as opportunities for building *intrigue*, where the theatrics and rhetoric of the radiological expert create conditions of puzzlement or curiosity.

In my video ethnography of radiologists teaching x-ray image interpretation to medical students, I recorded four different radiologists presenting their case studies in a meeting room (BRMR). Most radiologists began their first x-ray image presentation with an example of a structured approach to chest x-rays. However, during my fieldwork, I observed that from the first case presentation onwards, radiologists invited medical students to lead the discussion. This 'hot seat' approach allowed for a learning opportunity focused on the ambiguous character of the images, driven by student observations rather than the radiologist's input.

Medical students began the case by analysing the image in terms of its technique (anterior posterior [AP] or posterior anterior [PA]), demographics (age, gender), technical adequacy (lines and tubes, artifacts, exposure), and, finally, the anatomy. The length of each student's analysis was meticulously controlled by the radiologist, who allowed students time to observe and describe one finding at a time, often interrupting with prompts for corrections, checks, and diversions. This time management by the radiologist functioned as a kind of detective work, enabling students to find 'clues' and build a narrative of intrigue (Saunders, 2008). Managing the time of medical students' interpretive accounts in this way facilitated a cautious and vigilant approach to learning. It ensured that students did not rush through their analysis, fostering a deeper engagement with each aspect of the image. By controlling the pacing of the session through various types of interruptions—such as amending errors, redirecting inspections, and translating observations into proper terminologies—radiologists created a dynamic learning environment aimed at refining the description of findings through a process of regular interruption (Saunders, 2008).

During my video ethnography, radiologists frequently interrupted medical students when they paused or dwelled on locations or displayed uncertainty about what they were seeing and what to say next. In the extract below, Dr Delichon reads hesitation in the commentary of a medical student when faced with a case presentation and gently prompts them into seeing and saying the right thing:

Dr Delichon:	*Okay!* next one
Chloe:	[*nervous laugh*] So, this is, I'm assuming a PA film [*pause*] of a patient [*hesitates*] who [*pause*] [*moves head closer to the image*] oohhh [*exhales and rests elbows on the table to steady her gaze*] [*pauses*]. It's really hard to comment on either the rotation?
Dr Delichon:	Yeah, I would say it's fine
Chloe:	Or the penetration?
Dr Delichon:	So, it's okay? [*looks at Chloe and nods in encouragement*]
Chloe:	It's okay? Yeah, okay um so the trachea [sits up and straightens back], oohh again it's hard to comment on the trachea whether its central or not [*Chloe makes a thinking gesture that mimics Auguste Rodin's sculpture, The Thinker (*Le Penseur *in French)]*
Dr Delichon:	What are you going to do first before you comment on the trachea?

Chloe:	There are [*looks down and reads notes*] 'no external lines or metalwork'
Dr Delichon:	Good, 'no external lines or metal work'
Chloe:	[*nervous laugh*]
	[*Pause: six seconds of silent looking*]
Chloe:	Uhhhmmm
	[*Pause: six seconds of silent looking*]
Dr Delichon:	[*nods*] Yeah? Just making sure you're okay? Okay, good, so *trachea*?
Chloe:	Yeah, um it's hard to comment on whether the trachea is [*hesitates*] central?
Dr Delichon:	[*head moves closer to the computer screen to inspect it*] here [*Highlighting 1: cursor traces the trachea downwards*]
Chloe:	Uhh
Dr Delichon:	Yeah
Chloe:	So, oh yeah okay
Dr Delichon:	It's kind of here [*Highlighting 1: cursor traces the trachea downwards* (Fig. 7.2)]
Chloe:	So, it's deviated?
Dr Delichon:	Yeah
Chloe:	Um to the right
Dr Delichon:	Mhm

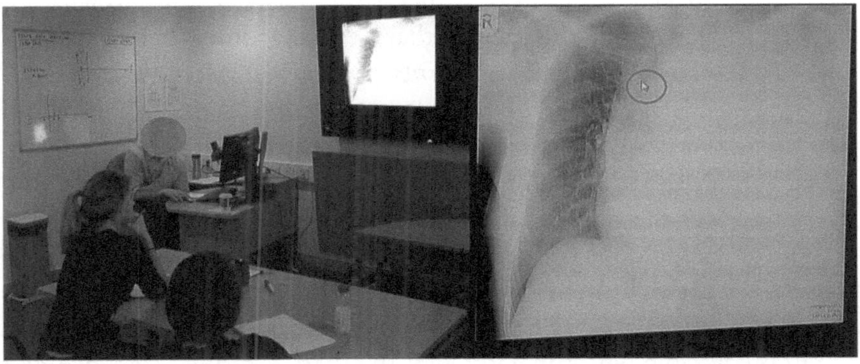

Fig. 7.2 Case 5: Pleural effusion

In the extract above, two voices are evident: the medical student's evocation of hesitancy, uncertainty, nervousness, and discomfort and the radiologist's rhetorical guiding of perception. The extract is typical of a radiologist reading features of speech delivery (pauses, hesitations, nervous laughter, elongation) and embodied conduct (silent looking, thinking gesture, gestures of frustration, corrective body movements) which interrupt a medical student's struggle with the image.

Another example of such interruption was provided by radiologist Dr Saury in his observation of the staccato-like pauses and gestures of frustration elicited by medical student Alexander while reading a case presentation:

Dr Saury: Okay, next person
Alexander: Um, I think he's got um, they've got an ECG on?
Dr Saury: Yeah, good
Alexander: Umm [*hesitates*] so there's opacity in the upper right *area*?
Dr Saury: Yeah
[*Pause: six seconds of silent looking*]
Dr Saury: So, you know about the consolidation last time? This one looks a bit different to me
Alexander: Mm
Dr Saury: Okay? And I think it looks *different* because I think this *trachea* is a bit further across [*Highlighting 1: Cursor floats up and down over the deviated trachea*], okay? I think it's being sucked across a bit further across this way but also what do you think this line is that's curving down here like that? [*Highlighting 1: Uses a smart pen to draw over the right horizontal fissure with an intermittent line* (Fig. 7.3)]. It's got a very well defined lower, lower limit in that area of opacity, hasn't it? What do you think that line might be? If I tell you: it's the horizontal fissure. So, this is left upper, sorry, right upper lobe collapse, okay? So, we've got increased density in the right upper zone.

Although radiologists in radiology seminars exhibited patience and allowed medical students time to analyse images, they often interrupted

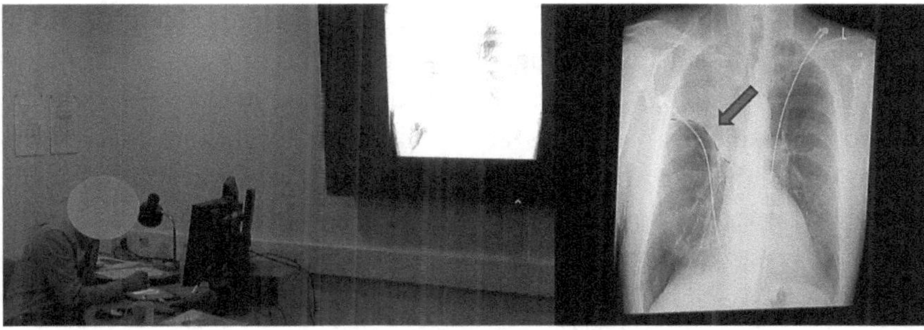

Fig. 7.3 Case 7: Right upper lobe collapse

with clues towards the 'right' things to see, engaging in a type of collaborative talk (Goodwin, 1994). Radiologists perceive medical students' commentary about images as that of an apprentice whose observations are long, drawn out, and arduous. In other words, radiologists see medical students as slow in their descriptions but not necessarily getting to the point: they are talking about the puzzle pieces instead of the key pieces of the puzzle. If medical students are to become effective junior doctors within the radiological hierarchy, as Dr Maxwell outlined earlier, they must learn how to identify abnormalities without wasting precious time actively searching.

I read this as an admission that radiology training does not readily lend itself to time efficiency. As such, radiologists must prioritise specific abnormalities and implicitly teach students that medical image interpretation, or seeing and saying whether something is abnormal or not, is a time-sensitive task. When radiologists interrupt medical students to speed up their interpretation, they perform a form of boundary work by helping students to focus on what is most important, ensuring they develop the ability to quickly identify and analyse key areas without getting bogged down by less critical details.

The same may be said of case presentations presented as 'never events.' According to NHS England (2018), 'never events' are "serious, largely preventable patient safety incidents that should not occur if healthcare providers have implemented existing national guidance or safety recommendations." Radiologists teaching case presentations to medical students deliver never events of all kinds. They not only are used to illustrate and communicate radiological errors but also help radiologists draw attention to problems of viewing, often formulated in terms of duplicity or peril (Winter, 2019). Such images are often used by teaching radiologists to warn medical students about different conditions that might induce uncertainty in their reading of images. Dr Maxwell often takes never event opportunities as an attempt to generate a sense of danger in dramatic ways: "every year there'll be a junior doctor in the press up before the GMC [General Medical Council] in trouble for saying 'yes, you can feed the patient' and the nasogastric tube was in the wrong place, so it's one of those never events." Delivering case presentations about never events and how they generate uncertainty is clearly important to radiologists.

Such boundary practices are not exclusively verbal or bodied. Timetables are also used as powerful resources to support time management. At the beginning of each rotation, the radiology lead handed out a timetable to mobilise a corridor walk that familiarised the students to the layout of the department, the location of each teaching session, and its duration. Although the timetable allotted fixed 'time slots' for teaching sessions (such as CXR image interpretation), the remainder were optional. Presented with a choice, medical students are the ones to decide what 'other' teaching attachments to attend. The professional's rhetoric of "direct your own learning [and] … if it's interesting, stay" emphasised during the departmental induction provides an informal network that shapes individual timetables and permits students to situate themselves in routine work scenarios making rotations as time economic as possible. Ad hocing, therefore, is an apt vehicle for organising 'self-directed' learning across the radiology department, not only because it fits in impromptu or idiosyncratic teaching at various junctures in the diagnostic workday (Saunders, 2008) but also because it falls within the autonomy of the medical profession. Most importantly for this chapter, ad hocing is a further type of boundary work strategy that deals with time and how it manifests in the organisation of opportunistic radiology teaching. This maximises time for both contextual clinical knowledge and technical knowledge, and allows space to teach while experts work. In other words, the timetable enables a mapping of clinical-radiology routines and academic activities into which the medical student is invited through fixed and ad hoc time zones—determining when the student learns, structuring the days, and allowing the very opportunity to extend their gaze across time and space (Frankenberg, 1992; Berg, 1996).

Spot Diagnosis and 'Obvious' Appearances for Accelerating Teaching

While prioritising chest x-rays and teaching a structured review of expected abnormalities played a significant role in managing time, spot diagnosis became an immediate strategy used by radiologists to focus on the most urgent and critical findings. In other words, when time was running out, radiologists prioritised teaching the immediate recognition of 'obvious' abnormalities.

In radiology teaching that includes chest x-rays, radiologists present 20 different cases, even when they have only one hour of fixed time to teach CXR image interpretation. The goal is to cover as many images as possible in each seminar. This is a time pressure that Dr Saury, at the beginning of a seminar, faces:

> So, all of these, don't worry about going through an order, because we just want to get through lots of pathology so you can start seeing stuff. But always do lines and tubes at the start and just tell me what you think the abnormality is. Dr Saury (BHRD radiologist)

Dr Saury's request may be read as a boundary strategy that places analytical focus squarely on the urgency of detecting pathology, thereby creating a distinct teaching practice from his colleagues. However, what begins as a quick attempt to spot abnormalities evolves into a diagnostic quest as the medical student encounters significant yet ambiguously unquantifiable findings, including interruptions and pauses. Nevertheless, focusing on immediate or urgent observations can be seen as an epistemic tactic, where novice eyes are trained to recognise certain appearances or 'patterns.' enabling them to accumulate knowledge of pressing abnormalities and become productive members of the diagnostic workforce. Additionally, although training emphasises abnormalities, the radiologist finds it important to allocate time for "lines and tubes at the start." While this may seem like a trivial observation, it is, in fact, meaningful against the backdrop of litigation concerns radiologists face, particularly in relation to 'never events' that Dr Maxwell mentioned earlier (such as the misinterpretation of nasogastric tubes, pacemaker lines, and surgical clips).

The neglect of a systematic approach in favour of a strong fixation on identifying abnormalities was a tactic shared by the other three radiologists. However, this deliberate neglect of 'order' tended to occur near the end of lessons. As the lesson progresses, medical students are given less time to read the image, provide relevant descriptions, and learn from mistakes in case of misinterpretation. Consequently, a thorough assessment of the case is not conducted, and knowledge about the patient is only partially reproduced, if at all. On the surface, this may seem reasonable and even typical of various types of teaching. However, given that junior doctors are often the 'first in line' to review chest x-rays, there is a heightened risk of misinterpretation. In fact, many studies assessing the visual expertise—or 'competency,' as they term it—of junior doctors emphasise a lack of knowledge and incomplete understanding of the CXRs they encounter (e.g., Eisen et al., 2006; Mehrotra et al., 2009; Satia et al., 2013; Christiansen et al., 2014). A major reason for this is the lack of teaching time. Studies continue to highlight the insufficient training opportunities junior doctors have with radiology trainees and consultants as a primary cause of misinterpretation errors, as well as faulty attitudes and practices (Lewis et al., 2016; Blazar et al., 2020; Ayesa et al., 2021).

This issue of 'lack of teaching time' leads radiologists to accelerate the identification of abnormalities through the strategic use of a 'spot diagnosis.' Radiologist educators use the term 'spot diagnosis' to describe a diagnostic task reduced to its most essential form, functioning as testing tool (Mort et al., 2003). This time-sensitive approach is often considered a professional diagnostic method, developed in response to immediate life-threatening risks in an increasingly fast-paced and litigious world:

Dr Delichon: Any *quick* abnormalities you can see?
Amit: Uh
Riya: Mm
Dr Delichon: Spot diagnosis!
Riya: Mm under the diaphragm?
Dr Delichon: Good
Riya: On the right side?
Dr Delichon: Yeah! Good one to pick out under the peritoneum [*Highlighting 1. cursor quickly hovers over the peritoneum* (Fig. 7.4)]

In this example, the radiologist, realising he only has five minutes left to present ten cases, encourages the medical students to quickly indicate if they 'spot' any abnormalities on the image. This approach of prompting a rapid interpretation is a common tactic used to manage the temporal rhythms and practices of teaching when time is running short. For example:

> *Okay!* [*looking at the clock on the computer screen*] uhh [*knocks down computer mouse*] so uh [*looks at the image on the computer screen*]. We've only got fifteen minutes and we've still got quite a few cases to go through so we'll kind of pick out the important bits. Dr Delichon (BHRD radiologist)

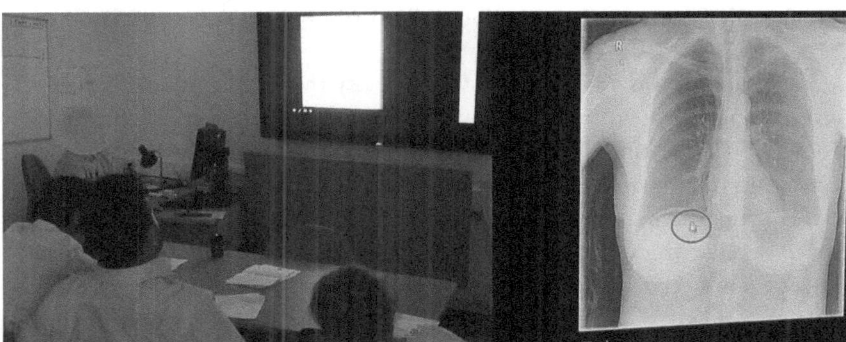

Fig. 7.4 Case 11: Pneumoperitoneum

Similarly, in another CXR image interpretation seminar, Dr Maxwell runs out of time after presenting 15 cases and delivers the next case with urgency. This time, however, the image is reduced to the principle of immediate recognition and the rule of 'seeing the obvious,' or, worse, it is entirely neglected or overlooked:

> Any obvious abnormalities on the film that you can tell me about? Dr Maxwell (BHRD consultant)

This hurried shift to a question-answer sequence that demands a quick or immediate response echoes Schuwirth et al.'s (2001) analysis of short case-based questions, where teaching is driven by mere pattern recognition. Pattern recognition has long been considered a form of 'non-systematic' reasoning, allowing learners to focus on whatever first captures their attention (Swinburne 1971; Corr et al., 2001). Being categorised in this manner reduces interpretation to simple size differences, like determining whether something is 'large' or 'big.' This contrasts sharply with the radiologist's earlier teaching practice, which created intrigue and puzzlement around the case (Saunders, 2008). However, as time runs short, spot diagnosis takes on increasing importance.

Just before the hour ends, Dr Delichon concludes his lesson by apologising to the students for the rushed 'whistle-stop' approach to teaching and suggests a more structured method of interpretation, hinting that it might compensate for the speed at which the material was covered:

> Okay, sorry, it was a bit whistle-stop. The key thing really to take home is to develop a strategy *now* for how you want to look at x-rays, write them down for all the kind of things you want to look at and then just repeat that over and over again. So, if you have it in a little book, just keep a note of where you, the system you want to use it until it becomes second nature to you. Because you will be looking at loads of chest x-rays on the ward, chest x-rays don't get reported particularly quickly by radiologists just because there's so many of them so you want to kind of be able to pick out the big things, so consolidations, infections, pneumothoraxes remember to pick out any big nodes, or masses if you think that might need further imaging. (Dr Delichon, BHRD radiologist)

Dr Delichon's remark that the lesson was "a bit whistle stop" suggests that teaching occurred within a limited timeframe. He further advises students to "develop a strategy" for examining x-rays, emphasising that having such a "system" will prove useful "on the ward." His focus on being systematic is crucial to avoid missing or overlooking important details: "you want to kind of be able to pick out the big things." Dr Delichon also reminds the students that they will often be the first to comment on chest x-rays, as "chest x-rays don't get reported particularly quickly by radiologists just because there's so many of them."

This account highlights the importance of recognising the big or obvious features in chest x-ray image interpretation seminars. While this may seem surprising, given that radiologists in their daily work are often concerned with subtle abnormalities hidden within the image (Saunders, 2008), they are accustomed to identifying more nuanced features and do not necessarily rely on pattern recognition alone to make a diagnosis. However, during the seminars I video recorded, prominent visual features such as 'big things' or 'big nodes or masses' in chest x-rays were clearly emphasised. All the radiologists included these significant abnormalities in their case presentations.

This demonstrates the importance of teaching obvious abnormalities to medical students—a point discussed at length by Kok et al. (2016) in the field of academic radiology. Their research suggests that the training of a systematic viewing approach may not be beneficial for medical students, as they "do not yet have the ability to catch smaller abnormalities from the corner of their eyes" (Kok et al., 2016, p. 201). While systematic teaching can promote systematic viewing, it is not directly linked to improved diagnostic performance. Given the focus on reducing workload, radiology teaching functions as a quality control measure for chest x-rays on the production line. It reinforces the priority of distinguishing major abnormalities from minor ones for medical students.

Conclusion

The rising demand for complex imaging technologies and the resulting workload in radiology have significantly altered the teaching landscape of radiological education, particularly in terms of time management and teaching practices. This chapter has explored how radiologists at Bridgestock Hospital navigate these pressures by employing boundary work strategies to manage their dual responsibilities of clinical practice and teaching. These strategies, particularly the emphasis on chest x-rays, structured reviews, and spot diagnoses, highlight the intricate relationship between time management and the reproduction of knowledge.

Boundary work strategies that prioritise the teaching of chest x-rays—which remains the most commonly performed x-ray examination in the United Kingdom (NHS England, 2020)—and the selection of compulsory case presentation knowledge by radiologists shed light on what images are included or ignored, with junior doctors treated as the first in line to cope with public demand. However, this could be an area for concern in the future as radiologists noticed that medical students were driven by preference for learning about CT rather than x-ray on the rotation.

Boundary work was also evident in the interactions between radiologists and medical students during case presentations. Following increases in 'never events' (White, 2022), the ambiguities of chest x-rays, and the limited image interpretation training that medical students receive, radiologists have responded by sharing structured or systematic approaches aimed at improving thoroughness and accuracy, and stabilising judgements under uncertainty (Van der Gijp et al., 2014; Kok et al., 2016; Winter, 2019). In their efforts to balance and give credit to important radiological knowledge, radiologists deployed several attention-grabbing techniques: the 'structured' approach cultivated expectations of abnormalities, while 'spot diagnosis' became a form of pattern recognition used by radiologists who ran out of time to conduct a comprehensive analyses of the available case presentations. Both expectant and obvious components of radiographic attention emerged as systematic and non-systematic tactics for boundary work, aiming to manage the challenging and time-consuming tasks of chest x-ray image interpretation.

The main issues I wish to highlight here is the danger of radiological teaching reducing the logic of abduction to mere pattern recognition, where processes of intrigue and uncertainty risk being lost due to time constraints. While this may be acceptable in expert-pedagogical situations, it can have unfavourable epistemic consequences for medical students learning to interpret medical images. My point is not to suggest that expectant observations and snap pattern recognition inherently cause interpretive errors but to show that they, like all radiological teaching, have diagnostic effects.

This chapter extends upon previous linkages between Gieryn's concept of boundary work and organising practices in medical work (e.g., Moreira et al., 2006; Burri, 2008; Reed et al., 2016; Lindberg et al., 2017) by explicitly framing boundary work as a time management strategy. Teaching chest x-rays to medical students is used as a boundary strategy to manage workload, allowing radiologists to focus on newer and more sophisticated imaging modalities. This practice not only preserves the prestige of the profession within the hospital or community but also addresses the immediate educational needs of medical students, albeit often at the expense of more comprehensive training.

This chapter also contributes to the literature on clinical reasoning for frontline radiology educators, particularly regarding the influence of the body and clinical culture on how and what information is received and put to use. It draws attention to the cognitive processes involved in clinical reasoning, such as analytical and non-analytical reasoning, as evidenced by the radiologists teaching medical students systematic (van der Gijp et al., 2014; Kok et al., 2016) and non-systematic (Swinburne 1971; Schuwirth et al. 2001; Corr et al., 2001) approaches; yet, it does so by recognising that cognition is not just a mental process but is deeply intertwined with the social and professional practices through which knowledge is constructed and communicated (Goodwin, 1994). In this way, clinical reasoning is not solely individual and psychological; it is distributed across people, objects, and time, such that reasoning and practice are dynamically produced and culturally constituted among groups of individuals working toward a shared goal (Goodwin, 1994, 2000; Alač, 2011; Winter, 2019, 2022).

The challenges for radiologists who teach medical students remain: to prioritise certain images over others, to interpret images comprehensively, and to ensure that harmful findings can be spotted in a short period of time. Boundary work practices help support a division of labour and time, and shape the delivery of radiological knowledge to medical students in matters of pressing concern to radiologists in the department.

Acknowledgements The research conducted for this chapter was supported by a PhD studentship in Sociology (STS pathway), funded by the Economic and Research Council (ESRC) (award: 149372004/1 awarded to Peter Winter) and sponsored by the University of Sheffield, UK. Special gratitude to the radiologists and medical students who kindly granted me access to video record their radiology teaching.

Competing Interests The author has no conflict of interest to declare that are relevant to the content of this chapter.

References

Alač, M. (2011). *Handling digital brains: A laboratory study of multimodal semiotic interaction in the age of computers*. MIT Press.

Atkinson, P. (1981). Time and cool patients. In P. Atkinson & C. Heath (Eds.), *Medical work: Realities and routines* (pp. 41–54). Gower.

Ayesa, S. L., Katelaris, A. G., Brennan, P. C., & Grieve, S. M. (2021). Medical imaging education opportunities for junior doctors and non-radiologist clinicians: A review. *Journal of Medical Imaging and Radiation Oncology, 65*, 710–718. https://doi.org/10.1111/1754-9485.13266

Barley, S. R. (1990). The alignment of technology and structure through roles and networks. *Administrative Science Quarterly, 35*(1), 61–103.

Berg, M. (1996). Practices of reading and writing: The constitutive role of the patient record in medial work. *Sociology of Health and Illness, 18*(4), 499–524. https://doi.org/10.1111/1467-9566.ep10939100

Blazar, E., Mitchell, D., & Townzen, J. D. (2020). Radiology training in emergency medicine residency as a predictor of confidence in an attending. *Cureus, 12*(1), e6615. https://doi.org/10.7759/cureus.6615

Burri, R. V. (2008). Doing distinctions: Boundary work and symbolic capital in radiology. *Social Studies of Science, 38*(35), 35–62. https://doi.org/10.1177/0306312707082021

Burri, R. V. (2013). Visual power in action: Digital images and the shaping of medical practices. *Science as Culture, 22*(3), 367–387. https://doi.org/10.1080/09505431.2013.768223

Care Quality Commission. (2018). *Radiology review: A national review of radiology reporting within the NHS in England*. The Care Quality Commission. https://www.cqc.org.uk/sites/default/files/20180718-radiology-reporting-review-report-final-for-web.pdf

Chew, C., O'Dwyer, P. J., & Sandilands, E. (2021). Radiology for medical students: Do we teach enough? A national study. *British Journal of Radiology, 94*(20201308), 1–6. https://doi.org/10.1259/bjr.20201308

Christiansen, J. M., Gerke, O., Karstoft, J., & Andersen, P. E. (2014). Poor interpretation of chest x-rays by junior doctors. *Danish Medical Journal, 61*(7), A4875. https://content.ugeskriftet.dk/sites/default/files/scientific_article_files/2018-11/a4875.pdf

Corr, P., Peh, W., Kune, W. S., Munro, L., Rae, W., Thoo, F. L., Chan, L. P., Goh, L. A., Hadley, L., Muttarak, M., & Quek, S. T. (2001). *Pattern recognition in diagnostic imaging* (No. WHO/DIL/01.2). World Health Organization. https://iris.who.int/bitstream/handle/10665/66843/9241546328_eng_LR_part1.pdf?sequence=25

Davies, K. (1994). The tensions between process time and clock time in carework. *Time & Society, 3*(3), 277–303. https://doi.org/10.1177/0961463X94003003002

Eisen, L. A., Berger, J. S., Hegde, A., & Schneider, R. F. (2006). Competency in chest radiography. A comparison of medical students, residents, and fellows. *Journal of General Internal Medicine, 21*, 460–465. https://doi.org/10.1111/j.1525-1497.2006.00427.x

Frankenberg, R. (1992). 'Your Time or Mine': Temporal contradictions of biomedical practice. In R. Frankenberg (Ed.), *Time, health and medicine* (pp. 1–30). Sage.

Gegenfurtner, A., Lehtinen, E., Helle, L., Nivala, M., Svedström, E., & Säljo, R. (2019). Learning to see like an expert: On the practices of professional vision and visual expertise. *International Journal of Educational Research, 98*, 280–291. https://doi.org/10.1016/j.ijer.2019.09.003

Gieryn, T. F. (1983). Boundary-work and the demarcation of science from non-science: Strains and interests in professional ideologies of scientists. *American Sociological Review, 48*(6), 781–795. https://doi.org/10.2307/2095325

Gieryn, T. F. (1999). *Cultural boundaries of science: Credibility on the line.* University of Chicago Press.

Goodwin, C. (1994). Professional vision. *American Anthropologist, 96*(3), 606–633. https://doi.org/10.1525/aa.1994.96.3.02a00100

Goodwin, C. (2000). Practices of seeing, visual analysis: An ethnomethodological approach. In T. van Leeuwen & C. Jewitt (Eds.), *Handbook of visual analysis* (pp. 157–182). Sage Publications.

Harrison, M., Rhodes, T., & Lancaster, K. (2023). Situating 'best practice': Making healthcare familiar and good enough in the face of unknowns.

SSM—Qualitative Research in Health, 4, 100343. https://doi.org/10.1016/j.ssmqr.2023.100343

Harrison, M., Smith, A. K. J., & Adams, S. (2024). Matters of time in health and illness. *Health Sociology Review, 33*(1), 1–9. https://doi.org/10.1080/14461242.2024.2319943

Heath, C., Hindmarsh, J., & Luff, P. (2010). *Video in qualitative research: Analysing social interaction in everyday life*. Sage. https://doi.org/10.4135/9781526435385

Higashi, R. T., Tillack, A. A., Steinman, M., Harper, M., & Johnston, C. B. (2012). Elder care as 'frustrating' and 'boring': Understanding the persistence of negative attitude toward older patients among physicians-in-training. *Journal of Aging Studies, 26*, 476–483. https://doi.org/10.1016/j.jaging.2012.06.007

Huang, B. K., Lubner, M., & Resnik, C. S. (2009). Balancing clinical service and education in the radiology residency. *Academic Radiology, 16*(9), 1161–1165. https://doi.org/10.1016/j.acra.2009.03.005

Ivarsson, J. (2017). Visual expertise as embodied practice. *Frontline Learning Research, 5*(3), 12–27. https://doi.org/10.14786/flr.v5i3.253

Joyce, K. A. (2008). *Magnetic appeal*. Cornell University Press. https://www.jstor.org/stable/10.7591/j.ctt7zfr6

Kok, E. M., Jarodzka, H., De Bruin, A. B. H., BinAmir, H. A. N., Robben, S. G. F., & Van Merriënboer, J. J. G. (2016). Systematic viewing in radiology: Seeing More, Missing less? *Advances in Health Science Education, 21*, 189–205. https://doi.org/10.1007/s10459-015-9624-y

Kwee, T. C., & Kwee, R. M. (2021). Workload of diagnostic radiologists in the foreseeable future based on recent scientific advances: Growth expectations and role of artificial intelligence. *Insights Imaging, 12*(88), 1–12. https://doi.org/10.1186/s13244-021-01031-4

Lewis, T. L., Sagmeister, M. L., Miller, G. W., Boissaud-Cooke, M. A., & Abrahams, P. H. (2016). Anatomy, radiology, and practical procedure education for foundation doctors in England: A National Observational Study. *Clinical Anatomy, 29*, 982–990. https://doi.org/10.1002/ca.22783

Lindberg, K., Walter, L., & Raviola, E. (2017). Performing boundary work: The emergence of a new practice in a hybrid operating room. *Social Science & Medicine, 182*, 81–88. https://doi.org/10.1016/j.socscimed.2017.04.021

Måseide, P. (2007). The role of signs and representations in the organization of medical work: X-rays in medical problem solving. In R. Iedema (Ed.), *The discourse of hospital communication* (pp. 201–221). Palgrave Macmillan. https://doi.org/10.1057/9780230595477_10

Maskell, G. (2022). Why does demand for medical imaging keep rising? *BMJ, 379*, o2614. https://doi.org/10.1136/bmj.o2614

Mehrotra, P., Bosemani, V., & Cox, J. (2009). Do radiologists still need to report chest x-rays? *Journal of Postgraduate Medicine, 85*, 339–341. https://doi.org/10.1136/pgmj.2007.066712

Moreira, T., May, C., Mason, J., & Eccles, M. (2006). A new method of analysis enabled a better understanding of clinical practice guideline development process. *Journal of Clinical Epidemiology, 59*, 1199–1206. https://doi.org/10.1016/j.jclinepi.2005.08.021

Mort, M., May, C. R., & Williams, T. (2003). Remote doctors and absent patients: Acting at a distance in telemedicine. *Science, Technology, & Human Values, 28*(2), 274–295. https://doi.org/10.1177/01622439022509

NHS England. (2018). *Never events policy and framework*. https://www.england.nhs.uk/wp-content/uploads/2020/11/Revised-Never-Events-policy-and-framework-FINAL.pdf

NHS England. (2020). *Diagnostics: Recovery and renewal. Report of the independent review of diagnostic services for NHS England, 2020.* https://www.england.nhs.uk/wp-content/uploads/2020/10/BM2025Pu-item-5-diagnostics-recovery-and-renewal.pdf

Price, R. C., & Le Masurier, S. B. (2007). Longitudinal changes in extended roles in radiography: A new perspective. *Radiography, 13*(1), 18–29. https://doi.org/10.1016/j.radi.2005.11.001

Reed, K., Kochetkova, I., & Molyneux-Hodgson, S. (2016). 'You're looking for different parts in a jigsaw': Foetal MRI (magnetic resonance imaging) as an emerging technology in professional practice. *Sociology of Health and Illness, 38*(5), 736–752. https://doi.org/10.1111/1467-9566.12398

Royal College of Radiologists (RCR). (2020, April). *Clinical radiology UK workforce census 2019 report.* https://www.rcr.ac.uk/media/2h1grjnz/clinical_radiology_census_report_2019.pdf

Samuels, E. (2017). Six ways of looking at crip time. *Disability Studies Quarterly, 37*(3). https://doi.org/10.18061/dsq.v37i3.5824

Sandell, K. (2010). Learning to produce, see and say the (ab)normal: Professional vision in ultrasound scanning during pregnancy. In E. Johnson & B. Berner (Eds.), *Technology and medical practice: Blood, guts, and machines* (pp. 29–50). Ashgate.

Satia, I., Bashagha, S., Bibi, A., Ahmed, R., Mellor, S., & Zaman, F. (2013). Assessing the accuracy and certainty in interpreting chest x-rays in the medical division. *Clinical Medicine, 13*, 349. https://doi.org/10.7861/clinmedicine.13-4-349

Saunders, B. (2008). *CT Suite: The work of diagnosis in the age of noninvasive cutting*. Duke University Press. https://doi.org/10.1215/9780822392002

Schuwirth, L. W., Verheggen, M. W., Van Vleuten, C. P. M., Boshuizen, H. P. A., & Dinant, G. J. (2001). Do short cases elicit different thinking processes than factual knowledge questions do? *Medical Education, 35*, 348–356. https://doi.org/10.1046/j.1365-2923.2001.00771.x

Snaith, B., Hardy, M., & Lewis, E. F. (2015). Radiographer reporting in the UK: A longitudinal analysis. *Radiography, 21*(2), 119–123. https://doi.org/10.1016/j.radi.2014.10.001

Swinburne, K. (1971). Pattern recognition for radiographers. *The Lancet, 297*(7699), 589–590. https://doi.org/10.1016/S0140-6736(71)91180-9

Twigg, J. (2000). Carework as a form of bodywork. *Ageing and Society, 20*(4), 389–411. https://doi.org/10.1017/S0144686X99007801

Van der Gijp, A., Schaaf, M. F., Schaaf, I. C., Huige, J. C. B. M., Ravesloot, C. J., Schaik, J. P. J., & ten Cate, T. J. (2014). Interpretation of radiological images: Towards a framework of knowledge and skills. *Advances in Health Sciences Education, 19*(4), 565–580. https://doi.org/10.1007/s10459-013-9488-y

Vavasseur, A., Muscari, F., Meyrignac, O., Nodot, M., Dedouit, F., Revel-Mouroz, P., Dercle, L., Rozenblum, L., Wanh, L., Maulat, C., Rousseau, H., Otal, P., Dercle, L., & Mokrane, F.-Z. (2020). Blended learning of radiology improves medical students' performance, satisfaction, and engagement. *Insights Imaging, 11*(61), 1–12. https://doi.org/10.1186/s13244-020-00865-8

White, J. (2022). *NHS never events on the increase.* https://www.pearsonlegal.co.uk/blog/news/nhs-never-events-on-the-increase/

Winter, P. (2019). *'Bodies of Seeing': A video ethnography of academic X-ray image interpretation in undergraduate radiology and radiography education* [Doctoral dissertation, University of Sheffield]. White Rose eTheses Online. https://etheses.whiterose.ac.uk/27904/

Winter, P. (2022). Lasers, screens and models: The material assemblages of learning pattern recognition in radiography education. In J. Nott & A. Haris (Eds.), *Making sense of medicine: Material culture and the reproduction of medical knowledge* (pp. 344–360). Intellect Books. https://doi.org/10.1386/9781789385779

Winter, P., & Linehan, M. (2014). Bernstein's theory of pedagogic discourse as a theoretical framework for educators studying student radiographers' interpretation of normality vs. abnormality. *Radiography, 20*(1), 58–64. https://doi.org/10.1016/j.radi.2013.09.004

8

Curative and Mad Futurities: The Temporal Implications of Peer Support Inclusion within Mental Health Systems

Aimee Sinclair

Peer support is commonly understood as the practice of drawing on shared experiences to support others through times of deep distress or adversity. As an organised political strategy within mental health contexts, peer support is often attributed to the consumer/survivor/ex-patient (C/S/X) movement, a social justice movement led by, and centring communities oppressed by psychiatric care. C/S/X activists have long highlighted the harms of psy-care, advocated for the right to self-determination, and upheld the value of experiential knowledge in conceptualising, and responding to, experiences labelled 'mental illness' (Epstein, 2013; O'Hagan, 2016). Peer support in this context is radical in its challenging of psy-logics that position individuals labelled mentally ill as lacking expertise and the ability to care for self and others. Instead, peer support asserts that through "the experience of being socially, politically, and

A. Sinclair (✉)
School of Allied Health, Curtin University, Bentley, WA, Australia
e-mail: aimee.sinclair@curtin.edu.au

K. Kenny et al. (eds.), *Timescapes of Health, Illness and Care*,
https://doi.org/10.1007/978-981-96-7055-0_8

materially shattered" individuals develop invaluable skills and expertise in navigating distress and care (Eales & Peers, 2021, p. 166).

Increasingly, peer support is drawn into contemporary mental health systems through the occupation of peer support work. On Whadjuk Noongar Boodja (known colonially as Perth, Western Australia), where much of the thinking, feeling, and writing for this chapter occurred, peers were first employed using government mental health funding in late 2000. Mahboub (2018) writes that, at the time, "… funders, and many mental health service providers … still held much confusion, fear and mistrust in the idea of having the 'mentally ill' provide services" (p. 208). Whilst often heralded for its potential to humanise mental healthcare, the inclusion of peer support within mental health systems, I argue, entangles such practices in psy-regimes of temporal surveillance and normalisation. Yet peer support relations; Mad time, Mad bodyminds,[1] and Mad care, also hold potential for disrupting normative (and often stifling) temporalities associated with progress, with productivity and with overcoming madness. I consider how peer support may foster temporal belonging; an acceptance and enactment of diverse timescapes including Mad futurities, where Mad existences, knowledges and practices are valued and enabled to flourish.

As part of a research project exploring the politics of peer inclusion, I met with fifteen individuals with experience facilitating peer support within the Australian mental health system (see Sinclair, Mahboub, et al., 2023; Sinclair & Mahboub, 2024 for further detail). Whilst the research focus was not explicitly on temporalities, temporal elements within these discussions affected me in unexpected ways. Some slowly niggled at me, prodding me to think differently. Others felt like a swift punch to the guts, unsettling my sense of worth. Throughout the writing of this piece, I continued to feel un-nerved, reflecting on normative temporal expectations and my 'failure' to meet them. It is these discussions and my responses to them, entangled with my own embodied responses to both Mad and psy-temporalities, that form the basis of this chapter. I am also indebted to many who have previously theorised on crip, Mad and care time. These works not only inform my analysis, they have also personally opened up

[1] I adopt the term *bodymind* from Price (2015) to signify the ways in which the physical and mental are often experienced as entangled rather than binary.

new ways of thinking and feeling about my own Mad existence/resistance. Leaning on Mad studies, I use and capitalise 'Mad' when referring to reclaimed politicised identities and practices that resist or subvert sanism (Diamond, 2013). Where I have used 'madness' as a descriptor for experiences often labelled as 'mental illness' or 'distress' it is not capitalised. In conceptualising madness, I draw on Bruce's (2021, p. 6) description of madness as both a dynamic social construction, and a lived reality. That is, madness as an "unruliness of will that resists and unsettles reigning regimes of the normal", as well as embodied experiences; feelings, perceptions, responses that may be painful or distressful, exhilarating or euphoric, the misfit of which often shatters us (Bruce, 2021, p. 6).

I anchor my writing for this chapter to a conversation between myself and peer support worker, Laura. Through our conversation, Laura's relationship with Eloise, someone she was employed to provide peer support to, became a central and prominent focus. My analysis, however, draws from across the discussions I had with all fifteen peer support workers from across multiple Australian states, as well as my own experiences. Thus, at points I share quotes from others and my own reflections alongside Laura's. I've chosen the conversation with Laura as a focal point for its rich demonstration of the productive forces that mandate recovery as a linear journey towards a curative future, with support contingent on individuals conforming to such temporal orientations. Simultaneously, the discussion between myself and Laura contains points of rupture; where peer support entanglements are affected by, and affect, diverse Mad temporalities and "queer crip Mad care" (Eales & Peers, 2021, p. 163). I share hesitantly, knowing the potential for Laura or Eloise to be the focus, reified as fixed in time and space, devoid of the shifting relations that produce these discourses, practices, and subjectivities. My intention is for Laura's reflections to provide a springboard for considering these relations, and how they produce particular ways of thinking, feeling, and becoming. I ask that you, as the reader, hold this in mind, knowing such forces affect all of us, albeit in different ways.

I begin with Laura's description of her relationship with Eloise, and a consideration of some of the material and discursive relations that shape their interactions, from their first "meet and greet" through to Laura's struggles with the "monotony" of long-term support. I then consider the effects of such relations, arguing that through psy-relations, peer support becomes part of mandating how time should be spent in the present to 'recover' in the future. I highlight how peer support practices, as configured within contemporary psy-regimes, enact some lives as worthy, others less so. I then return to Laura and Eloise, attending to the relations that intertwine with, and affect, their relationship in ways that produce possibilities beyond a curative future. Finally, I widen the story to consider the potential of peer support relations for producing temporal belonging, where diverse ways of being are supported and enabled to flourish.

Laura and Eloise

At the time of our discussion, Laura was employed by a peer-led organisation to provide community-based peer support funded by Australia's National Disability Insurance Scheme (NDIS). NDIS funding is allocated directly to the individual seeking support. This differentiates NDIS supports from other Australian community mental health supports, where organisations are block-funded under a commissioning model to provide collective welfare services. The aim of individualised funding is to maximise choice and control for 'participants' by enabling individuals to purchase services from a range of providers. Eloise, for example, having been approved for NDIS funding, would have potentially met with different providers to decide who she wanted to contract for supports. Laura was part of one of these initial meetings with Eloise, which Laura described as important to building rapport, "bringing up things that she mentioned she is into and things that she might know that I'm into". In this regard, some power sits with Eloise within the relationship with Laura, given she can choose whether Laura, and the organisation Laura is employed through, is contracted for services.

However in reality, multiple barriers exist that impact an individual's capacity to maximise choice within the NDIS (Wilson et al., 2022). One of these barriers, as highlighted through conversation with Laura, is that this 'choice' works both ways. That is, organisations providing NDIS services, such as the one Laura was employed by, have increased capacity to choose, or refuse, who they work with. Laura, for example, described how the organisation she works for "vet their clients" to ensure they are "recovery-focused". That is, they must "have the intention of wanting to be more well or wanting to change their life … or having some kind of goals". Laura described this as:

> an agreement between the individual and the peer support worker that recovery is on the cards… It's like we will aim for something … there's some agreement that we are on the same page that we all need to be more well.

This condition of peer support is not unusual; several peer support workers spoke of the ways in which organisations assessed and thus excluded those who were not "recovery-focused". Even within block-funded services, individuals were "transferred", excluded, or "exited" from supports if they were judged as uncommitted to a future-orientated temporality consisting of setting, progressing and measuring oneself against recovery goals. Several peer support workers, for example, spoke of gatekeeping practices, where clinicians (not the individual seeking support nor the peer worker), would determine who was "suitable" for peer support based on an assessment of whether the individual has "a very clear goal" and were not "too sick" to work towards this future self. As such, individuals, must perform a future-orientated, hopeful self to ensure they receive, and maintain, supports. Even those such as Eloise, who are NDIS-funded, and thus potentially have more control and choice, must demonstrate a commitment to "wanting to be more well" to maximise choice.

At their "initial meet and greet", Laura described how they discussed Eloise's goals. NDIS funding requires individuals to set and review goals towards "independence", with funds allocated to "help you overcome any disability-specific barriers that may be stopping you from pursuing your goals" (National Disability Insurance Scheme Agency, 2013, p. 1). Eloise, prior to meeting with Laura, would have engaged in NDIS interviews to set such goals, of which Laura is then expected to support Eloise to achieve.McWade (2015) describes such processes as "transforming the service user from chronic mental health patient into a neoliberal aspirational citizen" (p. 253). That is, through such processes, Eloise's desires are translated into "the language of aspirations, goals and hopes for the future" (p. 253). As such, Eloise and Laura's relationship was configured by the temporal register of future-orientation from the very start. Several peer support workers hinted at points where such translations faltered; where there was a mismatch between what the individual desired and what had been recorded as a 'suitable' goal towards independence. One peer support worker explained: "I think the NDIS made up, well not made up, but they set some goals with him but … when you talk to him, he doesn't aspire to do that kind of thing." Another stated: "I'll meet a client and find out that the goal that the community worker may have agreed upon with them is not the goal because they weren't able to say or … the worker didn't listen closely enough".

Laura's job, like most peer support workers, was to draw on her own experiences of recovery to orientate Eloise towards becoming McWade's 'neoliberal aspirational citizen' (2015). Enacted as role-models within Australian mental health policy, peer support workers are expected to symbolise triumph over madness, embodying hope for others that they too, through goal setting, self-management and personal responsibility may 'recover' (Sinclair, Fernandes, et al., 2023). Laura described this as giving someone "an idea of the fact that you can recover". Such work involves a delicate balance between relating to an individual's pain or distress, whilst also performing recovery as a linear journey in which madness only exists in the past; a performance that Laura described as putting on her "I've got my shit together façade". This need to *be* recovered, was a common feature of discussions with peer support workers. Entanglements of policies, job descriptions, storytelling training and organisational practices enact peer support workers as needing to be 'recovered' for an arbitrary period, enabling them to put their experiences "into perspective", shaping them into a linear temporal framing, where recovery consists of a past (being 'unwell', needing support), a present ('recovered', accepting personal responsibility, independent) and future ('recovered', but always with the risk of "relapse") (Costa et al., 2012). One peer worker described this as "a really neat coherent narrative of sickness to wellness".

Laura and Eloise's time together was governed by the goals set with/for Eloise, such that "the present is always in service to the future" (Robertson, 2015, p. 9). Within such logic, only certain ways of spending time are considered valuable, as one peer support worker described:

> What [the organisation] would consider working is having an appointment, generally going somewhere to do something, to achieve something. It might mean going to a Centrelink appointment or doctor's appointment or … maybe you might sit down and do some artwork with someone … a vision board.

Within this context, artwork is considered a worthwhile endeavour, but only if it is aspirational (such as a 'vision board'). Simply "passing time", such as "going out for coffee", is not considered "worthwhile" as "it's not goal-orientated, it's not something we can measure". Laura mentioned "healthy eating" as a goal of Eloise's, a common goal produced through an assemblage that attributes the poor physical health outcomes of people deemed mentally ill to "poor lifestyle habits" (Henderson & Fuller, 2011, p. 183). Laura is thus expected to work with Eloise to motivate her towards "healthy eating", supporting Eloise to independently meal plan, shop and cook.

Workers are expected to work alongside individuals to review progress against this futurity, using a variety of tools. Some of the tools mentioned by peer support workers involved clinical measures, such as the Kessler psychological distress scale (K10), aligning recovery with the reduction or absence of 'symptoms'. However, predominantly peers talked of outcome measurement tools such as 'recovery stars' (Onifade, 2011; Recovery in the Bin et al., 2019), 'wellness recovery action planning' (WRAP) (Scott & Wilson, 2011) and 'the collaborative recovery model and life journey enhancement' tools (CRM-JET) (Oades et al., 2005). Such tools require the setting of recovery goals aligned with 'overcoming' mental illness, planning the steps required to meet such goals, and measuring progress. WRAP, for example, involves identifying 'wellness tools', 'triggers' and 'early warning signs', documenting daily maintenance and crisis plans, undertaking self-surveillance and taking action in response to changes in one's mental health (Scott & Wilson, 2011). Through such tools, individuals develop a reflexive health habitus, enacted as personally responsible for 'overcoming' mental illness through discipline and future-planning (Scott & Wilson, 2011).

Laura had been supporting Eloise for almost a year when we talked and expressed disillusionment and frustration at the "chronicity" of Eloise's situation, suggesting Eloise's mental health had "gotten worse and worse and worse … and it's not showing signs of getting better". For Laura, there was a "heaviness" to the situation; it felt "monotonous … like a never-ending cycle of what she's going through". Laura partially attributed these affects to Eloise's seeming "refusal" to recover, describing Eloise as "recovery-focused when she first joined up with us" but not having "that intention anymore". Laura described Eloise as wanting "to live for reasons that are not recovery", describing that everything Eloise does "is pretty much the opposite of recovery":

> There's a lot of drugs involved, there's a lot of treating people badly and lying … all the things that we talked about that she wanted to do, she's kind of doing the opposite of them…
>
> There's like a lack on her part of actually wanting to, like she doesn't want us because she wants to recover, she wants us so she has someone to talk to and to not be lonely …. How do you keep supporting someone when it is almost like they don't want to recover?

The temporalities of Eloise's situation and her desires sit in tension with the normative temporalities of productivity produced through Laura's employment within the mental health system. Such temporalities suggest it is not enough for Laura just to 'be' with Eloise. For Laura and other peer support workers, there are goals to achieve, recovery stars to fill in, funding expectations to meet, clinical measures to improve upon. Peer support workers' time that they spend with someone is limited by funding allocations, programme requirements, organisational policies, inpatient bed availability, staffing numbers, recovery discourses; both in terms of total length of time they are funded to provide peer support, as well as temporally structured within the workday. For those not funded under NDIS, there is pressure to support someone to "become well" or at the very least adopt a future-orientated, aspirational temporality, before this time runs out. Support must be productive, future-orientated, efficient. When an individual fails to "progress" goals, this often impacts the worker. Laura, for example, was feeling less confident and "less inspired" in her role, questioning whether she was even doing peer support:

> It's definitely harder to feel confident in my role when I'm not seeing—even something that, when I first started working with her, was the smallest goal is now impossible.
>
> I'm not being a peer support worker when I'm with her. It feels like I'm just being like a sounding board .... I feel like a cross between a babysitter and a therapist rather than a peer support worker.

Talking and thinking through temporalities with peer support workers, I felt a stifling sense of limited time, of needing to progress faster, of time speeding up, and the misfit of bodyminds that refused, or were unable, to speed up or fit the normative temporalities required of them. In the next section, I draw on Mad theory to think about what these temporal affects mean for folks such as Laura, Eloise and myself, who don't always fit normative temporal expectations.

Psy-time, Curative Futures

Through Laura's descriptions, alongside those of other peer support workers, the temporal affects of the mental health system start to become visible. Goal setting and monitoring tools, practices of sharing one's lived experience of recovery, funding and programme requirements, psy-discourses regarding recovery, and organisational policies entangle to produce an aspirational, future-focused temporality, where "the present is governed ... as if the future is what matters most" (Adams et al., 2009, p. 248).

One way in which this future-orientated temporality could be read, is as a hopeful resistance to barren futures imposed by a "materially and symbolically violent psychiatric diagnostic temporality" (McWade, 2015, p. 248). That is, the ways in which psychiatric diagnoses construct madness as life-long and life-limiting, "extinguish[ing] a person's hopes and dreams for the future and replac[ing] them with a prospective lifetime of medicalisation and hospitalisation" (p. 248). Deegan (1998), a C/S/X activist, describes these lived experiences of temporal wasting:

> Our pasts deserted us and we could not return to who we had been. Our futures appeared to us to be barren, lifeless places in which no dream could be planted and grow into a reality. As for the present, it was a numbing succession of meaningless days and nights in a world which we had no place no use, and no reason to be (p. 13)

This sense, of "meaningless days and nights", of "barren futures", reflects an existence that sits outside of normative time, where one loses value; mad, unproductive and therefore useless within a colonial, capitalist system (McWade, 2015). I recall myself, a teenager on the brink of finishing high school, being told it was unlikely I would finish. I should take a year off, rest, certain futures erased. Many peer support workers had similar stories. Within the Australian mental health system, and in particular NDIS, the enactment of mental illness as a permanently disabling force lingers, with NDIS funding requiring a diagnosis of a 'permanent and significant disability'. Recovery, as cure, is seen as unlikely, and as such, a future devoid of meaning and citizenship. Within this context, peer support workers such as Laura, are predominantly understood as refuting such barren futures, embodying recovery by finding meaning and inclusion post-madness.

Whilst such may be read as a resistance to psy-logic, Laura's description of needing "to be more well", and the pressure she feels to be 'recovered', also hints at a curative imaginary; a compulsory orientation towards disability "that not only expects and assumes intervention but also cannot imagine or comprehend anything other than intervention" (Kafer, 2013, p. 27). That is, the only imaginable future for those deemed mad is one involving the "elimination of madness, or treatments to assimilate the disabled mind/body as much as possible" (p. 28). Recovery, within a curative imaginary, leaves little space for living well through or alongside madness. Rather, one must overcome madness as a mind condition through personal responsibility and effort (Clare, 2017). Through a curative imaginary, the barren futures that so many of us deemed mad have experienced are disrupted, but only for those willing to accept that such futures are barren because of our own mind deficits. Ironically, these 'recovered' futures are always unstable given that madness is enacted as internal, thus requiring the present to be constantly focused on monitoring and maintaining recovery into the future. Such futurities sit in stark contrast to the C/S/X movement's conceptualisation of recovery, as recovery from these oppressive effects of psy-logics (Voronka & Howell, 2012).

Tightly entangled with neoliberalist and capitalist notions of productivity, hope becomes an individualising imperative for service users to take personal responsibility, adopting self-care and self-management activities like 'vision boards' and 'healthy eating', to achieve independence in a timely fashion. Through contemporary mental health relations, peer support workers become "capacitated as inspirational, hopeful, and progressive success stories of neoliberal inclusion" (Fritsch, 2016, p. 12), enacting a "prudent, responsible subject who plans ahead, maintains control, and is constantly engaged in self-surveillance" (Scott & Wilson, 2011, p. 41). They do the right things, at the right pace, at the right times to be included. Only those who can perform wellness along normative temporal trajectories gain, and maintain, employment as peer workers. As such, peer support workers and 'service users' become divided along temporal lines, with the role of the peer support worker, as 'recovered', to orientate service users, as 'other', towards such normative temporal trajectories.

What becomes of those of us whose minds fail to 'recover' along these normative temporal trajectories? Whilst some may experience a period of extreme distress or madness, and then never again, many (myself included) will not. What happens to those who cannot fit neoliberal, aspirational futurities? Who do not have the capital or privilege to; who might not have access to affordable food, for example, or the time needed to "eat healthy"? Whose lack of material and social resources mean choice making is limited to daily needs, rather than future-planning (Wilson et al., 2022)? Or who refuse to, as an act of resistance? Those who desire peer support, not as a cure or support to overcome madness, but rather as someone to be with them in their present distress? Those who are working to survive deep, excruciating distress by remaining in the present, where acts of self-care and preservation (withdrawal, solitude, cutting, or in Eloise's situation, perhaps 'drugs' and 'treating people badly') may go unrecognised or be considered 'the opposite of recovery' by psy-logic? Those for whom the future feels hopeless or overwhelming, and thus staying in the present may be the safest place to be; when imperatives to futurity feel life-threatening? Within mental health systems, if 'progress' is not desired by the individual, or not made within a 'reasonable' timeframe, individuals are 'exited' from the service; deemed undeserving or unsuitable for peer support, or subject to increasing psychiatric intervention.

During my discussion with Laura, I was reminded of my own experience, as a 16-year-old inpatient of a psychiatric clinic, being threatened with involuntary treatment if I didn't put more effort into "becoming well". The inference then, as is produced now, was that I, and solely I, was responsible for becoming 'well', and in a timely manner. In the same way, Eloise is produced as refusing to recover due to lack of effort. It is not the wider assemblage that fails, it is Eloise herself. By failing to adopt a future-orientated, neoliberal subjectivity, Eloise becomes the "non-compliant subject", "unable or unwilling to take up a particular relationship to their mental health difficulties" (Blackman, 2007, p. 3; Rose, 2005). Reflecting such notions, one peer worker described individuals not wanting to "self-better" as "being a little bit stuck", lacking a "commitment to ongoing recovery". Another described their experience of only being invited to facilitate peer support when another worker called them up to say "so-and-so is really lazy; they need peer support". As mad subjects of curative regimes, our time is not ours to spend how we choose. Rather, if we desire care, support or inclusion, we must spend it in particular ways.

The effects of these temporal relations often deeply permeate our bodies and minds as mad subjects. Re-reading through the transcripts from my discussions with peer support workers, and reflecting on my own experiences, I felt exhausted. I was reminded of my ongoing desire for time-space to rest, not to be engaging in constant monitoring and self-betterment. No-one around me without a diagnosis of mental illness appeared to have such imperatives. A note I wrote to myself, scribbled on the side of a transcript, reads:

> The future governs my present. I haven't achieved enough today. I haven't been productive enough. It is rare for me to just sit and be. To survive. Is it not enough that I have survived? That I have stayed alive? That I have fed myself, stayed warm, been kind to others? What would it mean just to spend my day having a cup of tea with my neighbour? A day wasted.

Soldatic (2013) describes how, through socio-material practices of neoliberal capitalism, people's workless status becomes "inscribed not only on their bodies but also within, as they are forced to internalise social practices of morality that situate their bodies and minds as useless and waste" (p. 4). Those of us who 'waste time', who fail to meet normative temporalities of 'recovery', come to understand ourselves, as I often do, as a waste of time, "a waste of life" (McWade, 2015, p. 250). Far from relieving distress and valuing Mad lives, these temporalities and subjectivities intertwine to enact some lives less worthy. Alternative ways of understanding, and being in relation to, our experiences, our Mad selves, time, and others, are erased.

What I have argued thus far, is that through inclusion within the mental health system, peer support becomes part of the regime of curative futurity. Whilst such a futurity disrupts a narrative of 'barren futures' by challenging the permanency of mental illness, its dominance erases the futures of those who 'fail' to overcome madness. However, to stop here would tell only part of a complex story, leaving forces such as neoliberalism and psy-logic "looking like dead effects imposed on an innocent world" (Stewart, 2007, p. 1). Whilst the inclusion of peer support produces potential for mandating curative futurities, the discussions I shared with peer support workers revealed more complexity, highlighting potentials of becoming "an elsewhere and elsewhen of disability" (Fritsch, 2016, p. 11). Thus, I return now to Laura and Eloise to consider how their relations produce potential for maddening time, care and futures.

Returning to Laura and Eloise

Choosing to talk predominantly about her relationship with Eloise, Laura seemed pulled in several directions. The curative futurity produced through the mental health system, becomes visible in Laura's sharing because, rather than imbricating smoothly and going unnoticed, it was hitting up against other forces entangled with and through her relationship with Eloise. One of these forces was Laura's own temporal pacing. Laura described herself as having a naturally slow pace, unenthused by neoliberal aspirations, and unable to work with others who she described as "go-getters":

> I really struggle with working in the community when people want to go, go, go. When they want to; "'I've got to go to this appointment' … We're going to do this task…" And I can't work with clients like that, that are really busy and want to get a lot done in the shift time.
>
> I've never been a goals-focused peer support worker. I've always been very, "'Let's just do day-to-day"… I don't think that goals are as useful as the system makes them out to be or as important as the system makes them out to be.

Laura also described how "chill" Eloise is. They had similar temporal pacing and both valued living in the present:

> She goes at the same pace as I do … Eloise will literally be like, " 'What do you want to do today?': I want to sit in the lobby … because it's dark." And we will sit there for two hours … And half the time… we'll make one or two phone calls to book an appointment for her… And then some of the time we'll just be laughing about memes or something.
>
> The way that she moves in such a slowish pace and stuff kind of just works for me, like we're just chilling doing nothing. And in some ways, that's really good for me.

Laura also spoke to how her personal values, and what she understood as the values of peer support, contrasted with the idea that one should stop receiving support "because they've gone backwards":

> I don't think that that's ethical and that's not what I think peer support is either, is to drop someone because their mental health has gotten worse … my value as a peer support worker is that mental health has its ups and its down and that people deserve support just as much when they're in relapse or whatever than they do as when they're in recovery.
>
> I'm proud of myself for sticking to my values, which is that she deserves support even if she doesn't seem like she wants it or even if she's not acting like she even cares… as long as she's still saying, "'Yes, come on Saturday.'" Then I'm going to go on Saturday.

Another important element involved the support Laura received from her organisation. Laura described being able to partially work through "moments" of feeling "stuck" through peer supervision, and the support of her "bosses", who were experienced peer workers. She also described adopting a practice of "balancing out" her time with Eloise with supporting other individuals, such that her entire workload did not involve supporting Eloise.

A curative temporality sits in tension with these relations. Laura and Eloise's temporal rhythms, desires, peer support values, the relationship and affects between them, peer-led organisational culture and practices interact to produce ambivalence, and a thinking-feeling-becoming otherwise. Reflecting on how she doesn't feel like she is doing 'peer support' as enacted through mental health systems, Laura considered how instead her practice is increasingly becoming "like an act of service". She drops the expectation or desire for a particular outcome and instead the connection becomes important:

> I'm just doing my duty as a human to put something out there that has some kind of effect that can help another person…
>
> even when I'm struggling to have, like, hope for that person … I still am grateful for human connection.

Laura questioned the usefulness of peer support workers "inspiring" others to be future-focused, suggesting that sometimes when people are in deep distress, the present is more pressing:

> I think that sometimes when people are struggling with their mental health they don't even have the capacity … to feel inspired… And I think that often when people are struggling with their mental health … it comes from desperation, not inspiration.

Laura had also started thinking and feeling differently "about recovery even as a term", suggesting rather the importance of learning "to live with it [distress]", accepting her "own distress is like an everyday part of my life" and "just trying to… live as well as we can with what's going on". This last statement sits in tension with the positioning of Eloise, who is denied the contextual specificity of what is going on in her life that might shape how well she can live within that. Laura was, however, feeling less pressure to put her "'I've got my shit together'" façade on, challenging the idea of distress or madness needing to exist solely in the past. Rather, it felt safe for her to surface her vulnerability within the peer relationship:

> I didn't want them to know that if I had just been crying that day or whatever... building this relationship ... has also broken that down for me a bit. I've cried a little bit in front of her and I've gone to work and just been like, "'I'm really sorry if I don't seem present today'.

Mad Time, Mad Futurities

Crip time has been theorised as a refusal to embrace a non-disabled future, time outside of productivity, flexible time, departure from straight time; "whether straight time means a firm delineation between past/present/future or an expectation of linear development" (Kafer, 2013, p. 34; Sheppard, 2020). Building from such notions, the concept of Mad time encapsulates temporal orientations tied more specifically to embodied experiences of madness and mental healthcare. Cosantino's (2022) powerful poetic meditation on Mad trans time, describes Mad trans time as "a deeply embodied theorizing, challenging and actively disrupting normative temporalities, blurring the artificial boundaries between past, present, and future; knowing and (un)knowing; being and becoming" (p. 1). Rather than seeing Mad bodyminds as needing discipline, Mad time invites us to consider madness as a productive force for re-imagining time and futures otherwise. What if we were to consider Eloise's 'failure' to recover in the right way, at the right pace, for what it can tell us about normative temporalities and the possibilities of Mad time and Mad care?

We might consider, for example, how the "chronicity" of Eloise's situation, her desires to "just be", entangled with Laura's own desires and experiences of distress, prompts alternative relations to care. Baraitser and Brook (2021) talk about a temporality of endurance, of 'waiting with', underpinned by timelines of madness having "a life span, one that unfolds an eventual burning out over time" (p. 10). As they explain, the 'chronicity' of one's situation prompts a thinking-doing otherwise:

> [T]he task of care then becomes those pragmatic measures needed to keep a person alive... for that subsidence. Maintaining a position of hovering and adjusting over decades entails a series of concrete prosaic interventions: keeping vaccinations up to date, timely housing letters to prevent eviction, trying to enable adequate diet, parenting support. Care in this context is simply the tacit agreement to remain present, in touch, and to go on taking these vital, ordinary steps. The hope is that enough of a life remains intact at the 'end' for something to be reclaimed (p. 10).

There is something about Laura's descriptions of her time with Eloise that reflects this "hovering and adjusting". Laura and Eloise sit alongside one another, literally, in a dark lobby, laughing at memes, whilst also working together to book appointments: taking on these "vital ordinary steps". I think about my own experiences of distress and how in these moments I need a hovering, not cure, but rather someone to wait patiently with me, knowing this too shall pass. Puig de la Bellacasa (2017) describes how care both takes time, as well as "making time of an unexceptional particular kind", in which "nothing much appears to happen other than the ordinary maintenance work that enables the sustenance of liveable and lively worlds" (p. 206). Read within this context, everyday activities of "going to a Centrelink appointment or a doctor's appointment" don't have to be part of a curative futurity, but rather could be read as enacting Mad time—stretching out or producing time "in situations that otherwise felt to be stuck or 'chronic'" (Baraitser & Brook, 2021, p. 1). Such practices involve "a capacity to go on knowing about crisis without attempts at manic repair, through fostering forms of connection that consist of waiting with, enduring with, staying with, staying alongside, and through the continual offer of simply seeing someone again" (Baraitser & Brook, 2021, p. 11). As Laura states, "as long as she's still saying, '"Yes, come on Saturday'." Then I'm going to go on Saturday".

The vital importance of this connection, forged through making time with people, was threaded throughout conversations with peer support workers. It involved a witnessing of people's pain alongside an acceptance of where someone is, at that moment; "just being there". A sense of slowing down, or suspending time, to be with people, to listen. Reflecting this importance, when I asked Laura what she thought Eloise got from her, she responded: "I think I'm the person in her life who listens to her the best".

This slowing down or suspending time, being present and refusing to motivate someone towards a curative future—or a refusal *to be* motivated, enacts madness not as something to be fixed, but rather something to be in relation with. Blackman (2007, p. 19), describing the approach adopted within the peer-based hearing voices network, speaks to "making friends with", rather than overcoming, one's experiences of hearing voices. Such practices involve, as Laura hints at, a suspension of judgement and expectations; a letting go of needing someone to be different, to be "more well". In doing so, individuals deemed mad are no longer positioned as problems that need fixing, but rather as acceptable and valuable as they are, with their own desires and temporalities seen as valuable, too. Peer support becomes not about orientating someone towards the future, but rather being present and building connection, and negotiating time together. Laura's description of "laughing at memes" with Eloise reflects these moments of joy and connection spent in the present as articulated by several peer support workers. Together, they "carelessly meander" (perhaps care-fully meander), pushing back on a curative futurity, allowing time to feel, to grieve, to do nothing but survive (Barlott & Setchell, 2022, p. 102).

Such slowed temporal orientations resonate with those produced through ally assemblages as documented by Barlott and Setchell (2022). Such assemblages "carelessly meander", disregarding efficiency, structure, and the rapid pace usual to mental health relations (p. 102). Freely given, these relationships were not contained within a set number of hours, nor do they have an end-point. There are no performance indicators, no temporal reporting measures. Within such relations, the connection itself forms the reason for connecting, with no goals set for the relationship other than the relationship itself. A timeless connection, perhaps, outside of normative temporal pressures.

Such capacities are formed through relations, not in or by the autonomous subject. The relations that Barlott and Setchell (2022) describe 'endure' over time because they sit outside of mental health policies, goal-setting technologies, reporting measures. Similarly, peer support workers described being able to give time, spend time, stretch time, more freely *outside* of the mental health system. Laura described her and Eloise's relationship as being able to 'endure' because of their matched temporal pacings, care for one another, peer values, training, and supervision. Attending to these entangled relations allows us to consider what produces potential to madden time and care.

When peer support workers talked of making or suspending time, there was sometimes discussion of the future with those they supported. Whilst this could be partly attributed to a curative imaginary, I sensed something else emerging; an opening of possibilities, of becoming. Such practices involved an imagining of a different relationship to self and madness than that prescribed by normative psy-logics, as well as an imagining of alternative futures to that underpinned by a curative imaginary. They involved a refusal to 'stop' time until one had been cured or overcome madness, to resist the messaging, as one peer support worker described, of having to "disinvite myself from citizenship for a period of time and do the sanctioned tasks that are required of me to get to this place so that I am a citizen again". Rather, space was created for "dreaming" (Cosantino, 2022, p. 4); opening up futures inclusive of madness.

In doing so, we may recognise the fluctuating, ebbing and flowing, often unpredictable temporalities of madness, that, through its entanglement with wider relations, may enable us to do some things, in some moments, and not in others. In some ways, Laura's comments about relapse/recovery highlight normative forces, producing recovery as a linear journey, albeit with bumps, towards 'wellness'. However also in her comments can be read a recognition of this ebbing and flowing: 'its ups and downs', as our bodyminds intra-act with the world around us. Mad bodyminds may, at various times, slow time down, or panic in a way such that linear time unravels, "making time seem simultaneously to speed up and slam shut, leaving one behind" (Kafer, 2013, p. 38). It sometimes folds time back on to itself, where the past/present/future become blurred. Rather than 'cure' this unpredictability, ebbing and flowing, we might learn to work with it, perhaps even embrace it. For peer support workers, this ebbing and flowing is often what enables a connection with others, knowing what it is like to "misfit" normative time, to be 'out of time' (Garland-Thomson, 2011). An embodied knowing, for example, of what it means to struggle to work in a system that demands uniformity in pace and scheduling, or struggling to attend appointments because they are scheduled when bodyminds may refuse to move, or the rage/grief/fear of not qualifying for certain income supports because of the sometimes-intermittent nature of madness. These embodied experiences of madness hold potential for developing strategies and resources for managing such temporal misfitting; knowledges, where supported, that can be used to resist and re-arrange temporalities, environments, and practices, enabling an accommodation, and valuing of, diverse and fluid temporal needs and desires.

Conclusion

Within formal mental health systems, individuals are diagnosed according to time, must attend appointments within certain timeframes, articulate their 'illness' story according to a particular timeline, are allocated time-delimited funding for support of particular duration, and expected to recover within certain timeframes. Mad bodyminds rarely fit within these normative temporal demands. We take 'too much time' or 'not enough time', we fail to be 'on time'. We are considered "too slow, too fast, too uncontrolled, too reliant, too different, too much and also not enough" (Sheppard, 2020, p. 39). Consequently, we are subject to disciplinary practices through the mental health system. Drawing on the experiences of Laura and Eloise, entangled with my own experiences and that of other peer support workers, I have argued that through inclusion, peer support becomes entangled in this temporal disciplining, specifying how time should be spent, enacting curative futurities and deeming certain existences a 'waste of time'. Yet simultaneously, the Laura–Eloise assemblage demonstrates the productive potential of peer support relations; entanglements of Mad bodyminds, desires and care that may produce a thinking-feeling-becoming other than that aligning exclusively with normative temporalities and a curative futurity. Such relations have potential to produce Mad futurities; in which Mad existences and practices may be valued in the present rather than banished to the past. Attending to this complexity, where the inclusion of peer support workers both enables and constrains such futures, is important if we are to continue moving towards more liveable worlds for individuals deemed mad, and for those who choose to embrace their madness.

Acknowledgements The thinking I share here is only possible because of those who have gone before me, and who shared and theorised alongside me as part of this research. This includes (but is not limited to) my supervisory team: Dr Christina Fernandes, Dr Sue Gillieatt, Lyn Mahboub, and the folks with experience as peer support workers who so generously shared their thinking, feeling and experiences through discussions with me.

Competing Interests This research was in part supported by an Australian Government Research Training Program (RTP) Scholarship. The author has no conflict of interest to declare that is relevant to the content of the chapter.

References

Adams, V., Murphy, M., & Clarke, A. E. (2009). Anticipation: Technoscience, life, affect, temporality. *Subjectivity, 28*(1), 246–265. https://doi.org/10.1057/sub.2009.18

Baraitser, L., & Brook, W. (2021). Watchful waiting: Temporalities of crisis and care in the UK National Health Service. In L. Baraitser & W. Brook (Eds.), *Vulnerability and the politics of care* (pp. 230–247). British Academy. https://doi.org/10.5871/bacad/9780197266830.003.0015

Barlott, T., & Setchell, J. (2022). *Edge entanglements with mental health allyship, research, and practice: A postqualitative cartography* (1st ed.). Routledge. https://doi.org/10.4324/9781003286486

Blackman, L. (2007). Psychiatric culture and bodies of resistance. *Body & Society, 13*(2), 1–23. https://doi.org/10.1177/1357034X07077770

Bruce, L. M. J. (2021). *How to go mad without losing your mind: Madness and Black radical creativity*. Duke University Press.

Clare, E. (2017). *Brilliant imperfection: Grappling with cure*. Duke University Press.

Cosantino, J. (2022). 'Now don't say we didn't warn you': A poetic meditation on the (im)possibilities of Mad trans time. *International Mad Studies Journal, 1*(1), 1–14. https://doi.org/10.58544/imsj.v1i1.5240

Costa, L., Voronka, J., Landry, D., Reid, J., McFarlane, B., Reville, D., & Church, K. (2012). Recovering our stories: A small act of resistance. *Studies in Social Justice, 6*(1), 85–101.

Deegan, P. (1998). Recovery: The lived experience of rehabilitation. *Psychosocial Rehabilitation Journal, 11*(4), 11–19.

Diamond, S. (2013). What makes us a community? Reflections on building solidarity in anti-sanist praxis. In B. A. LeFrançois, R. Menzies, & G. Reaume (Eds.), *Mad matters: A critical reader in Canadian mad studies* (pp. 1–22). Canadian Scholars' Press.

Eales, L., & Peers, D. (2021). Care haunts, hurts, heals: The promiscuous poetics of queer crip Mad care. *Journal of Lesbian Studies, 25*(3), 163–181. https://doi.org/10.1080/10894160.2020.1778849

Epstein, M. (2013). *The consumer movement in Australia: A memoir of an old campaigner*. https://www.ourcommunity.com.au/files/OCP/HistoryOfConsumerMovement.pdf

Fritsch, K. (2016). Cripping neoliberal futurity: Marking the elsewhere and elsewhen of desiring otherwise. *Feral Feminisms, 5*, 11–26.

Garland-Thomson, R. (2011). Misfits: A feminist materialist disability concept. *Hypatia, 26*(3), 591–609. https://doi.org/10.1111/j.1527-2001.2011.01206.x

Henderson, J., & Fuller, J. (2011). 'Problematising' Australian policy representations in responses to the physical health of people with mental health disorders. *Australian Journal of Social Issues, 46*(2), 183–203. https://doi.org/10.1002/j.1839-4655.2011.tb00213.x

Kafer, A. (2013). *Feminist, queer, crip*. Indiana University Press.

Mahboub, L. (2018). The world according to me: A Western Australian peer work journey, some history, reflections and thoughts. In J. Meagher, F. Jackson, A. Stratford, E. Jayakody, & T. Fong (Eds.), *Peer work in Australia: A new future for mental health* (pp. 202–215). RichmondPRA and Mind Australia.

McWade, B. (2015). Temporalities of mental health recovery. *Subjectivity, 8*(3), 243–260. https://doi.org/10.1057/sub.2015.8

National Disability Insurance Scheme Agency. (2013). *Setting goals*. https://www.ndis.gov.au/participants/creating-your-plan/setting-goals

O'Hagan, M. (2016). Responses to a legacy of harm. In J. Russo & A. Sweeney (Eds.), *Searching for a rose garden: Challenging psychiatry, fostering mad studies* (pp. 9–13). PCCS Books.

Oades, L., Deane, F., Crowe, T., Lambert, W. G., Kavanagh, D., & Lloyd, C. (2005). Collaborative recovery: An integrative model for working with individuals who experience chronic and recurring mental illness. *Australasian Psychiatry, 13*(3), 279–284. https://doi.org/10.1111/j.1440-1665.2005.02202.x

Onifade, Y. (2011). The mental health recovery star. *Mental Health and Social Inclusion, 15*(2), 78–87. https://doi.org/10.1108/20428301111140921

Price, M. (2015). The bodymind problem and the possibilities of pain. *Hypatia, 30*(1), 268–284.

Puig de la Bellacasa, M. (2017). Soil times: The pace of ecological care. In *Matters of care: Speculative ethics in more than human worlds*. University of Minnesota Press.

Recovery in the Bin, Burgess, R., & Thomas, E. (2019, September). *Neorecovery: A survivor led conceptualisation and critique [Transcript]*. 25th International Mental Health Nursing Research Conference, The Royal College of Nursing, London, UK.

Robertson, R. (2015). Out of Time: Maternal time and disability. *Studies in the Maternal, 7*(1). https://doi.org/10.16995/sim.194

Rose, N. (2005). In search of certainty: Risk management in a biological age. *Journal of Public Mental Health, 4*(3), 14–22. https://doi.org/10.1108/17465729200500020

Scott, A., & Wilson, L. (2011). Valued identities and deficit identities: Wellness Recovery Action Planning and self-management in mental health: Valued identities and deficit identities. *Nursing Inquiry, 18*(1), 40–49. https://doi.org/10.1111/j.1440-1800.2011.00529.x

Sheppard, E. (2020). Performing normal but becoming crip: Living with chronic pain. *Scandinavian Journal of Disability Research, 22*(1), 39–47. https://doi.org/10.16993/sjdr.619

Sinclair, A., Fernandes, C., Gillieatt, S., & Mahboub, L. (2023). Peer work in Australian mental health policy: What 'problems' are we solving and to what effect(s)? *Disability & Society, 1–26*. https://doi.org/10.1080/09687599.2022.2160926

Sinclair, A., & Mahboub, L. (2024). Maddening post-qualitative inquiry: An exercise in collective (Mad) theorising. *Qualitative Health Research*, 10497323241231896. https://doi.org/10.1177/10497323241231896

Sinclair, A., Mahboub, L., Gillieatt, S., & Fernandes, C. (2023). 'You just treat me like a human being': Using Lived Experience to (re)imagine boundary practices in mental health settings. *The British Journal of Social Work, 53*(3), 1408–1425. https://doi.org/10.1093/bjsw/bcad044

Soldatic, K. (2013). Appointment time: Disability and neoliberal workfare temporalities. *Critical Sociology, 39*(3), 405–419. https://doi.org/10.1177/0896920511430168

Stewart, K. (2007). *Ordinary affects*. Duke University Press.

Voronka, J., & Howell, A. (2012). Introduction: The politics of resiliance and recovery in mental health care. *Studies in Social Justice, 6*(1), 1–7.
Wilson, E., Campain, R., Pollock, S., Brophy, L., & Stratford, A. (2022). Exploring the personal, programmatic and market barriers to choice in the NDIS for people with psychosocial disability. *Australian Journal of Social Issues, 57*(1), 164–184. https://doi.org/10.1002/ajs4.154

Part III

Challenging Chrononormativities

9

Resting, Waiting and Other Forms of Resistance: The Chronopolitics of Chronic Illness

Mara Pieri

Lia is sitting on a bench in a public park in the city of Porto. Peacocks and birds stroll around freely, seagulls fly over us, kids play with rocks close to a fountain, and a group of young people sit on the grass, smoking and laughing. It is a beautiful afternoon in the Portuguese springtime and I have just asked Lia whether she thinks her illness has taught her something she would not have known before. She pauses, looks over the horizon, then smiles and says: "It donated me a different notion of time. I think illness created a stronger urgency, in life, to pursue living the life I truly want, you know?". She smiles, pauses, and continues: "It is basically this. Everything is so ephemerous,

> I do need to give importance to what is really important. And for me it is love, human relationships".[1]

[1] The interview is part of a study conducted on the experiences of LGBTQ+ people with chronic illness between 2017 and 2021 (Pieri, 2023). The original Portuguese text has been translated into English by the author.

M. Pieri (✉)
Centre for Social Studies, University of Coimbra, Coimbra, Portugal
e-mail: marapieri@ces.uc.pt

K. Kenny et al. (eds.), *Timescapes of Health, Illness and Care*,
https://doi.org/10.1007/978-981-96-7055-0_9

Lia's words offer a glimpse of the importance of time in the experience of illness: as she underlines, living with a chronic illness changes the perception of one's present and future. In her case, being ill offered a new urgency in pursuing happiness, as if time resulted both accelerated and more intense. Experiencing illness as a matter of time is not uncommon and there are various ways in which time defines the journey of a chronically ill person like Lia. Chronic illness may surge as an unexpected disruption of the pace of normalcy (Bury, 1997; Larsson & Grassman, 2012); or it may intervene to accelerate pre-existing processes (Pieri, 2023). As Kafer underlines, "familiar categories of illness and disability—congenital and acquired, diagnosis and prognosis, remission and relapse, temporarily able-bodied and 'illness, age, or accident'—are temporal; they are orientations in and to time" (2013, p. 26).

In this chapter, I aim to explore the bond between time and illness in the experience of chronicity. Following the hint suggested by Lia, I am interested in discussing to what extent chronicity creates a different notion of time and how this process happens. In particular, I will discuss how the chronicity of illness shapes how we experience time in the long run, how we reflect on the past and imagine the future, and how we reconcile the impermanence of the everyday with long-term horizons. In the first section, I analyse the concept of "chrononormativity" (Freeman, 2011) as a theoretical framework that looks at time as both regulating and producing normalcy. The contributions of crip studies (Kafer, 2013; Samuels, 2017; Sheppard, 2020) are particularly important in providing shape and context to this analysis. In the second section, I reflect on the temporal dimensions of chronic illness, focusing on three aspects: chronicity, rest, and waiting. Finally, I present concluding reflections on how the temporal experience of chronic illness suggests possible ways out of compulsory normalcy and what alliances—both political and imagined—can emerge based on a shared experience of time.

Before moving into the theoretical exploration of time and chronic illness, it is necessary to interrupt the linear progression of this chapter to introduce a parenthetical pause—a diversion similar to Lia's deep breath and reflective gaze before responding to my question. This interruption relates both to the methodology and the content of this chapter: a pause of recognition, reflection, and positioning. As a chronically ill academic,

I continuously reflect upon and make choices regarding the clashes between time and illness. Every day I grapple with the pressures to meet deadlines, deliver presentations, write, and seize opportunities, while simultaneously adhering to the slower pace dictated by my body—a rhythm that is, unsurprisingly, misaligned with the fast-paced demands of academia. In the form you read it now, this chapter shows a linear reflection. However, the visible text is underpinned by countless hours spent mustering the energy to write a few sentences, numerous interruptions for rest, and repeated requests to extend deadlines and accommodate delayed submissions. By making these hidden processes visible, I acknowledge that academic time is structured around ableist assumptions (Rodgers et al., 2023; Samuels & Freeman, 2021) and argue that dismantling them requires a critical examination of how we contribute to its perpetuation. In her insightful analysis of crip spacetime in academia, Price asserts that time can be both harmful and healing, noting that "academic time is composed not only of a fast-moving, bell-ringing present, but also of histories of inequality and abuse, as well as uncertain futures" (2024, p. 79). As I write, I simultaneously experience the temporal disruptions imposed by chronic illness and struggle to conform to academia's expected timelines. This meta-process deeply informs this chapter and I deem important that readers are aware of it. Inevitably, I carefully considered whether to disclose my chronic illness in this work—as I have done in other publications (see Pieri, 2023). There are costs associated with both coming out and remaining closeted about one's illness, just as coming out also as queer taught me. Nevertheless, a serious discussion of time in the context of health and illness, particularly within an academic framework, needs transparency about the standpoint from which I speak. My position is one of continual temporal struggle. This parenthetical reflection sets the stage for the subsequent sections, emphasising that this discussion pertains to lived, rather than abstract, experiences of time.

The Power of Time: Chrononormativity

One of my favourite books has always been Alice's Adventures in Wonderland by Lewis Carroll (1865). From a child's perspective, it is the story of a curious girl, Alice, who wanders in different spaces and times, meeting all sorts of weird characters. However, through an adult's perspective, the book offers surprising layers of interpretation about social norms, language, people and, most of all, time. In one of the most interesting episodes, Alice dialogues with a character called Mad Hatter:

> "I dare say you never even spoke to Time!"
> "Perhaps not," Alice cautiously replied; "But I know I have to beat time when I listen to music." "Ah! That accounts for it" said the Hatter. "He won't stand a beating. Now, if only you kept on good terms with him, he'd do almost anything you like with the clock." (Carroll, 1865)

This exchange reveals many insights: the elusive nature of time, its omnipresence in our daily lives as a universal constant, the challenge of maintaining a harmonious relationship with it, and the illusion that we can control it according to our will. It is also a fruitful starting point to discuss how we can interpret the experience of time through chronic illness. This starting point is the recognition that time is the product of social definitions: it does not exist in itself, it is what we make of it (Adam, 1995). As such, time is also a powerful regulatory force that governs societies and how we live. Freeman coins the term "chrononormativity" to highlight this specific meaning of time:

> Chrononormativity is a mode of implantation, a technique by which institutional forces come to seem like somatic facts. Schedules, calendars, time zones, and even wristwatches inculcate what the sociologist Evitar Zerubavel calls "hidden rhythms," forms of temporal experience that seem natural to those whom they privilege. (2011, p. 3)

The internalisation of normative timelines and rhythms is thus crucial to guarantee access to social legibility, power, and privileges. The concept of chrononormativity shows that time is the result of social, cultural, and economic constructions that are flexible, changeable, and exposed to instability. The politics of distribution, definition, and delimitation of time are based on the same axes of oppression that regulate social life, like heteronormativity, racism, ableism, and ageism. As I have argued elsewhere (Pieri, 2023), chrononormativity reproduces all the forms of oppression around which societies are structured. In particular, it is bound to normalised notions of able-bodiedness and health. In a specular way to the compulsory heterosexuality identified as a marker of oppression by Adrienne Rich (1980), crip studies analyse how the idea of a compulsory able-bodiedness (McRuer, 2006) is a crucial structuring axis of social organisation. As such, able-bodiedness is a form of normativity that assumes that all body-minds are inherently similar and functioning in equal ways and that sanctions deviations from this supposed normality. In this sense, not only physical disabilities but also chronic illness, mental health issues, neurodivergence and other health conditions fall outside the normativity of able-bodiedness, hence producing a deviation from the norm (Kafer, 2013; Sheppard, 2020). In the past two decades, crip has comes to identify a vast array of experiences, conditions, political stances, and practices. For the purpose of this chapter, though, I follow the suggestion of Margaret Price, according to whom:

> Crip theory works with identity but is primarily methodological rather than identitarian. In other words, its aim is not to shore up rights or representation of bodyminds labeled disabled but, rather, to disrupt ideas that are mediated through bodyminds, including normalcy, fitness, health, and "ability" itself. (2024, p. 11)

In the disruption of ideas around what is normal, what is health, what is ability, crip as a methodology offers precious instruments to elaborate reflections on time as a crucial axis through which these ideas as reproduced. Hence, chrononormativity is not only a matter of time, it is also a matter of crip time: a concept that takes us into the core of how able-bodiedness and health are constructed around specific understanding of rhythms and timing.

The Expectations about Generativity

In the study I conducted with LGBTQ+ people with chronic illness (Pieri, 2023), some recurrent topics emerged with insistence. They all had to do with some form of societal expectation towards individuals to be productive of something for the general good: whether they spoke about children, money, success or health, people would refer to an underlying, all-encompassing expectation towards "being productive". Amongst the many domains in which time intervenes as a normative force, I consider interesting to focus on three in particular that are significant for they represent nuances of this underlying expectation of generativity: reproduction, productivity, and happiness.

The first is the regulation of reproduction as an issue of time. Reproduction holds a pivotal role in societal organisation: it allows the continuation of linear genealogies, the link between past, present, and future. Societies shape their future by ensuring that reproduction happens in regulated ways, for example through the legislation on abortion, adoption, or access to medically assisted reproduction (Roseneil et al., 2020). However, as Halberstam notes, "reproductive time and family time are, above all, heteronormative time/space constructs" (Halberstam, 2005, p. 10). The heterosexual and gender-normative couple model moulds the expectation of reproduction. The struggles for LGBTQ+ parenting and adoption, the shifting regulation of abortion rights, and the difficulties women encounter in having their self-determination recognised continue to highlight how reproduction is not only a matter of who gets to reproduce but also when and how. In this context, Roseneil et al. (2020) introduces the concept of "repronormativity", which refers to the societal expectation that reproduction is central to social life and serves as a key criterion for full citizenship. Consequently, individuals are deemed "good citizens" if they reproduce within culturally accepted timelines, which align with the conventional markers of adulthood. In many societies, teenage pregnancy is stigmatised, while pregnancy beyond a certain age is often viewed as inappropriate or even obscene. Public health policies frequently reflect these norms, as they may discourage or restrict reproductive access for women with disabilities and chronic illnesses, effectively making reproduction a privilege for some and an impossibility for others (Hassan et al., 2023). In several countries, practices such as selective abortion of fetuses with disabilities or the forced sterilisation of disabled women remain accepted (Kafer, 2013).

The underlying motivation behind many reproductive policies is the preservation of an able-bodied, heterosexual, and gender-normative lineage. Within this framework, crip time represents a divergence from straight time, understood as either a rigid separation of past/present/future or the expectation of linear progression from dependent childhood to independent, reproductive adulthood (ibid., p. 34). The experience of chronic illness disrupts this linear trajectory, introducing a non-linear and complex timeline for reproduction. It challenges naturalised boundaries such as menopause and menstruation and often turns the reproductive process fraught and difficult. Moreover, individuals with chronic illnesses face societal suspicion and shame for disrupting the expected able-bodied lineage, especially when there is a risk of passing on an illness to their children (Hassan et al., 2023). They also endure unspoken doubts about their capacity to fulfil parental roles.

A second relevant domain of chrononormative dynamics is productivity: emerged during early capitalism and enhanced in neoliberal economies, the push to productivity is at the core of what we nowadays may consider "time well spent". The idea that for every minute spent working something needs to be produced was a crucial gear in the consecration of the human exploitation of resources (Adam, 1995). The notions of disability and illness are also intrinsically connected to a long-standing tradition of thinking about health and able-bodiedness as the capacity to work and, hence, to produce (Shildrick, 2005; Tremain, 2015). Contemporary neoliberalism enforces time well beyond the mere division of labour and regulates every part of the day and every phase of life through a relation to productive work. This division of time is, again, founded on racism, sexism, and ableism. For example, queer subcultures that celebrate fun through night parties are deemed morally deviant not only because of their gender and orientation but also because they commit to leisure in times in which proper workers are sleeping: by subverting clock times, they threaten the social order (Halberstam, 2005). People with disability or chronic illnesses face enormous difficulties in entering the job market because workplaces are centred around standard rhythms and are not flexible in accommodating other timescapes (Sheppard, 2020). The times of chronic illness are largely incompatible with the productivity expected in neoliberal rhythms: as I will argue later, they prefigure chronic illness as an experience out-of-time.

A third interesting aspect of chrononormativity is the expectation to have a good life, or what is generally included in the broad notion of "happiness". Whilst the orientation to a state of well-being is inscribed in what makes us human, in the past two decades a new narrative has been gradually growing: supported by an exploding industry around wellness and by the performative demands of social media, the idea of self-improvement and individual success has progressively transformed the idea of "happiness" (Petersen, 2015). Having a purpose and working to express one's potential fully has become a sort of moral duty (Cederström & Spicer, 2015): the pressure to individually achieve the best possible life constitutes a mantra where all responsibilities weigh on the individual and their capacity to be the best version of themselves. This sort of compulsory happiness is generally based on a performative tautology: "by finding happiness in certain places, it generates those places as being good, as being what should be promoted as good" (Ahmed, 2010, p. 6). What Cederström and Spicer call "the duty to be happy" (2015) insists that happiness lies in symbolic places where we are expected to look for it: for example, coupledom, parenting, health, and success in our professional career. This way, happiness becomes a question of following rather than finding (Ahmed, 2010). Achieving (or following) happiness means being well-oriented in time towards the directions considered inherently right and it depends on the ability to stay in line with this orientation without deviations. The happiness duty is also declined towards the expectation to take care of our wellness and actively be healthy. A good citizen, a good person, commits to be positive, to self-improve, and to take care of their well-being. The pressure over taking care of our bodies and minds is ever-present to the point of becoming a "wellness syndrome" (Cederström & Spicer, 2015): a moral demand to be constantly focused on our wellness in every aspect of our lives. As Petersen also points out, "increasingly, citizens are expected to assume a 'positive outlook', to remain 'hopeful', and to play an active role in the project of advancing and optimising health" (2015, p. 4). The remarkable growth of the industry connected to wellness, fitness, and beauty, together with the expansion of services linked to mindfulness, meditation, and therapy confirm this tendency. Implicitly and explicitly, the imperative of healthism depreciates the non-conforming, such as disabled, overweight, ill or depressed people, and condemns unhealthy practices, like smoking, drinking alcohol, or eating irresponsibly. Moreover, it obscures the intersections of class, gender, race, and able-bodiedness that influence the way individuals have access to a good life (Kim & Schalk, 2021): the narrative of the individuals as creators of their destiny eclipses the social causes of oppression and blames the single for their shortcomings. Therefore, everyone as an individual is expected to make any effort possible to feel better, live better, and be better, despite the socio-economic oppression they face. It is a regime of bio-morality and bio-citizenship, a modern disciplinary power (Tremain, 2015). The profound consequences of this logic are the de-politicisation of choices and the individualisation of responsibility. Within this regime, disability becomes an obstacle to be overcome through the right attitude, an extraordinary love for life, or an acceptable performance of gender and sexuality. Similarly, chronic illness represents the result of unhealthy choices that can be either prevented through responsible choices or overcome with a positive attitude (Pieri, 2023).

As discussed so far, chrononormativity is thus a powerful normalising force that indicates normative ways to reproduce, produce, and be happy. These spheres are not separated one from the other: on the contrary, the imperative of health and success is shaped by specific expectation on productivity; or, the boundaries of acceptable reproduction are defined by ideals of health and able-bodiedness. Chrononormativity is pervasive and ubiquitous in establishing a correct form of living time. On the contrary, chronic illness works through bumpy trajectories and unpredictable rhythms (Sheppard, 2020). In this sense, we cannot analyse the time(s) of chronic illness without confronting the pressures of chrononormativity; however, as I will explore in the next section, we may also find examples of resistance and subversion to normativity in this apparent clash of rhythms.

The Time(s) Of Chronic Illness

Literature on critical disability studies and, in particular, crip studies, offer a wide range of perspectives that can help us develop this perspective further. As Sheppard notes,

> There are as many forms of crip time as there are crip bodyminds, crip ways of being in the world and being in/through time. Crip time, therefore, is defined […] as a failure to be on time and in straight-able time, albeit in a myriad of possible ways; rather than being defined by what it is, crip time is defined by being in opposition to straight-able time. (2020, p. 40)

In Sheppard's work, crip time works counter-normatively to able-bodied time: the "myriad of possible ways" to navigate time is both a form of failure to comply with normative rhythms and a possibility to foresee alternatives to them. From a crip perspective, we could argue that chronic illness is a litmus test that unveils the normativity inherent to the time we live in: everytime chronically ill people need a break or claim their right to slow down, they are denouncing that the time they happen to be forced into is not adequate to their functioning and is inherently ableist (Price, 2024).

Crip time creates a shift in the perspective for how illness and disability order the body: it decentres notions of the 'normal' body and instead presents illness and disability as temporally governed ways of being (Kafer, 2013). More than explaining how illness is, the temporal categories we use to define it say much about how we think health should be: they speak more about able-bodiedness than illness.

A similar perspective on the temporality of illness and disability is offered by feminist disability studies scholar, Rosemarie Garland-Tomson (1997), who describes ageing as a gradually disabling process and argues that for anyone who lives long enough, disability is only a matter of time. In a compelling essay about crip time, Ellen Samuels (2017) suggests six ways of looking at crip time and how they shape the time of chronic illness both as liberating and oppressing. For example, crip time involves grief: in the case of chronic illness, it is a time to elaborate the loss of health and able-bodiedness. The chronicity of a condition repeatedly presents signs of what life would be without the limitations imposed by the illness. Or, crip time is sick time, as the time in which we stop to let our body-minds heal despite the pressures that the world would ask to comply with. As it is the case of this very chapter, crip time is also writing time: as I discussed in the introduction, writing is an opportunity to make sense of chronic illness both from my embodied experience and from an academic-informed perspective. Doubtlessly, the many interruptions forced by illness to this process configure the time spent writing this piece as a form of crip time. Additionally, though, thinking about this time is also retrieving the importance of making room for silenced experiences to emerge and be heard—again, prefiguring crip time as a form of resistance.

As these contributions suggest, it is more insightful not to focus on what crip time *is*, but rather on what crip time *does*: how it defies chrononormativity; how it alters the normative perceptions of reproduction, productivity, happiness; how it expands or distorts the pace and the rhythms of ordinary life; how it eventually changes the way illness and disability are shaped. Looking at chronic illness through this lens offers the opportunity to interrogate, for example, how chronicity is shaped by chrononormativity; how the simple act of resting unveils a political importance; how waiting wrinkles the notion of normative rhythms. In the discussion that follows, I focus on each of these aspects.

Deriving from the Ancient Greek word "*kronos*" (time), chronicity is essentially a condition of embodied time, where time is engrained in the body. Chronicity is defined by two different forms of time: durability and unpredictability. Durability refers to the fact that any health condition that lasts for more than six months and has no favourable prognosis—that is, it is not expected to disappear—is considered chronic: in this sense, very different conditions may be all considered under the common category of "chronic" only by the fact that they are long-lasting (Bury, 1997; Lerum et al., 2015). In contrast to this medicalised definition, as a chronically ill person, it always struck me how my chronic illness has been the most stable element of my adult life: in a world of short-term contracts, fleeting relationships, and changing trajectories, chronic illness always remained, unchanged, as a perpetual companion. Besides durability, however, chronicity also involves an almost opposite form of time: unpredictability (White, 2023). The appearance of symptoms, the burst of flares, the timing of crisis, as well as the duration, the intensity or the gravity of pain and impairment, do not follow any linear rule: chronically ill people learn to navigate the unpredictable, bumpy, irregular rhythms of illness in their daily life.

The co-existence of both durability and unpredictability characterises chronic illness as an experience of time that deviates from the chrononormative logic of linearity and reproducibility, instead producing a sort of time travel. As Samuels (2017) points out:

> Disability and illness have the power to extract us from linear, progressive time with its normative life stages and cast us into a wormhole of backward and forward acceleration, jerky stops and starts, tedious intervals and abrupt endings.

Indeed, literature on the lived experiences of chronic illness show that illness does not only alter one's relationship with their body but also their notion of time. In a study of the narratives of people living with IBS (Irritable Bowel Syndrome), White (2023) explores how ill people adopt multiple strategies to contain the unpredictability of their symptoms and play along with the irregularity of their bodily functions. White argues that their body works as a metronome that beats time through multiple signs and figurations that become central to the management of everyday life. For example, one of the interviewees speaks of "the eleven o'clock rule" to indicate the time around which her family would know what kind of day she was to have. The ability to read patterns, anticipate flares, and navigate the unexpected encourages the formation of a "crip wisdom" (Krebs, 2022): a knowledge of bodies and time harnessed on intimate experiences of bodily instability rather than social or normative expectations. In the previously mentioned study I conducted with LGBTQ+ people with chronic illness (Pieri, 2023), participants presented similar narratives about their capacity to learn to follow the pace of chronic illness against external pressures: whether by educating friends and family around the need to leave always open the possibility of opting out until the last minute or by tattooing the motto "Twenty minutes at a time" on the wrist, interviewees show how the process of chronicity is also a process of learning a different *tempo*, both in the short term and in the long-run.

It is exactly in this understanding of chronic time as a form of wisdom that the act of resting emerges as close to subversive. In the contemporary healthist notion, resting is often considered a form of self-care which needs to be optimised, controlled, and improved: the industry has been flooded with apps to monitor the quality of sleep, devices that remind us when to take a break and for how long, and platforms that promise to help us reach complete relaxation (Petersen, 2015). However, the weaponization of rest by the industry of wellness (Cederström & Spicer, 2015) reinforces the neoliberal ideas of time as a precious resource that needs to be optimised and exploited to its maximum. If chronic illness reveals a different way to occupy time, it does so also in the way it unveils the profound pressure existing around rest and its neoliberal, colonial roots. Black radical thought and disability justice movements propose critical contributions to resting, discussing it as a form of resistance to the white, capitalist, healthist oppressive rules (Campt, 2017; Piepzna-Samarasinha, 2022). Activist examples such as "The Nap Ministry—Rest is resistance" (Hersey, 2022) show the importance of reframing rest as a tool to opt out, to refuse, and to resist the dominant pressures to productivity. The experiences of chronically ill people resonate with a similar necessity to withdraw from normative rhythms in favour of different paces. Chronic pain forces to stop and rest in unpredictable moments and for unpredictable periods: besides the physical suffering it causes, chronic pain alters the possibility of following the supposed linearity of days, activities, and schedules.

In this sense, Sheppard reflects on pacing as an active strategy elaborated by chronically ill people to accommodate, navigate, and follow the unpredictable rhythms of pain:

> Pacing is the activity of scheduling a daily life, particularly rest and low-activity periods, to either reduce the likelihood of a period of high pain or fatigue from occurring, or to enable them to do other higher-energy tasks and, significantly, to conceal the impact of those high-energy tasks as much as possible. Pacing may be forced upon the bodymind by pain or fatigue as well; it can be the time and inactivity needed to rest and recover. (2020, p. 43)

Sheppard collected narratives from people with chronic pain, who manage their everyday through countless choices of compromise between the social demands of productivity and the fatigue expressed by the inner body/self. Indeed, if considered through neoliberal lenses, activities such as pacing, napping, resting, and sleeping, are strictly non-productive: they require a suspension, a disengagement from the rest of the world, and a detachment from the rhythms of the others. The act of separation of one's rhythms constitutes both a need and a conscious act of crip self-care. The inability to perform within the expected timelines can generate a sense of loss and mourning, particularly in the (often long-lasting) phases in which illness is not diagnosed or recognised (Sheppard, 2020; Pieri, 2023). However, when the choice of opting out from certain demands is consciously taken, it epitomises a wilful deviation from expectations, in the queer way suggested by Ahmed (2010). It may also indicate a precise desire to mould the rhythms of existence on a different tune, thus holding a promising, transformative power for the relationship between the chronically ill person and their body: as Lia suggested at the beginning of the article, for example, a change in the intensity of life. This form of radical care is at the centre of activist practices based on intersectionality (Chazan, 2023). A growing debate is also bringing the reflection on academia and practices of knowledge production: contemporary academics are expected to work faster and harder in a competitiveness-driven and ultra-monitored environment based on tight schedules and performance audits (Brown & Leigh, 2020). Reflections on ableist structures in academia and chrononormative pressures in the knowledge production chain are crucial in unfolding an understanding of time that encompasses disabled, chronically ill, neurodivergent thinkers (Apelmo & Nordgren, 2021; Chazan, 2023; Richards, 2019).

The ability to pace, slow down, and trace more liveable rhythms of life extends to another crucial element in the experience of chronicity: waiting. Chronically ill people spend a considerable amount of their time waiting: at the doctor, in clinics, laboratories, and hospitals, they wait to be treated; in bed, they wait for the medication to produce effects or for pain to soar; at home, they wait for a flare or a crisis to pass, to be temporarily better; in their families, they wait to be recognised in their invisible conditions and not be asked again "Have you tried yoga?"; in the public space, they wait for improvements in accessibility and accommodation for their needs. Moreover, they wait for the result of tests or the arrival of new sanitary equipment; they wait for the approval of new healthcare protocols or the acceptance of special requirements to make their workplace or school accessible; they wait to know how their condition evolves or their body reacts to new therapies in the long run; they wait for scientific progress and experimentations to improve. Waiting is intrinsically constitutive of the crip time of chronic illness, from the everyday level to the most overarching life-long perspective. The neoliberal healthist paradigm interprets waiting as a form of wasted time: unproductive and immobile. However, exactly because of its unproductiveness, waiting time can be a surprisingly fruitful condition of anticipation and reflection. Krebs (2022) notes how during the COVID-19 pandemic, especially in the months in which social isolation was implemented in most countries in the world, "what many non-disabled people experienced as a 'collective disorientation' was, in many ways, a reorientation toward crip/sick ways of life" (p.19). Although the dominant narrative pointed to waiting for the return to normal (Pieri, 2022), the collective suspension from the everyday temporal logic showed that disabled and chronically ill people were better equipped to manage the anticipation and the frustration of waiting because they had been doing it for years:

> In the time of COVID-19, those who had lived previously with the privilege of normative ability began to learn what sick and disabled people have known forever: that crip time isn't easy, it isn't fair, it cannot be reasoned with. (Samuels & Freeman, 2021, p. 247)

Although it did not last long, the universalisation of crip time showed to many a glimpse of how we could live if we followed crip rhythms—however unfair—instead of chrononormative ones. A particularly intriguing aspect of imagining crip time at work would be, for example, its connection to creativity and self-determination. As discussed earlier, Samuels (2017) identifies in crip time the opportunity to make room for creative action (what she defines as 'writing time'). Again, we could thus imagine crip time as a time in which suspending every other activity (letting them wait) to write is a way to make space for the unheard and the invisible. Waiting time can become a moment to create room for speaking, registering, remembering, collecting experiences, and weaving intersectional connections: to create new archives of crip living. Moreover, the anticipation of what is to come, the anticipatory scheduling (Kafer, 2013) highlights a capacity to wait for the right time to do something, that is: the capacity to act exactly when it is not harmful to the body-mind and thus, once again, of performing self-care through a deep understanding of the complexities of time. Contrary to the notion of *Kronos*, that defines chronicity as a "unstable terminality" (Lerum et al., 2015), the concept of *Kairos* appears to be the most adequate to describe this understanding of crip time. In fact, in ancient Greek, Kairos is the time of opportunity, a fleeting, almost ineffable, instant when everything is possible and doable. A crip Kairos would mean the ability to know when the conditions are right to seize the moment; and the resilience in transforming waiting times into meaningful (and not necessarily productive) times.

Imagination, Resistance, and Alliances on Time

The use of a crip perspective on the time(s) of chronic illness opens important questions on the pervasiveness of chrononormativity in shaping notions of health and illness. Chrononormativity is key to understanding how the experiences of chronic illness are shaped and can be transformative. The perspective on crip time offers an important key to understanding how we can shape a different future:

> Crip time can be some, or all of: a refusal to embrace a (non-disabled) future; a failure to have a future; a failure to move from past to present to future in a straight line or at the required pace; a failure to progress from dependence to normatively-defined independence; a failure to progress through some, or all, developmental stages, at the right pace or in the right order; and/or a failure to 'do' gender, sexuality, race, class, age in temporally-dependent ways. (Sheppard, 2020, p. 40)

The notion of crip time as a site of transformation that sprouts from failure, resonates with the "queer art of failure" proposed by Halberstam (2011): according to the author, failure is the site where exceptional resources and surprising outcomes can happen, when we are open to embrace them; also, it is something that queer people (and, as argued in this chapter, chronically ill and neurodivergent people) have always done well. Failing expectations and deviating from them is a promise for different futurities, a potential for alternative worlds where the subjectivities who do not fit in rigorous labels can thrive. Failure can happen at any time and with every expectation ingrained in certain rhythms: indeed, queer theory offers a wide articulation of metaphors and images that place queerness in the role of defying chrononormativity (Edelman, 2007; McBean, 2016; Muñoz, 2009). Recently, the works on trans temporalities highlighted how trans and non-binary people defy the very notion of future and past, by occupying a sort of incessant nowness between imaginaries of the future and silences from the past (Malatino, 2019). Retrieving the hidden stories behind oppression, constructing archives, listening to the voices of the past is a form to redefine trans silence and propel its potential as a temporal dimension, "a different clock or a thousand clocks or an anticlock that explodes trans temporality beyond the barometer of transition" (Smilges, 2022, p. 151).

The preoccupation with chronopolitics that integrate alliances and intersectional experiences is also at the centre of critical ageing studies, which reflect on the intersections of ableism, heteronormativity, and ageism in the construction of the temporalities for older people. As Sandberg and Marshall (2017) point out, spectres of dementia and disability in ageing futures reproduce chrononormative preoccupations: "If the success of hetero-aging futures lies partly in its links to generativity, then dementia—through loss of memory—threatens to disrupt that generativity and represents as such a form of queer crip temporality" (2017, p. 5). Leahy (2021) also reflects on the impact that constructions of able-bodiedness/health have in prescribing normative (and supposedly successful) ageing patterns for older people. In their poignant book about the promises and failures of cure, Clare reminds us that "we cannot afford to forfeit imagination" (2017, p. 256), since it still is the most important instrument to build different paths towards the future. In this chapter, I explored how experiences of time through chronic illness reveal alternatives to the temporally dependent notions of success and health. These experiences unveil practices of resistance to normative time that cannot be restricted to mere observation of the present but need to be located in a broader temporality. Imagination is key to recognising that body-minds considered "too slow, too fast, too uncontrolled, too reliant, too different, too much and also not enough" (Sheppard, 2020, p. 39) are great at tweaking temporal rules and opening unexpected paths. Waiting, resting, stopping, and managing both the long-term chronicity and the short-term unpredictability are all examples of practices where the pressure to reproduce, produce, and be happy is deconstructed, dismantled, and overcome in the everyday.

Reaching the conclusion of this chapter, I am compelled to go back again to Ancient Greek—a resource from the past that helps me in shaping the future. In this language, the union of "*kronos*", time, and "*manteia*", divination, creates the word "chronomancy". It defines the capacity to foresee the right time to do something. In some ways, it designates a sort of supernatural ability to manipulate time or, as in the excerpt from *Alice's Adventures in Wonderland* mentioned at the beginning of this chapter, "to do whatever you want with the clock". Living in the anticipatory scheduling, learning to navigate the unpredictable, knowing when to turn the back to productivity pressures and pause: the experiences of people with chronic illness show that chronomancy is a way of doing crip time and indicate potential directions outside of the normativity imposed by the social clock. Therefore, when looking at the horizon, in the midst of a sunset, Lia states that "Everything is so ephemerous, I do need to give importance to what is really important", she is also showing us one of these directions and leading the way to alternative understandings of time.

Acknowledgements The author would like to acknowledge funding received by the FCT—Fundação Pela Ciência e a Tecnologia (https://doi.org/10.54499/2021.03925.CEECIND/CP1698/CT0004).

Competing Interests The authors have no conflicts of interest to declare that are relevant to the content of this chapter.

References

Adam, B. (1995). *Timewatch: The social analysis of time*. Polity Press.
Ahmed, S. (2010). *The promise of happiness*. Duke University Press.

Apelmo, E., & Nordgren, C. (2021). Still waiting for the hand to be raised. On being crip killjoys at an ableist university. In H. Egard, K. Hansson, & D. Wästerfors (Eds.), *Accessibility denied. Understanding inaccessibility and everyday resistance to inclusion for persons with disabilities* (pp. 107–122). Routledge.

Brown, N., & Leigh, J. (Eds.). (2020). *Ableism in academia*. UCL Press.

Bury, M. (1997). *Health and illness in a changing society*. Routledge.

Campt, T. M. (2017). *Listening to images*. Duke University Press.

Carroll, L. (1865). *Alice's adventures in wonderland*. Macmillan.

Cederström, C., & Spicer, A. (2015). *Wellness syndrome*. Wiley.

Chazan, M. (2023). Crip time and radical care in/as artful politics. *Social Sciences, 12*(2). https://doi.org/10.3390/socsci12020099

Clare, E. (2017). *Brilliant imperfection: Grappling with cure*. Duke University Press.

Edelman, L. (2007). *No future. Queer theory and the death drive*. Duke University Press.

Freeman, E. (2011). *Time binds: Queer temporalities, queer histories*. Duke University Press.

Garland-Thomson, R. (1997). *Extraordinary bodies: Figuring physical disability in American culture and literature*. Columbia University Press.

Halberstam, J. (2005). *In a queer time and place: Transgender bodies, subcultural bodies*. New York University Press.

Halberstam, J. (2011). *The queer art of failure*. Duke University Press.

Hassan, A., Yates, L., Hing, A. K., Hirz, A. E., & Hardeman, R. (2023). Dobbs and disability: Implications of abortion restrictions for people with chronic health conditions. *Health Services Research, 58*(1), 197–201. https://doi.org/10.1111/1475-6773.14108

Hersey, T. (2022). *Rest is resistance. A manifesto*. Little Brown Spark.

Kafer, A. (2013). *Feminist, queer, crip*. Indiana University Press.

Kim, J. B., & Schalk, S. (2021). Reclaiming the radical politics of self-care: A crip-of-color critique. *South Atlantic Quarterly, 120*(2), 325–342. https://doi.org/10.1215/00382876-8916074

Krebs, E. (2022). A sour taste of sick chronicity: Pandemic time and the violence of "returning to normal". *Communication and Critical/Cultural Studies, 19*(2), 119–126. https://doi.org/10.1080/14791420.2022.2063354

Larsson, A. T., & Grassman, E. J. (2012). Bodily changes among people living with physical impairments and chronic illnesses: Biographical disruption or normal illness? *Sociology of Health & Illness, 34*(8), 1156–1169. https://doi.org/10.1111/j.1467-9566.2012.01460.x

Leahy, A. (2021). *Disability and ageing. Towards a critical perspective*. Bristol University Press.

Lerum, S. V., Solbraekke, K. N., Frich, J., & Holmoy. (2015). Unstable terminality: Negotiating the meaning of chronicity and terminality in motor neurone disease. *Sociology of Health and Illness, 37*(1), 81–96. https://doi.org/10.1111/1467-9566.12182

Malatino, H. (2019). Future fatigue: Trans intimacies and trans presents (or how to survive the interregnum). *TSQ: Transgender Studies Quarterly, 6*(4), 635–658. https://doi.org/10.1215/23289252-7771796

McBean, S. (2016). *Feminism's queer temporalities*. Routledge.

McRuer, R. (2006). *Crip theory: Cultural signs of queerness and disability*. New York University Press.

Muñoz, J. E. (2009). *Cruising utopia the then and there of queer futurity*. New York University Press.

Petersen, A. R. (2015). *Hope in health: The socio-politics of optimism*. Palgrave Macmillan.

Piepzna-Samarasinha, L. L. (2022). *The future is disabled. Prohecies, love notes and mourning songs*. Arsenal Pulp Press.

Pieri, M. (2022). When vulnerability got mainstream: Reading the pandemic through disability and illness. *European Journal of Women's Studies, 29*(1). https://doi.org/10.1177/13505068221090424

Pieri, M. (2023). *LGBTQ+ people with chronic illness: Chroniqueers in Southern Europe*. Springer International Publishing.

Price, M. (2024). *Crip space time: Access, failure, and accountability in academic life*. Duke University Press.

Rich, A. (1980). *Compulsory heterosexuality and lesbian existence*. Antelope Publications.

Richards, R. (2019). Shame, silence and resistance: How my narratives of academia and kidney disease entwine. *Feminism & Psychology, 29*(2), 269–285. https://doi.org/10.1177/0959353518786757

Rodgers, J., Thorneycroft, R., Cook, P. S., Humphrys, E., Asquith, N. L., Yaghi, S. A., & Foulstone, A. (2023). Ableism in higher education: The negation of crip temporalities within the neoliberal academy. *Higher Education Research & Development, 42*(6), 1482–1495. https://doi.org/10.1080/07294360.2022.2138277

Roseneil, S., Crowhurst, I., Hellesund, T., Santos, A. C., & Stoilova, M. (Eds.). (2020). *The Tenacity of the couple-norm. Intimate citizenship regimes in a changing Europe*. UCL Press.

Samuels, E. (2017). Six ways of looking at crip time. *Disability Studies Quarterly, 37*(3), 10.18061/dsq.v37i3.5824.

Samuels, E., & Freeman, E. (Eds.). (2021). *Crip temporalities*. Duke University Press.

Sandberg, L. J., & Marshall, B. L. (2017). Queering aging futures. *Societies, 7*(3). https://doi.org/10.3390/soc7030021

Sheppard, E. (2020). Performing normal but becoming crip: Living with chronic pain. *Scandinavian Journal of Disability Research, 22*(1), 10.16993/sjdr.619.

Shildrick, M. (2005). The disabled body, genealogy and undecidability. *Cultural Studies, 19*(6). https://doi.org/10.1080/09502380500365754

Smilges, J. L. (2022). *Queer silence: On disability and rhetorical absence*. University of Minnesota Press.

Tremain, S. L. (2015). *Foucault and the government of disability*. University of Michigan Press.

White, L. (2023). Like clockwork? (Re)imagining rhythms and routines when living with irritable bowel syndrome (IBS). *Sociology of Health & Illness, 45*(6), 1259–1275. https://doi.org/10.1111/1467-9566.13504

10

Redefining Time, Energy, and Expectation with Spoon Theory

Imogen Harper

Spoon theory is a well-established and popular metaphorical description of the ways in which energy levels can be unpredictable and management-intensive for those who live with chronic illness. It forms the foundation of many lay descriptions of the experience of chronic illness, and it is also related to the popular online identity label of 'spoonie'. While its prominence has at times been noted in academic literature, there is little (if any) discussion of what, conceptually, has made spoon theory resonate with so many people over time. This chapter will use spoon theory to think through the temporal dimensions of chronic illness as both an everyday reality and an existentially destabilising event. Further, it will ask how the description of energy as existing in discrete allotments, which can be both taken away and replenished, destabilises normative conceptions of chronological time.

Spoon theory was created in 2003 by Christine Miserandino as a way to describe how she, and others living with chronic illnesses, are often

I. Harper (✉)
Sydney Centre for Healthy Societies and Charles Perkins Centre, University of Sydney, Sydney, NSW, Australia
e-mail: imogen.harper@sydney.edu.au

K. Kenny et al. (eds.), *Timescapes of Health, Illness and Care*,
https://doi.org/10.1007/978-981-96-7055-0_10

required to plan their days and futures with limited and unpredictable energy levels. On her blog, *But You Don't Look Sick?*, Miserandino wrote a post which used spoons as a metaphor for energy. She explained that her life with lupus involved a constant awareness of her fluctuating and often limited physical capacity, and she described her energy concerns as living with a finite set of spoons. Each day she considered not only how the activities she had planned would deplete those spoons, but also the fact that tomorrow she may wake up with fewer spoons than anticipated, or to something unanticipated that will demand their use (Miserandino, 2003).

For many who live with chronic physical and mental illness, spoon theory has become a well-known idea. The label of 'spoonie' has also become a way that people living with chronic illness, mental illness, or neurodivergency may refer to themselves. At the time of writing, 99,300 posts on Instagram are tagged with #spoontheory, and 3.2 million posts are tagged with #spoonie. Popular medical advice websites, such as WebMD, Healthline and Cleveland Clinic also have blog posts explaining the theory (Cleveland Clinic, 2021; Cristol, 2021; Schultz, 2019). It has further been brought into the popular vocabulary through articles published by media outlets such as *Slate* and *The Washington Post* (Hess, 2016; Latifi, 2023).

Despite this popularity, the theory has received less attention than one might expect from chronic illness, disability, or mental health scholars. Where it is discussed, the focus is on how this terminology creates a sense of group identity and experience, rather than a consideration of what it is that spoon theory is saying about the lived experience of illness and pain (Gonzalez-Polledo, 2016; Gonzalez-Polledo et al., 2020; Isika et al., 2020; Sendra & Farré, 2020).

Spoon theory is very much tied up in digital technologies—it was shared originally in a blog post, later popularised through social media platforms such as Facebook and Twitter, and is now cemented in its importance as a frequent reference point through content shared on applications such as Instagram and TikTok. The important role of social media in spoon theory's development and spread is not surprising, and it reflects existing literature on the ways in which illness and disability politics, identities, and knowledges are influenced by the affective capabilities of social media and online communication. Forms of solidarity between those with shared illness experiences have been expanded and reshaped by these technological affordances, as one's own experiences of illness have become easier to share (Conrad & Stults, 2010). This has resulted in the rapid creation of online spaces where knowledge and care can be provided (Ask & Abidin, 2018; Foster, 2016; Whooley & Barker, 2021). However, social media does not just bring people together—online spaces have the capacity to demonstrably reshape what it means to be ill, and to create a new 'world' for those living with illness, pain, and disability (Ginsburg & Rapp, 2013; Gonzalez-Polledo, 2016).

So, what does it mean that many online spaces concerned with chronic illness have defined themselves in part through identifications with spoon theory? The relevance of spoon theory goes beyond its role in evidencing the significance of individual and group identity in online spaces. Its popularity highlights the experiences of energy depletion and instability that people with chronic health conditions want to explain and bond over. The theory—as it exists as a phenomenon, rather than just in the original blog post—demonstrates an autonomous rethinking of how time is conceptualised for those living with chronic illness.

This chapter is based on the belief that ideas and theories created in everyday, online spaces should be taken as serious contributions to academic understandings of whatever the community is concerned with. In this case, the argument is that spoon theory is not just the idea that founded the label of 'spoonie', but instead a theory that offers insight into the lived experience of illness, pain, and disability. In particular, this chapter is interested in the ways in which spoon theory describes and validates the disruption of linear or 'clock(ed) time' (Adam, 2006; Zerubavel, 1982) that chronic illness can instigate and perpetuate.

The Evolution of Spoon Theory

In its original iteration, spoon theory comes from Miserandino's attempts to explain to her friend "what it felt like to be me, to be sick." On her instruction, her friend holds 12 spoons, which act as a physical representation of energy. Different tasks (such as getting out of bed or making breakfast) and different oversights (such as skipping lunch, or spending too much time at the computer) cost spoons. Miserandino has her friend walk her through a hypothetical day, spending spoons as she goes. The crux of the exercise is demonstrating the ever-present weight of contending with finite and changeable energy levels:

> The difference in being sick and being healthy is having to make choices or to consciously think about things when the rest of the world doesn't have to. The healthy have the luxury of a life without choices, a gift most people take for granted.

By 2013, Christine Miserandino had posted a YouTube video of 75 photos of spoon tattoos that had been sent to her, and the BBC had published a short explainer article on the theory (BBC, 2013). At this point the badge of spoonie (a label that does not appear in the original blogpost) was also in popular use on social media. The details of this history are not recorded, and it can be difficult to track the spread of this Internet phenomenon—today, people's understanding of spoon theory and its origins is largely shaped by the contexts that they are now seeing it in. For example, while this chapter focuses on its origins and discussion in chronic illnesses spaces, there are differences in the way it is discussed and applied in neurodiverse communities and research (see, e.g., McGuinness, 2021).

Spoon theory is not ubiquitous in all online chronic illness spaces, but where it does exist, it often reflects the concepts used elsewhere in digital cultures literature to describe online communities. For example, spoon theory is a way to symbolise a culture of shared experience and care (Byron, 2021), and often represents a form of "everyday activism" (Vivienne, 2016), as the decision to share personal stories or patient-centred information challenges medical supremacy and norms around visible, acute illness. The affordances of each social media platform are different, but people access them in an integrated, polymedia landscape where they can move freely and frequently between platforms (Madianou & Miller, 2012). On each platform there exist "affective publics" where *connective* (rather than *collective*) gestures bring people together (Papacharissi, 2020). In the case of chronic illness, there is a shared sense of physical and mental struggle, along with a common feeling of being misunderstood and disbelieved. Connective gestures show support and demonstrate that one is not alone, while also providing resources and tools that allow people to seek help elsewhere, manage their own conditions, and better describe their circumstances.

While academic work should take seriously the tools that online spaces use to understand life with a chronic health condition, we must also remember that one important function of these spaces is protecting experiences and knowledge from the expert systems that may otherwise dismiss them (Kelleher, 2001; Whelan, 2007). Given this, appropriating their content and work into the research sphere can be problematic. Spoon theory exists in a space of resistance, and is also itself a form of resistance to normative expectations about productivity and to assumptions about what different tasks require. This chapter does not seek to detract from those qualities, or appropriate it unthinkingly into academic nomenclature. Instead, my intention is to draw attention to the power and resonance of its ideas, with the aim of creating a better appreciation for the experience of energy and capacity instability and depletion that often accompanies chronic illness.

Methodological Considerations

As digital worlds and social technologies have ingrained themselves in society, there has been a proliferation of various innovative digital research methodologies. This chapter is based on a two-part qualitative study: semi-structured interviews with 19–29 year-olds living with a chronic illness, and a digital ethnography of Instagram pages which talk about chronic illness and disability. The digital ethnography is of most relevance to this chapter.

Instagram is a photo and video sharing social media application, where users can browse their own 'feed', which contains mostly posts (with captions) by accounts they follow, and an 'explore' page of posts by algorithm recommended accounts. There are many features of the app that allow for various forms of content creation and inter-account interaction, and they all serve a different purpose and cater to different types of content. There are a wide variety of public accounts on Instagram that offer representation, information, and support for those with chronic illnesses and disabilities. Any user can consume or connect with the content of any number and combination of these accounts.

For this study, I sought a methodology that allowed me to immerse myself in the dynamic and social environment of this chronic illness community. To do this I created an Instagram account that made and interacted with content relating to chronic illness and disability. Instagram was selected not only for its own popularity, but also because it offered some insight into other social medias—many Instagram users repost their own and others' TikTok content, and Instagram also allows creators to link to external blogs or YouTube channels.

My account served three purposes. First, as an ethnographic approach, it offered real-time observation of content and a comprehensive observation of Instagram's different social features (Gonzalez-Polledo, 2016). Second, it utilised the benefits of parallel vulnerability in ethnography (Winkler, 2017; Zizzo et al., 2021) and in turn allowed for a better understanding of the political power of mutual vulnerability (Vachhani, 2024). Given this, I felt a third benefit arose from it as an ethical practice—I was engaged with the relevant social media community by posting excerpts of academic and popular literature (and related ideas) that I was thinking about, while also reading and interacting with others' posts not just as a 'researcher' but also as an online community member.

There are significant ethical and analytic dilemmas when attempting to research the content of, and behaviour in, an online space (Barker, 2008; Burles & Bally, 2018; Lester, 2020; Ravn et al., 2020). I put on my profile that I was "a PhD candidate studying the experiences of people with chronic health conditions" and only followed public accounts. All elements of the digital ethnography (and interviews) received university ethics approval.

Participating in this online world revealed the ways in which a digital ecosystem incorporates common cultural touchstones like spoon theory. It became clear that there was a disconnect between academic and medical literatures and the ideas and language of online spaces. Specifically for this chapter, what I observed was the strangeness of academic and medical attempts to explain chronic energy concerns failing to take the well-established vocabulary of spoon theory more seriously.

Spoon theory is a core concept that appears online in a variety of ways. The label of spoonie exists both as a practical way of finding relevant content and as a symbol of connectedness. In some cases, people may explicitly understand themselves as belonging to the 'spoonie community', but there is also an implicit sense of membership that comes through understanding the meaning of an otherwise opaque label. Accounts focusing on chronic illness frequently have posts that explain spoon theory and what it means to be a 'spoonie'. The terms are also used in memes and other light-hearted or comedic content about chronic illness experiences.

The online environment itself shapes the behaviours and feelings expressed on digital platforms, and 'offline' understandings of identity and belonging do not necessarily transpose onto the online space (Poletti & Rak, 2013a). For example, the constraints of a social media mean that mentioning key words or tagging content with #spoonie is a highly practical gesture, since it allows people to find your content and helps the algorithm identify who you see as your people. While spoon theory explains what happens in the offline everyday, the label of spoonie helps construct an online world for people with shared experiences and interests, making it potentially an affective indication of care and understanding rather than necessarily an ever-present identity label. That said, the spoonie label does extend beyond the digital space. For example, one interview participant had attended support groups run by The Spoonie Society, which until recently was a business that began by selling heat and cold packs, and which had has over 40,000 followers on Instagram.

Interview recruitment was done through physical and online flyers which sought participants who had been living with a chronic health condition (diagnosed or undiagnosed) for at least six months. While the study was titled "young peoples' experience of chronic illness in the digital age" there was no requirement for participants to be engaged in online chronic illness spaces, and the flyer did not mention digital technologies or online media. That was important because it helped put this social media content into an everyday 'real world' context. For many participants, chronic illness content was a portion of their social media consumption. Participants valued content that helped them feel in some way supported, which included content that provided practical advice, evidence that they were not alone, humorous angles on their situations, and ways to politically situate their experiences. In my sample, there was a strong gendered division, as women more often spoken about content on Instagram and TikTok, while men more often spoke, sometimes exclusively, about Reddit. There is more work to be done in this area—further research could look more closely at a greater variety of online environments, and, through digital ethnography and interviews, seek to better understand how different vocabularies function across these spaces.

In my study, this methodology helped identify that the vocabulary of online illness communities can strongly diverge from academic literature, and spoon theory was the primary example of this. The remainder of the chapter will focus on how spoon theory might signal the extent to which one's sense of time and biography are disrupted by illness.

Thinking with Spoon Theory

Time, and how it is experienced and discussed, plays an important role in sociology of health and illness (Harrison et al., 2024). This is particularly true in regards to the temporal disruptions of chronic illness (Green & Lynch, 2022; Morris, 2008; Saunders, 2017; White, 2022). The prominence and resonance of spoon theory is instructive for inquiries related to this, especially given that the comments it makes about life (and time) with chronic illness differ in some ways from vocabulary and concepts that are more commonplace in academia. Below I use spoon theory as a conceptual lens with which to think about the experience of chronic illness, while also considering how it deviates from and/or extends other ways of framing these experiences.

Storytelling about the Healthy and Ill Self

> Most people start the day with unlimited amount of possibilities, and energy to do whatever they desire, especially young people. For the most part, they do not need to worry about the effects of their actions. […] When you are healthy you expect to have a never ending supply of "spoons". But when you have to now plan your day [when chronically ill], you need to know exactly how many "spoons" you are starting with. It doesn't guarantee that you might not lose some along the way, but at least it helps to know where you are starting.
>
> […] I explained that some days were worse then others; some days I have more spoons then most. But I can never make it go away and I can't forget about it, I always have to think about it. I handed her [my friend] a spoon I had been holding in reserve. I said simply, "I have learned to live life with an extra spoon in my pocket, in reserve. You need to always be prepared."
>
> (Christine Miserandino, 'The Spoon Theory', 2003)

Spoon theory was born from a story about what the everyday looks like for someone with chronic illness. It is, in part, a way to narrate and bind together the story of fluctuating energy levels. The additional label of spoonie takes these experiences and uses them in the description of a group identity, elevating this everyday story as a key component of one's 'narrative'. In this regard, spoon theory helps interrogate the potentials and pitfalls of narrative analysis in stories of time and energy in chronic illness.

Narrative analysis in the social sciences responds to the fact that stories of self are a key component of how individuals understand who they are and how they exist in their communities and cultures. It examines the meanings of specific events as an *episode* in larger relational and temporal networks, and argues that "struggles over narrations are thus struggles over identity" (Somers, 1994, p. 631). In the case of chronic illness, narratives can help draw together the frequent struggles individuals go through when asking both themselves and medical professionals what symptoms like pain or fatigue mean. How one narrates, for example, a sick day, has implications for the relationship between illness, productivity, and identity.

Stories are also a crucial component of understanding the disruptive nature of illness. Illness disturbs the expected present, and in turn may cast questions over both the past and the future. Recognising the way illness disturbs one's expected life-story is important for appreciating illness's emotional toll, and those who are sick often find themselves expending energy to create and come to terms with new stories. Arthur Frank's *The Wounded Storyteller* goes into detail about the process of narrativising illness, and he argues that people with serious illness

> learn by hearing themselves tell their stories, absorbing others' reactions, and experiencing their stories being shared. [...] The body sets in motion the need for new stories when its disease disrupts the old stories. [...] The personal issue of telling stories about illness is to give voice to the body, so that the changed body can become once again familiar.
> (Frank, 1995, pp. 1–2)

More recently, the emphasis on narrative construction has been problematised. Narratives provide both a 'message' and a 'completeness' that may not accurately depict how life is experienced, particularly in cases of trauma (Andrews, 2010; Hyvärinen et al., 2010). The desire for narrative coherence can also unduly elevate a point of destruction (e.g., when illness 'hits'), and it can focus analysis on how individuals seek to understand their past, rather than how they continue to develop their sense of self in the present (Kenny et al., 2017). In the case of chronic illness, the literature surrounding Michael Bury's 1982 concept of biographical disruption demonstrates these tensions (Bury, 1982, 1988; Larsson & Grassman, 2012; Locock & Ziebland, 2015; Monaghan & Gabe, 2015; Williams, 2000). This work highlights that researchers need to be cautious when trying to find a narrative in participant testimony. That said, researchers must also recognise that many are still often drawn to trying to find or construct a story surrounding events and emotions in their life (Thomas, 1999, 2010).

The online world has in some ways made it easier for autobiographical content to exist outside of narrative form (Poletti & Rak, 2013b, p. 10). This is a helpful observation when considering how spoon theory functions online. The role of narrative provides useful insight into the function of a shared vocabulary that quickly references a way of life—identifying as a 'spoonie', or referencing spoon theory in another way, makes familiar the experience of challenging and unpredictable energy levels. However the shortcomings of narrative analysis are also instructive, as spoon theory is built around incoherence and a need to focus on the present, which undermine traditional narrative constructs. It therefore exists as a narrative refrain for making sense of one's struggles, and as a short-hand for indicating that these struggles are a difficult-to-explain, but shared, experience.

Illness Over and Across Time

> You don't just get up. You have to crack open your eyes, and then realize you are late. You didn't sleep well the night before. You have to crawl out of bed, and then you have to make your self something to eat before you can do anything else, because if you don't, you can't take your medicine, and if you don't take your medicine you might as well give up all your spoons for today and tomorrow too.
>
> [...] When your "spoons" are gone, they are gone. Sometimes you can borrow against tomorrow's "spoons", but just think how hard tomorrow will be with less "spoons". I also needed to explain that a person who is sick always lives with the looming thought that tomorrow may be the day that a cold comes, or an infection, or any number of things that could be very dangerous. So you do not want to run low on "spoons", because you never know when you truly will need them.
>
> (Christine Miserandino, 'The Spoon Theory', 2003)

Spoon theory explains that it is wrong to assume that someone will always have enough energy to perform the expected chronology of a day. It challenges the automatically generated to-do lists that structure much of our time, helps us appreciate how many things throughout a day require energy expenditure, and argues that capacity limits are not defined by available minutes and hours.

For timescales that stretch across days, months, and years, chronic illness highlights just how many assumptions there are in expected biological chronologies. Two assumptions that spoon theory explicitly challenges in this regard are that rest can be delayed until convenient, and then that rest can be reliably utilised to refresh the body and mind. It also challenges the expectation that the young are healthy and carefree, and our expectation that any kind of recovery period will be linear. These beliefs about the ability to bend the needs of the body to a convenient schedule (across periods of fatigue, youth, or recovery) are wrong for everyone—another form of story which simplifies our bodies and minds into predictable machines. That said, the symptoms and risks of chronic health conditions do give a clear and high-stakes cost to neglecting the body.

The use of spoon theory to organise these experiences of chronic illness into an accessible narrative speaks to the central role of time in explaining illness experiences. One argument in Alison Kafer's book, *Feminist, Queer, Crip*, is that the experience of illness and disability is tied closely with a number of temporal constructions: temporal medical terminologies such as 'chronic' or 'intermittent' are an important component of medical labels, while temporal expectations are disrupted by both the practicalities of various disabilities, and ableist interactions with people or built environments (Kafer, 2013, pp. 25–26). Kafer further argues that we need to "wrestle with the ways in which 'the future' has been deployed in the service of compulsory able-bodiedness and able-mindedness," where "curative time" is often imposed such that there is "an understanding of disability that not only *expects* and *assumes* interventions but also cannot imagine or comprehend anything other than intervention" (Kafer, 2013, p. 27). The very nature of chronic illness challenges these acute, curative models, but day-to-day experiences of sudden, unavoidable fatigue also challenge ideas around short-term 'cures' in the form of either a quick break or, perhaps more often, pushing through.

These observations and arguments exist because of the particular social constructions of time that are embedded in our lives (Cipriani, 2013; Southerton, 2020; Zerubavel, 1982). Time is increasingly understood as a commodity that we can spend, save, or waste, and health has become a crucial component in 'evaluating' how effectively one's time is utilised (Kenny, 2015). Along with this, a (pre)occupation with what is to come—and how we best prepare for it—brings the future to the present as both individually and societally we are primed to 'anticipate' (Adams et al., 2009). When one is managing a chronic health condition, it is both the everyday social standardisation of time and the assumptions around the rhythm of life that are disrupted.

In the medical sphere, people living with either limited energy and/or the need to not significantly deplete that energy are told to engage in 'pacing'. Gavin Francis explains the need to pace in his book *Recovery: The Lost Art of Convalescence*, in which he argues for us to rethink our expectations around recovery. He explains that those recovering from illness or injury "acquire a new language of the body. [...] Someone in recovery needs to learn to listen to their own body so that they can begin to slow down and stop an activity *before* they begin to exhaust their energies" (Francis, 2022, pp. 20–21).

Descriptions of pacing also appear in informative content spread in the online space. Why, though, does spoon theory persist as a separate idea? Pacing clearly explains the requirement to not let one's available energy drop below a certain level, but in some ways this keeps the focus on energy stores and expenditure as a continuum one must be aware of throughout the day (or week, or month, or year). It is also often used as a way to impose productivity back onto a person who is ill or in pain, in an attempt to bolster and prioritise their participation in, for example, the workforce. That is not to say that pacing cannot be used to empower decision making, or to justify 'politicised self-care' (Sheppard, 2020). However, potentially because of its roots in neoliberal and biomedical healthcare, it does not provide an alternative and subversive structure to the conception of time, and it rarely confronts the truly 'chronic' nature of chronic illness.

Spoon theory, by contrast, gives people a binary and binding 'thing', instead of time, to mark the progression of a day with. This is highlighted in Miserando's own description: when she recounts her decision to use spoons, she explains to the reader that "I wanted something for her to actually hold, for me to then take away." So, if ordinarily time has become the commodity that we save, spend, waste, or loose, spoon theory allows energy to be commodified in a similarly structural sense. This allows it to tap into other temporal structures that proliferate throughout society. For example, spoon theory demonstrates the tension that those with a chronic illnesses face when they must live with a heightened anticipatory regime, while also having a heightened sense of hopelessness in relation to planning and predicting the future. That is, they cannot risk depleting their spoons for short-term purposes, given the possibility of long-term pain, and yet each day one's number of spoons is reset unpredictably. This is in contrast to standardised time, where you are supposed to have the same number of hours in each of your days, and the same number of hours compared to others' days.

This sense of chronic illness fundamentally restructuring time exists also in historical accounts of convalescence. Most relevantly, Hosanna Krienke argues that 'convalescent time' is a structural narrative component of many Victorian novels (Krienke, 2021). She demonstrates that medically and socially the period of convalescence was understood as a state between medical crisis and cure—as a period that was not static, but that embraced the precarity and ambiguity of a pause in usual life. As Krienke explains, convalescence "represented a timescale removed from the pressure of efficiency and productivity" and therefore "was not an identity but a temporality" (Krienke, 2021, pp. 4, 8). Spoon theory does not relate specifically to a period of convalescence, but it does do something similar in giving ill-bodies a different timescale on which to operate. Spoon theory therefore helps satiate the desire for narrative structure in what is otherwise a period defined by ambiguity. It gives meaning and form to the constant and perpetually uncertain struggle for energy—a task other conceptions of time can struggle to do.

Discussion

Narrative and time are in many ways two sides of the same coin—they are both tools we use to make sense of what happens in our lives, and they are both so deep in our nature it can feel impossible to imagine life without them. While we may recognise that our current understanding and use of time is constructed, it can still be difficult to escape the pressure to tie what has happened to what is happening to what will happen. Likewise, we can know that not everything can be made sense of as a narrative, but we may still be drawn to the act of storytelling and struggle to escape its confines, particularly when we seek to access and consider our own pasts, presents, and futures.

Spoon theory does not necessarily deliberately speak to these issues, but its persistence is telling, and the ideas it contains are an important springboard for further discussion. These discussions include how chronic illness challenges dominant conceptions of time, and the kinds of storytelling that can help make sense of illnesses that manage to be both highly unpredictable and exhausting in their tedium.

The essential move of spoon theory is to create a model of daily structure that replaces energy with spoons. Ordinarily, our energy and capacity for various tasks answers to time: Do we have time to do some additional work? Did we leave enough time to sleep and replenish our energy levels? For how long can we neglect our bodies and minds while we prioritise other commitments? Spoons, however, do not answer to time.

We can do things to deplete our spoons—like not take medication—just like we can do things to deplete our time, but spoons become the defining unit of a day, and the number of spoons we have has nothing to do with the time told by a clock. This theory not only helps reclaim how one plans their day looking forward, but it provides the narrative structure required to make sense of behaviours that do not fit well with a story that otherwise would be built around time passing. It is worth noting here that the usual narrative introduction to, say, a day in bed—"I was sick and/or exhausted"—does not cut it for chronic illness. Sickness, and often exhaustion, are chronic states, and it is useful to suggest that some different unit is shifting when tasks feel impossible.

Understanding this has implications for the ways in which illness experiences are discussed in social, academic, and healthcare settings. One simple recommendation is that healthcare professionals feel confident in the language of spoon theory, and consider directing their patients to spaces where these ideas are discussed by people also living with chronic illness. Another takeaway is that discussions of chronic illness, including in social and research settings, should adopt ways of talking about illness experiences that are not tied to linear time or binary states of health and illness. Spoon theory sees chronic illness as the addition of an organising dimension of life – one that goes beyond both timescales and discrete periods of illness. Its success implies that people might be grasping for different conceptualisations of time as they try to explain what it means to be constantly conscious of their capability amidst unpredictable energy loss and regeneration. Imposing the framework of clocked time could make these discussions more alienating, and communication more difficult.

Conclusion

Time takes on new meanings when someone lives with a chronic illness. On the one hand, it is a crucial organising component of both their healthcare and how their condition is understood, while on the other hand, there is often immense disruption to the feeling of time passing and the expectations that come with that. This complicates the use of stories that rely on linear models of time.

The way spoon theory has resonated with many demonstrates the desire to turn away from time as an organising structure to the daily experience of chronic illness. The invention of a different vocabulary to describe the perpetual struggles of managing energy and fatigue highlights that these experiences are understood as in some way fundamentally different from the usual patterns of energy expenditure and recovery. The even greater popularity of the label generated from spoon theory—spoonie—suggests that these experiences are ones that are understood as a potentially defining aspect of chronic illness, the recognition of which can form a foundation for community support. In taking seriously the ideas and metaphors generated in autonomous and online spaces, we can (and should) be inspired to think through the experiences of chronic illness with language that we know resonates with people over time and space.

Competing Interests Imogen is supported by the Charles Perkins Centre Jennie Mackenzie Research Fund and School of Social and Political Sciences at The University of Sydney.

References

Adam, B. (2006). Time. *Theory, Culture & Society, 23*(2–3), 119–126.

Adams, V., Murphy, M., & Clarke, A. E. (2009). Anticipation: Technoscience, life, affect, temporality. *Subjectivity, 28*, 246–265. https://doi.org/10.1057/sub.2009.18

Andrews, M. (2010). Beyond Narrative: The shape of traumatic testimony. In M. Hyvärinen, L.-C. Hydén, M. Saarenheimo, & M. Tamboukou (Eds.), *Beyond narrative coherence* (pp. 147–166). John Benjamins Publishing Company.

Ask, K., & Abidin, C. (2018). My life is a mess: Self-deprecating relatability and collective identities in the memification of student issues. *Information, Community & Society, 21*(6), 834–850. https://doi.org/10.1080/1369118X.2018.1437204

Barker, K. (2008). Electronic support groups, patient-consumers, and medicalization: The case of contested illness. *Journal of Health and Social Behaviour, 49*, 20–36. https://doi.org/10.1177/002214650804900103

BBC. (2013). Explaining low stamina levels—With spoons. *BBC*. https://www.bbc.com/news/blogs-ouch-22972767

Burles, M. C., & Bally, J. M. G. (2018). Ethical, practical, and methodological considerations for unobtrusive qualitative research about personal narratives shared on the Internet. *International Journal of Qualitative Methods, 17*, 1–9. https://doi.org/10.1177/1609406918788203

Bury, M. (1982). Chronic illness as biographical disruption. *Sociology of Health & Illness, 4*(2), 167–182. https://doi.org/10.1111/1467-9566.ep11339939

Bury, M. (1988). Meaning at risk: The experience of arthritis. In R. Anderson & M. Bury (Eds.), *Living with chronic illness. The experience of patients and their families*. Unwin Hyman.

Byron, P. (2021). *Digital media, friendship and cultures of care*. Routledge.

Cipriani, R. (2013). The many faces of social time: A sociological appraoch. *Time & Society, 22*(1), 5–30. https://doi.org/10.1177/0961463X12473948

Cleveland Clinic. (2021, November 16). What is the spoon theory metaphor for chronic illness? *Cleveland Clinic: Health essentials*. https://health.clevelandclinic.org/spoon-theory-chronic-illness

Conrad, P., & Stults, C. (2010). The internet and the experience of illness. In C. E. Bird, P. Conrad, A. M. Fremont, & S. Timmermans (Eds.), *Handbook of medical sociology* (6th ed., pp. 179–191). Vanderbilt University Press.

Cristol, H. (2021, July 7). What is the spoon theory? *WebMD*. https://www.webmd.com/multiple-sclerosis/features/spoon-theory

Foster, D. (2016). Keep complaining "til someone listens": Exchanges in tacit healthcare knowledge in online illness communities. *Social Science & Medicine, 166*, 25–32. https://doi.org/10.1016/j.socscimed.2016.08.007

Francis, G. (2022). *Recovery: The lost art of convalescence*. Profile Books.

Frank, A. (1995). *The wounded storyteller: Body, illness, and ethics*. University of Chicago Press.

Ginsburg, F., & Rapp, R. (2013). Disability worlds. *Annual Review of Anthropology, 42*, 53–68. https://doi.org/10.1146/annurev-anthro-092412-155502

Gonzalez-Polledo, E. (2016). "Chronic Media Worlds" Social media and the problem of pain communication on Tumblr. *Social Media + Society, 2*(1), 1–11. https://doi.org/10.1177/2056305116628887

Gonzalez-Polledo, E., Tarr, J., & McCracken, A. (2020). Spoonielife: A conversation about chronic pain expression and alternative social worlds on tumblr. In A. McCracken, A. Cho, L. Stein, & I. N. Hoch (Eds.), *A tumblr book: Platform and cultures* (pp. 307–314). University of Michigan Press.

Green, J., & Lynch, R. (2022). Rethinking chronicity: Public health and the problem of temporality. *Critical Public Health, 32*(4), 433–437. https://doi.org/10.1080/09581596.2022.2101432

Harrison, M., Smith, A. K., & Adams, S. (2024). Matters of time in health and illness. *Health Sociology Review, 33*(1), 1–9. https://doi.org/10.1080/14461242.2024.2319943

Hess, A. (2016, March 4). *The social media cure*. https://slate.com/technology/2016/03/how-spoonies-people-with-chronic-illnesses-use-memes-selfies-and-emojis-to-soothe-their-suffering.html

Hyvärinen, M., Hydén, L.-C., Saarenheimo, M., & Tamboukou, M. (2010). Beyond narrative coherence: An introduction. In M. Hyvärinen, L.-C. Hydén, M. Saarenheimo, & M. Tamboukou (Eds.), *Beyond narrative coherence* (pp. 1–15). John Benjamins Publishing Company.

Isika, N. U., Mendoza, A., & Bosua, R. (2020, February). "I need to compartmentalize myself": Appropriation of Instagram for chronic illness management. *ACSW '20: Proceedings of Australasian Computer Science Week Multiconference*. https://doi.org/10.1145/3373017.3373040

Kafer, A. (2013). *Feminist, queer, crip*. Indiana University Press.

Kelleher, D. (2001). New social movements in the health domain. In G. Scambler (Ed.), *Habermas, critical theory and health* (pp. 119–142). Routledge.

Kenny, K., Broom, A., Kirkby, E., Wyld, D., & Lwin, Z. (2017). Terminal anticipation: Entanglements of affect and temporality in living with advanced cancer. *Subjectivity, 10*(3), 374–392. https://doi.org/10.1057/s41286-017-0034-x

Kenny, K. E. (2015). The biopolitics of global health: Life and death in neoliberal time. *Journal of Sociology, 51*(1), 9–27. https://doi.org/10.1177/1440783314562313

Krienke, H. (2021). *Convalescence in the nineteenth-century novel.* Cambridge University Press.

Larsson, A., & Grassman, E. (2012). Bodily changes among people living with physical impairments and chronic illnesses: Biographical disruption or normal illness? *Sociology of Health & Illness, 34*(8), 1156–1169. https://doi.org/10.1111/j.1467-9566.2012.01460.x

Latifi, F. (2023, January 14). Spoon theory: What it is and how I use it to manage chronic illness. *The Washington Post.* https://www.washingtonpost.com/wellness/2023/01/14/spoon-theory-chronic-illness-spoonie/

Lester, J. N. (2020). Going digital in ethnography: Navigating the ethical tensions and productive possibilities. *Cultural Studies - Critical Methodologies, 20*(5), 414–424. https://doi.org/10.1177/1532708620936995

Locock, L., & Ziebland, S. (2015). Mike Bury: Biographical disruption and long-term and other health condition. In F. Collyer (Ed.), *The Palgrave handbook of sociology theory in health, illness and medicine* (pp. 582–598). Palgrave Macmillan.

Madianou, M., & Miller, D. (2012). Polymedia: Towards a new theory of digital media in interpersonal communication. *International Journal of Cultural Studies, 16*(2), 169–187. https://doi.org/10.1177/1367877912452486

McGuinness, K. (2021). An evaluation of a tool, based on spoon theory, to promote self-regulation and avoidence of burnout in autistic children and young people. *Good Autism Practice, 22*(1), 59–72.

Miserandino, C. (2003). The spoon theory. *But you don't look sick?* https://butyoudontlooksick.com/articles/written-by-christine/the-spoon-theory/

Monaghan, L. F., & Gabe, J. (2015). Chronic illness as biographical contingency? Young people's experiences of asthma. *Sociology of Health & Illness, 37*(8), 1236–1253. https://doi.org/10.1111/1467-9566.12301

Morris, D. (2008). Diabetes, chronic illness and the bodily roots of ecstatic temporality. *Human Studies, 31*, 399–421. https://doi.org/10.1007/s10746-008-9104-y

Papacharissi, Z. (2020). Affective publics: Solidarity and distance. In D. A. Rohlinger & S. Sobieraj (Eds.), *The Oxford handbook of digital media sociology.* Oxford University Press.

Poletti, A., & Rak, J. (Eds.). (2013a). *Identity technologies: Constructing the self online.* University of Wisconsin Press.

Poletti, A., & Rak, J. (2013b). Introduction. In A. Poletti & J. Rak (Eds.), *Identity technologies: Constructing the self online* (pp. 3–22). University of Wisconsin Press.

Ravn, S., Barnwell, A., & Neves, B. B. (2020). What is "Publicly Available Data"? Exploring blurred public-private boundaries and ethical practices through a case study on instagram. *Journal of Empirical Research on Human Research Ethics, 15*(1–2), 40–45. https://doi.org/10.1177/1556264619850736

Saunders, B. (2017). "It seems like you're going around in circles": Recurrent biographical disruption constructed through the past, present and anticipated future in the narratives of young adults with inflammatory bowel disease. *Sociology of Health & Illness, 39*(5), 726–740. https://doi.org/10.1111/1467-9566.12561

Schultz, K. (2019, April). I'm a "Spoonie." Here's what i wish more poeple knew about chronic illness. *Healthline.* https://www.healthline.com/health/spoon-theory-chronic-illness-explained-like-never-before#5

Sendra, A., & Farré, J. (2020). Communicating the experience of chronic pain through social media: Patients' narrative practices on Instagram. *Journal of Communication in Healthcare, 13*(1), 46–54. https://doi.org/10.1080/17538068.2020.1752982

Sheppard, E. (2020). Performing normal but becoming crip: Living with chronic pain. *Scandinavian Journal of Disability Research, 22*(1), 39–47. https://doi.org/10.16993/sjdr.619

Somers, M. (1994). The narrative constitution of identity: A relational and network approach. *Theory and Society, 23*(5), 605–649. https://doi.org/10.1007/BF00992905

Southerton, D. (2020). *Time, consumption and the coordination of everyday life.* Palgrave Macmillan.

Thomas, C. (1999). Narrative identity and the disabled self. In M. Corker & S. French (Eds.), *Disability discourse* (pp. 47–55). Open University Press.

Thomas, C. (2010). Negotiating the contested terrain of narrative methods in illness contexts. *Sociology of Health & Illness, 32*(4), 647–660. https://doi.org/10.1111/j.1467-9566.2010.01239.x

Vachhani, S. J. (2024). Networked feminism in a digital age—Mobilizing vulnerability and reconfiguring feminist politics in digital activism. *Gender, Work & Organization, 31*(3), 1031–1048. https://doi.org/10.1111/gwao.13097

Vivienne, S. (2016). *Digital identity and everyday activism: Sharing private stories with networked publics.* Palgrave Macmillan.

Whelan, E. (2007). "No one agrees except for those of us who have it": Endometriosis patients as an epistemological community. *Sociology of Health & Illness, 29*(7), 957–982. https://doi.org/10.1111/j.1467-9566.2007.01024.x

White, L. (2022). Like clockwork? (Re)imagining rhythms and routines when living with irritable bowel syndromes. *Sociology of Health & Illness, 45*(6), 1259–1275. https://doi.org/10.1111/1467-9566.13504

Whooley, O., & Barker, K. K. (2021). Uncertain and under quarantine: Toward a sociology of medical ignorance. *Journal of Health and Social Behaviour, 62*(3), 271–285. https://doi.org/10.1177/00221465211009202

Williams, S. (2000). Chronic illness as biographical disruption or biographical disruption as chronic illness? Reflections of a core concept. *Sociology of Health & Illness, 22*(1), 40–67. https://doi.org/10.1111/1467-9566.00191

Winkler, I. (2017). Doing autoethnography: Facing challenges, taking choices, accepting responsibilities. *Qualitative Inquiry, 24*(4). https://doi.org/10.1177/1077800417728956

Zerubavel, E. (1982). The standardization of time: A sociohistorical perspective. *American Journal of Sociology, 88*(1), 1–23. https://doi.org/10.1086/227631

Zizzo, G., Warin, M., Zivkovic, T., & Maher, J. M. (2021). Productive exposures: Vulnerability as a parallel practice of care in ethnographic and community spaces. *The Australian Journal of Anthropology, 32*(2), 150–165. https://doi.org/10.1111/taja.12404

11

"My Health Sucked the Future Right Out of Me": Time and Temporality in Life with Intracranial Hypertension

Kelly Moes

This chapter explores the temporal dissonance of living with chronic Intracranial Hypertension (IH).[1] I highlight the complex interplay between the fluctuations and uncertainty of the temporal experience of living with IH alongside the more structured and linear temporality experienced through healthcare encounters. These two competing temporal dimensions shift perceptions of past and present experiences and give new meaning to future possibilities and plans. I argue that conceptualising the illness experience through medicalised perspectives significantly shapes a view of the future based on able/healthy-bodied normative expectations.

Intracranial Hypertension is a systemic neuro-metabolic disorder. Clinically characterised by increased intracranial pressure, IH typically involves chronic headache, visual impairment, and cognitive dysfunction

[1] IH is also known as Idiopathic Intracranial Hypertension (IIH) and Pseudotumor Cerebri. While I have elected to use the general nomenclature IH, participants in this study relate to and are quoted using a variety of terms used in their medical system.

K. Moes (✉)
Centre for Culture and Technology, Curtin University, Perth, WA, Australia

K. Kenny et al. (eds.), *Timescapes of Health, Illness and Care*,
https://doi.org/10.1007/978-981-96-7055-0_11

(Grech et al., 2020; Thaller et al., 2023). IH is considered a rare disease, with an increasing global incidence of around 1.2 per 100,000 per year. Incidence is significantly higher for females aged 18 to 44, and racial differences have been noted (McCluskey et al., 2018; Shaia et al., 2024). The majority of IH research concentrates on biomedical factors, although considerable clinical uncertainty remains. People who live with the condition also highlight considerable negative impacts on their daily lives, yet few articles have focused on sociological, environmental, and personal factors (Lehman, 2003). The temporality of IH has not been previously addressed. By examining the nature of time in IH, this chapter thus offers a deeper understanding of the lived experience of IH.

In this chapter, I draw on survey data and asynchronous online discussion from adults living with IH to examine the experience of IH across three key temporal stages: past, present, and future. The experience of IH affects how people with the condition perceive and understand time. We can situate the temporal layers of the IH experience by drawing on notions of 'crip-time' in the context of chronic illness, as discussed by Kafer (2013) and Sheppard (2020), which highlights how normative understandings of time are disrupted. The ebbs and flows of seeking medical validation and treatments further contribute to this altered temporal experience, creating a feeling of uncertainty in the everyday illness experience. Building on Kafer's notion that crip time has a non-linear time progression and encompasses 'extra time' (2013, p. 34), I show how study participants express the present through this 'extra time'. People with IH (pwIH) demonstrate a temporal dissonance as they attempt to balance the uncertainty of their everyday experience while living in and through medical time. The medicalised experience of IH develops a deep ambivalence in past, present, and future narratives, which encompass experiences of lost time and loss of oneself and the dissonance between a hope for a cure and desire to lead a 'normal' life and hopelessness towards a future with IH. I argue that these ambivalent expressions of time in IH demonstrate the "complexities of crip lives" (Sheppard, 2020, p. 45). Additionally, I show how adopting research methods informed by my own lived experience with IH to accommodate 'crip-chronic' temporality opens space for those of us with chronic illness to meaningfully engage in research and promote the role of experiential expertise in disability and medical humanities futurities.

Temporal Dissonance and Crip Time

The experience of Intracranial Hypertension (IH) and its disruption to planned life events are closely intertwined. Bury's notion of chronic illness as "biographical disruption" suggests that the meaning we ascribe to the chronic illness experience is "situated in a temporal and life-course context" (Bury, 1997, p. 124). Charmaz (1995) extends this by contextualising temporal disruption in terms of the intrusiveness of the illness experience. These well-developed concepts are particularly significant for women diagnosed with IH in early adulthood, as their diagnosis and illness trajectory may influence their future choices and life events. In an effort to realign past and present selves with societal and taken-for-granted expectations of a 'normal' life trajectory, chronically ill people undergo a process of "narrative reconstruction" (G. Williams, 1984, p. 197; S. Williams, 2000). This adaptation is often a lifelong process for pwIH, made difficult due to the uncertainty of their illness experience (Wyckoff, 2007). Wyckoff reveals uncertainty as a prominent theme in the IH experience, generated by a disruption to quality of life and a sense of enforced life changes. Margaret Price (2016) describes the sense of not knowing what to expect in terms of outcomes and future events that occur unpredictably and unavoidably as "ambient uncertainty". Price emphasises how this connects the context and ascribed meanings as people with chronic illnesses navigate this changing temporal landscape, adding to the burden of the lived experience (Brown, 2018). In IH, clinical uncertainty spans multiple aspects of the condition (Mollan et al., 2019). This medical uncertainty, expressed diagnostically through the term 'idiopathic',[2] exacerbates a lack of knowledge and understanding about IH among treating professionals (Witry et al., 2021). This makes it difficult for pwIH to comprehensively understand their condition and the factors that contribute to it, reinforcing ambient uncertainty and complicating the lived experience.

[2] Chronic IH can be caused or triggered by an identifiable cause, such as an underlying condition, or specific drugs, however the most commonly cited form is known as 'Idiopathic Intracranial Hypertension' (IIH), where 'idiopathic' refers to its unknown causal mechanisms. Recent literature (see, e.g., Yiangou et al., 2023) suggests that the condition may no longer be idiopathic, with an increasing understanding of its driving mechanisms as a neuro-metabolic disorder.

We can further unpack this uncertainty and a temporal landscape built around normative healthy/able-bodied frameworks in the context of living through crip time. Crip theory's usage of 'crip' separates conceptualisations of disability based on societal and legal definitions and medicalised frameworks (Chen et al., 2023, p. 3). Crip acknowledges all non-normative ways of supporting the inclusion of individuals who may not identify as disabled or lack a medical diagnosis. Crip time, an aspect of Crip Theory, can help explore the complexities of the disability experience and deepen our understanding of the temporal experiences of chronic illness. Crip time embraces ambient uncertainty, adjusting to varying temporal rhythms rather than forcing people with chronic illness-disability to adhere to healthy/able-bodied expectations. Sheppard (2020) contends that crip time is a "messy, expansive, vague-but-specific" way to explore and challenge notions that time is linear, sequential, predictable and productive. For Sheppard, crip time is defined by its departure from, or failure to conform to, normative time conventions and expectations (2020, p. 40). Crip time acts as a non-linear temporal mode encompassing multiple timelines and draws attention to the fluctuating nature of chronic illness lived experiences. Daily routines and cycles of illness (including relapses and remissions) contribute to this variable pace. Crip time therefore provides a useful framework to understand the temporal dissonance of the IH experience, where many individuals with IH navigate a life characterised by "*good days*" or "*bad days*", that demands a flexible approach to normative timeframes.

Our perception of time is intrinsically linked to notions of normalcy (Pieri, 2023), influenced by sociocultural expectations that dictate the acceptance of sick or disabled people. This normativity is particularly evident in the context of the Parsonian 'sick role' requirement to be economically productive citizens (Parsons, 1951). As highlighted by Foucault, time is essential for understanding the clinical gaze and disease progression through recovery and rehabilitation (Foucault, 1975 as cited in Lupton, 1997, pp. 98–99). Time is explicit in medical terms such as 'chronic', 'acute', or 'in remission', just as it influences diagnosis and treatment. Consequently, 'medical time' plays an integral role in chronic illness experiences and shapes our understanding of them. The non-linear experience of crip-chronic time challenges this dominant, medicalised concept of time and thus influences the way those with chronic illness respond.

Inviting a deeper understanding of the complexities of 'IH Time', these competing temporal landscapes create what Larsson and Grassman call a "double time-table" (2012, p. 1164). While attempting to manage the day-to-day reality of the illness, individuals with IH attempt to situate their identity, relationships, and plans for the future over a longer period. We see this through their temporal expressions of past, present, and future IH selves.

Researching in 'IH Time'

This discussion of time and temporality in the context of Intracranial Hypertension (IH) is drawn from research conducted as part of a larger doctoral project focusing on the perspectives of adults living with IH.[3] In this section, I examine how a deep understanding of crip time, informed by my own lived experience of Intracranial Hypertension, has shaped the research design and blended the varying temporal needs of the research group and researcher. Insider research is an established and valued method in Critical Disability Studies. 'Disability as Method' centres Disability and disabled ways of thinking, knowing, and telling in the research (Inckle et al., 2023; Kitchin, 2000; Mills & Sanchez, 2023; Price & Kerschbaum, 2016). The methods and methodologies of this project are therefore an important aspect in this exploration of time and temporality in IH.[4]

The project consisted of an online and international qualitative survey of 563 adults living with IH. The survey supported open expression from participants and provided a diverse baseline to explore the variables of

[3] Ethics approval for this study was granted by Curtin University Human Research Ethics Committee in January 2022 (HRE2022-0037). All participants provided informed consent for this doctoral project. The primary data collection was conducted throughout 2022, with members of the 'IH Voices Research Discussion Group' providing ongoing clarification and feedback.

[4] Framed by a shared positionality, this chapter uses inclusive 'us' and 'we' pronouns when discussing the lived experience, while discussion drawn from research participants are reflected as 'their' expressions.

health and sociocultural experiences in IH and IH-identity. All participants were then invited to join an asynchronous research discussion group, mediated through the familiarity of the Facebook 'group' environment; 101 individuals engaged in this participant-led discussion over six months in 2022, enabling deeper exploration of illness narratives and collective discourse about needs, desires, joys, and challenges for pwIH.

The participant pool, drawn from a global pool of IH-specific groups on Facebook, included adults (18+ years) diagnosed with, or seeking a diagnosis of, IH. Participants' illness experiences ranged from those newly diagnosed to those who have lived with IH for more than 30 years. In line with the clinical literature noting a predominance of females of reproductive age, most participants belonged to this group (Toshniwal et al., 2024). Participants represented 37 geopolitical locations and self-identified from a broad range of sociocultural and ethnoreligious categories, although the majority (75%) identified as White or Western European. This depth of representation supported my argument that the experience of IH is largely the same despite differences across healthcare systems. While acknowledging that the experience of IH is variable, I have used verbatim quotes (*in italics*) from participants selected as representative of the collective narrative. It is also important to note that many participants did not identify with 'disability' or as 'crip'. Most saw their identity framed in complexity, particularly in relation to time and the fluctuations of their non-normative bodies, emphasising that their identity (as disabled, chronically ill or sick) "*depends on the day*". Examining their experiences through the lens of crip-chronic time helps us explore and comprehend the non-normative approaches to living with IH.

Drawing on the researcher's lived experience with IH, this study was designed to support and accommodate flexible and non-normative temporal participation. The importance of centring disability in the research design is highlighted by Price and Kerschbaum, who argue that "disability crips methodology" (2016, pp. 20–23). This approach seeks to ensure inclusivity by focusing on collective access rather than making accommodations as an afterthought. A key dimension of this methodology is time, whereby attentiveness to how disability can shape time enables its adaptive integration into research practices. My use of Facet Methodology (Mason, 2011) recognises the multiplicities and complexity of the experience of IH, whereby different facets of a phenomenon can be seen differently depending on how they are examined. Facet methodology facilitates researchers in identifying interwoven patterns that impact one another and supports flexible play with methods to explore the lived experience. This enabled me to 'crip' the research space to blend participant and researcher needs. Embracing my experiential knowledge in designing research methods, I acknowledged the labour-intensive nature of conducting research and its potential impact on my own health and disability needs (Price & Kerschbaum, 2016). An openness with my peers about my temporal requirements built rapport and trustworthiness as research partners. I was attentive to the 'extra time' of IH lives, including unpredictable and varying energy limitations and shifting temporalities, including fast and slow thinking, accommodating unproductive time and attendance to medical time, and working asynchronously and across different time zones. Emphasising Crip Spacetime (Price, 2016), my research methodology also leaned on my insider understanding of how pwIH adapt to temporal changes in IH and their need for information, connectedness, and legitimacy by coming together in virtual spaces. By leveraging the strong network and global community on social media and replicating that environment, this study facilitated a research community across multiple sociocultural contexts.

Adopting a long-form online and asynchronous group format facilitated collective narrative exploration while accommodating participants' individual needs, including allowances to dip in and out of the study as dictated by their health and energy fluctuations or other personal circumstances. In contrast to face-to-face or synchronous methods (including online meeting platforms), this approach was more accessible in terms of demanding less energy and supporting greater opportunities to engage around time zone differences. The slowed pace permitted by asynchronous engagement and threaded conversations enriched narrative responses by providing ample time for reflection, enabling more profound insights into the questions posed. Using visual imagery as conversational prompts further accommodated slowed cognition, and modified photo voice techniques supported those struggling to find words for self-expression. The use of qualitative surveys as an additional method allowed for a broad range of perspectives and social demographic representation and accommodated and facilitated the inclusion of participants who may have found online group formats too demanding or lacked adequate time. Facet Methodology also afforded time and space to explore the rich collective narrative. Thought-provoking lines of inquiry illuminated in survey responses were discussed in greater depth in the Facebook group.

A broad view was applied to examine the multiple contextual layers of living with IH to identify the underlying themes and critical 'flashes of insight' across multiple sociocultural contexts, particularly those that 'trouble' existing knowledge and assumptions about IH (Mason, 2011, p. 82). Rather than a descriptive summary, the critical analysis of data was insight-driven as I sought to identify the most powerful representation of the collective perspective through a process of constant comparison. Participants were not asked directly about time or temporalities, although one participant-led discussion thread centred on the question '*What happens as we age?*'. Despite this, the non-normative temporal landscape of IH is evident in the collective narrative.

In outlining my research methodology, I demonstrate how a research design that has been consciously 'cripped', as informed by crip time, thoughtfully accounts for the specific needs and characteristics of chronically ill and disabled participants, ensuring a more inclusive, engaging and accessible research experience.

Present

Intracranial Hypertension (IH) is mainly experienced in the present, characterised by daily fluctuations and changes in pace dictated by medical time. People with IH (pwIH) demonstrate a temporal dissonance in the constancy of daily, never-ending symptoms affecting their daily lives *("it never goes away")*, contrasting with the linearity of medical time, including a sense of waiting for a cure and recognition by healthcare professionals. This misalignment highlights a need to examine how medical interpretations shape our understanding of disability in IH (Linton, 1998), supporting Pieri's argument that 'cripping' chronic illness requires questioning medical knowledge and its authority over disabled individuals (2023). Factors such as diagnostic waiting times, living with poor health and in pain, deferring present lives hoping for improvement or curative treatments, and envisioning an endpoint (or lack thereof) all contribute to a non-linear, non-normative progression of crip time, with its "jerky stops and starts [and] tedious intervals" (Samuels, 2017). While acknowledging the difficulty in managing the fluctuating severity of IH, many experience IH as "*debilitating*" and often perceive it as "*unfair*". They view life with IH as a burden, expressing hopelessness and exhaustion as they navigate the present. While good and bad days exist, an overall sense of uncertainty is ever-present.

IH Time is Good Days and Bad Days

The day-to-day management of IH involves navigating the complexity of unpredictable episodes and fluctuations in symptom severity, where those living with the condition express, "*you never know if it's going to be a good day or bad day*". Good days are marked by the ability to complete daily tasks with minimal effort. This may be a short period of symptom relief or periods of remission lasting for months or years. Participants explain that 'good days' are far from an absence of symptoms, but "*even with mild to moderate IH symptoms*", they can complete most daily tasks. Bad days, characterised by loss of functionality or significant pain, are experienced in slow motion, attending only to basic needs, if at all. One participant described the fine line between a good and bad day as "*a drop of water*", noting they are "*always on the edge of breaking down*". Participants highlighted that these fluctuations and the unpredictable nature of IH significantly impact their daily lives, including their ability to plan and manage time. Rather than living by 'clocked time' (Cluley et al., 2024), pwIH live to a schedule dictated by their condition. The irregular passage of time this generates is emphasised by statements like "*Sometimes … it feels like déjà vu*". This suggests that the present experience of IH is often structured through non-normative ways of being. Emphasising the importance of living in the present moment and taking "*each day as it comes*", a determination to maintain balance despite the challenges of IH is clear: "*I refuse to let IIH define my life completely and be sick all the time … I hurt every single day [but] I will downplay it, so we won't change plans*"; and "*My goal is to get through each day."* This helps explain how, for some, the dynamic and uncertain nature of IH impacts their experience of the present.

Demonstrating the somatic reality of IH time, participants emphasise that managing fluctuating levels of energy impairment and pain is a daily challenge. Participants demonstrate a desperation to maintain a 'normative temporality', yet their health condition and medical time force them to submit to a different pace of life. A common sentiment among participants is that trying to keep up with normative time expectations is exhausting and overwhelming, with many demonstrating how even the simplest tasks can impact their anticipated routines. Expressions of debilitating physical fatigue, neuro-fatigue, pain, and other fluctuating symptoms highlight how IH is an "energy-limiting chronic illness" (Hale, 2021). Individuals with energy-limiting conditions need to carefully ration their limited energy, commonly referred to as 'spoons' (Miserandino, 2003), to accomplish basic tasks and minimise the exacerbation of other symptoms. This energy limitation and associated rest and recovery time are expressed by participants who note that even on good days, they are easily exhausted and often require extended periods of rest and recovery after relatively brief activity, noting that "*It's frustrating … my days are so unpredictable and sometimes all my energy goes to just making sure I bathe and eat.*"

It is clear that even though they may recognise their limitations, pwIH struggle to align their experience of time with personal and societal expectations of normalcy. This is amplified by the feeling that they need to justify their non-normative time to others. Bê (2016) found that women with chronic illness often had to negotiate their embodiment with others who expected them to behave as they did before their symptom onset, with little acknowledgement of the changes in their lives. Echoing this sentiment, participants highlight how their own and others' expectations of productivity are misaligned with their illness experience: "*[friends] just think I'm supposed to get on with life and not be sick*". Many participants also demonstrated the competing normative productivity expectations of the workplace with their fluctuating and unpredictable temporalities, for example, where standard allowances for sick leave do not account for the time needed to attend to their health needs. As a result, many report having to reduce work hours or seek alternative employment or education options that offer remote access or flexible scheduling: "*I now work from home and have a very flexible schedule. I stay ahead in my work so that when I'm having bad days, I can … be less than productive, and I don't get in trouble.*" Others report giving up work/education altogether—often against their will. For example, "*At first I tried to continue working, but … it soon became obvious that as my condition deteriorated, I wasn't going to be able to keep up with work and I had to quit.*"

Individuals with IH emphasise the importance of a flexible social framework that accommodates their varying experiences of time. Many participants explained how significant rest and recovery time is required, noting they learn to build rest periods into their routines, particularly after energy-expending activities: "*I learned to readjust my life to this illness. I do try make the most of what I can and rest on the hard days. Sometimes those days last weeks.*" Participants also highlighted the additional time needed to recover after treatments and interventions such as lumbar punctures or surgeries. While many said that it is impossible to predict either good or bad days, paying close attention to potential triggers, such as weather or menstrual cycles, means they can attempt to plan their lives around them: "*I am very wary of going anywhere, I'm constantly checking the weather, or … how many people are attending family events.*" Participants explained they need to rest before and after travel or social gatherings, with several admitting they cancel or avoid making plans due to discomfort or stigma and environmental obstacles in social situations: "*I don't go out and casual shop with friends anymore … it's a waste of my energy or 'spoons'*" and "*I try not to plan too far in advance in case I will be in too much pain*", resulting in social isolation.

Overall, the pervasiveness of the lived experience of IH is clear: "*It's exhausting. The appointments, the pain, the always having to advocate for yourself, the lack of support, the feeling alone, it wears me down.*" Their expressions demonstrate the difficulty pwIH have in navigating normative time schedules and the role of these external influences as a key factor in the careful management of IH crip spacetime as individuals readjust temporal expectations for their present selves.

IH Time is Medical Time

The uncertainty and unpredictability associated with living with IH can be attributed, at least in part, to its embeddedness in medical systems. Endless appointments and management of objective health measures typically consume the experience of the present. Although different spacetimes are generated by varying illness severity and the radical inequality of availability of, and access to, healthcare resources, participants in this project illustrate that the global experience of IH is largely the same and rooted in systemic issues. The medical system reinforces sickness (Charmaz, 1991, p. 263), and there exists a duality between medical "clocked" time and lived, crip time (Cluley et al., 2024). By considering the IH experience in the context of 'medical time', we can begin to unpack how the medicalisation of IH might orient the way we think about and experience chronic illness-disability.

People with IH experience speeding up and slowing down of time on the basis of severity and treatment urgency. The health system is primarily structured to treat and respond to acute conditions, typically characterised by rapid onset and short duration. In contrast, chronic conditions such as IH persist over time and may fluctuate or reoccur in varying severity. The health system triages need, dictating treatment urgency, meaning that IH is experienced through this 'triage time'. The high variability in time to receive a diagnosis or treatment based on clinical criteria is seen in the collective narrative of participants in this study. For example, participants note how time speeds up when their initial symptoms are treated as an emergency, only to subsequently slow down as they are forced into a 'wait and see' phase between treatments (*"I was taken by ambulance to the hospital… diagnosed… then literally nothing for 7 months"*). Despite these often long medicalised 'waiting times', for the person, there is still an urgency to be fixed or treated (*"have been waiting over a month for the neurologist and neurosurgeon to review my results and get back to me. Nobody takes this illness seriously, nobody"*). Participants also said they experienced delays in diagnosis or treatment, particularly when they did not match the expected clinical picture. Many individuals also express experiences of dismissal and delayed treatment until they develop acute symptoms such as vision loss or shunt infection. Comparatively, some participants explained how the positive and negative effects of medical interventions and treatments altered their time experience. For example, while some participants highlighted that surgical intervention was *"life-changing"*, noting an improvement in good days after procedures such as shunt placement, they still had to contend with fluctuations in functionality due to factors like shunt malfunctions or bad days during seasonal changes, demonstrating that even with the intervention of medical time uncertainty in IH time is omnipresent.

The experience of time in IH is also influenced by the substantial time spent managing medical appointments and treatments, which can be time-consuming and exhausting (Jowsey et al., 2012). The siloed nature of the medical system, where different doctors and specialists are required for different aspects of healthcare and medical management in IH, exacerbates this. Participants relate this drawn-out and slowed time to the variable and unpredictable nature of IH, whereby some treatments require frequent attendance and others have a lengthy wait. Participants emphasised the prolonged waiting times for referrals across multiple specialties, noting,

> *It's hard to sit in front of a doctor and tell them how sick you 'were'... a referral to a specialist here can sometimes take months. By the time I go I usually don't have the same symptoms or they are less severe. One time I had actually forgotten why I was referred to a certain specialist at all.*

Additional time needs to be factored in based on the accessibility and availability of specialised healthcare providers in their locality and the time required to travel to appointments, especially given the impact of IH on driving capabilities, mobility, and energy levels. Extended travel time is also common due to geographic distance from specialist facilities, particularly when seeking specialists with expert knowledge in IH. Many participants also expressed the inconvenience of appointment schedules and the unpredictability of treatment needs, highlighting that "*a flexible schedule is essential*". Many say this involves managing normative allowances for 'sick time' off work, noting they "*can't afford to be sick*" when they have exhausted all their sick leave benefits early. Noting the time burden of the sick role, pwIH express that this creates difficulty fitting a life they consider 'normal' around the demands of medical time.

In addition to scheduling and maintaining a complex appointment schedule, 'IH Admin time' includes the organisation of medications, accessing pharmacies, managing medication, and treatment side effects. For some, attending to insurance matters also consumes a significant amount of time. This temporal dimension also includes the extra time pwIH spend preparing for their appointments and curating documentation and evidence that legitimises their experience. As a rare and medically uncertain condition, participants express they often meet with healthcare professionals with limited, if any, knowledge of the condition. Medical authority generates 'epistemic invalidation' (Carel & Kidd, 2014; Fricker, 2007; Wendell, 1996) whereby healthcare professionals often discount the lived realities and testimonies of IH. People with IH often express a strong negative sentiment about the misalignment of their lived experience and the clinical interpretation of their condition. They expressed frustration at the time spent on medical interventions, particularly where there was little to no therapeutic gain. This is demonstrative of crip time experienced as disbelief (Sheppard, 2020, p. 41). Clementine Morrigan (2017) raises the 'trauma time' generated by these negative experiences in the healthcare system, including being devalued or dismissed, often with regularity. Participants voice this sense of medical trauma through expressions such as:

> *It really bothers me how the indifference and lack of empathy, just the cold-hearted way that my doctors ... handle me ... continues to add to my medical trauma ... It's traumatic enough already, don't f**king add to it by being an arse.*

The testimonial invalidation highlighted by most participants, underpinned by how they move in/through medical time, therefore characterises the experience of the present in IH.

Past

The temporal dimension of the past in IH can be best understood through the experience of time lost and the grief of their former selves prior to the illness experience. In their representation of crip time, Samuels (2017) describes this memory of a healthier body and the process of mourning the way we 'used to be' as 'grief time'. Emphasising this, participants in this study tended towards an intensity in their language to express this loss and disruption, such as *"its brutal"* and *"it stole my life"*. A loss of the identity they held prior to illness onset is evident in expressions such as *"I'd give anything to feel like myself again"* and *"I often find myself thinking of the 'old' [name] but I'm very different now"*. Participants also demonstrate time lost: *"I think I missed out on so much because I was forced to grow up when I got diagnosed"* and demonstrate frustration in a disrupted life course: *"I feel quite cross that my lifelong plans have been scuppered"*. This suggests that their expectations of anticipated and planned temporality have been altered by their experience of IH.

The chronicity of IH and perception of time lost demonstrated by participants in their expressions of their past and present selves presents a need to look at IH across the lifespan and explore how people think about and manage IH as they age, as well as the impact of the lived experience on their future goals and plans.

Future

Disruptions in time and anticipated temporal cycles also impact future life choices for pwIH, and individuals demonstrate they struggle to plan for or envision a future. Uncertainty in their present lives reinforces their apprehension of the future. Participant descriptions of living with the constant threat of relapse or worsening symptoms, including loss of eyesight, could be considered an "ambient sense of potential consequences" (Price, 2016). The chronicity of the lived experience is a significant factor for many pwIH, generating a future narrative that typifies the chronic illness phraseology 'no end in sight' (Benness, 2019). While hope for the future is evident in their chase for remission or curative treatments to regain a sense of 'normalcy' in their lives, they demonstrate strong ambiguity in their expressions of their future selves. Underpinned by its medical framework, pwIH *"dream about a future free of IIH, a cure [but] the grim reality has settled in that IIH is an uninvited guest in this game of life"*. This sense of resignation highlights an impact on mental well-being and perception of IH as a burden (for themselves and their loved ones), raises questions about their morbidity and mortality, and requires complex decisions about the future. Life with IH, framed by pathologised perspectives, might then be characterised as living in a state of 'ill-being' (Woodard, 2022) where future hope and hopelessness are intricately intertwined.

This duality is shaped by medical frameworks and sociocultural norms surrounding health. The treatment and recovery-focused approach of the (Western) medical system, alongside normative expectations for wellness, generates "curative imaginaries" for chronically ill-disabled people (Kafer, 2013, p. 27). This is evident in the hopeful expressions of those who live with IH, where they demonstrate a desire for a cure: *"We need a cure. Everyday functions are an uphill battle and life is harder because not much is known about IIH"*, or at least, improvement in symptoms, *"Though my IIH symptoms have improved immensely and seem to only flare around … my triggers. I am very hopeful that I'll be able to reach remission again before this time next year"*. The notion of remission in IH is complex and is perhaps a narrative fostering false hope for pwIH. The concept of remission implies recovery. It offers an attractive prospect of pain relief and a return to normality, yet its temporary nature is often marred by inevitable failure. In the context of IH, remission usually refers to clinical improvement in papilledema (optic nerve swelling) and intracranial pressure levels, although a "persistent post-IIH headache" remains (Mollan, Grech, et al., 2021).

Similarly, emphasising normative 'wellness' standards, a focus on weight and weight loss as a potential solution or modifiable factor for IH (Mollan, Mitchell, et al., 2021) individualises the 'problem' of IH. When attempts at weight loss fail or do not lead to a reduction in symptoms, it suggests there is no reliable way to minimise the person's pain or regain their lost function, fueling disappointment and frustration: "*It feels like it is considered a 'fat person condition'. Losing weight is the only option available. Until they are satisfied with weight loss then they see no other option. They often brush off my concerns, symptoms and fears.*" Under this pathologised framework, the hope for remission is often tied to an imagined future in which weight loss has been successful. People with IH therefore grieve their lost functioning and capacity alongside their imagined healthy/able-bodied futures (Kafer, 2013). I contend that this perspective could contribute to negativity when reframing life narratives. For pwIH, while the perception of remission amounts to an end of the disruption to their daily life and a return to planned futurity, in actuality, this may only ever be partial and temporary and therefore only serves to maintain the ambient uncertainty of the IH lived experience.

A life bounded by normative definitions of health and wellness may ultimately trap people in a state of ill-being bounded by the sick role. Demonstrating how pwIH think deeply about this potentially endless state of ill-being, one participant wrote, *"I assume I will always be disabled and living with the pain from IIH. And finding a way to accept that was really hard … the thought of living this way another 30–40 years feels impossible."* Charmaz argues "feeling trapped by an uncontrollable future also traps one in a dialectic of negative emotions", where the state of ill-being becomes the dominant factor in life and contributes to a time perspective of a dreaded future (1991, p. 251). Generating ambivalence towards a future with IH, this challenges pwIH to consider issues related to their mortality, including premature death: *"I honestly don't see much of a future now I have IIH … Every day I try with this illness, I ask for help and I'm still sitting here wondering if life is even worth living anymore."* Literature shows that individuals with IH have a 50% higher likelihood of dying from unexpected circumstances than their non-IH counterparts (Hermes et al., 2020). While this suggests lower health outcomes, participants also raise mental health concerns and a perception that IH is a burdensome life, suggesting a higher risk of suicidality for pwIH: *"It may not be life threatening, but it is a huge cause of suicide in the IIH community. We need more treatment options; we need to not feel alone". "Our healthcare is terrible… The specialist refused to see me and said nothing was wrong. I was in the hospital constantly, treated terribly, left in pain and going blind. I tried to take my own life and will have that scar both physically and mentally forever."* The importance of quality of life also leads pwIH to consider factors such as disability support systems, housing options as they age, and their end-of-life options: *"I hope that I have mostly good days still and remain stable as I age. If I have negative health outcomes … I have been considering every option including the MAID program."* As Wendell points out, these decisions may be made on a perceived situation of hopelessness due to "inadequate support services and poor opportunities" (1996, p. 159) rather than the person's physical condition. Wendell compels us to consider whether under different circumstances, such as social support and coordinated care/management, the same life/death decisions would be made.

While the hope for a future free of IH is clear, it is juxtaposed with an underlying sense of resignation and acceptance as participants acknowledge that IH is a chronic condition that is unlikely to change significantly. Responses show that negative experiences and a sense of 'no end in sight' generate strong expressions of despair towards their future and fear about ageing with IH with a constant threat of worsening or recurring symptoms: *"Can't bear to think of the future. Endless years ahead of this pain, fatigue and empty life is not appealing…Frankly the future is bleak so it's better not to consider it."* People with IH express that they feel trapped by IH (*"Each day feels like I am surviving and I hate that I can't seem to get myself out of this stuck place"*), with little prospect for relief or improvement:

> *It's incredibly difficult for me to think about my future with chronic illness as I am still coming to terms with the fact that I even am chronically ill, there is no cure, there likely won't be in my lifetime, there won't be relief, there won't be an end, I just need to learn to cope.*

Many also note that anticipation of a lifetime with IH has altered their career choices and anticipated work trajectories; for example, *"My career ended due to this condition and I'm not sure I will ever go back to it, but I wouldn't mind being able to work part time or even volunteer."* For many, it has also shaped their imagined parental futurity, for example, *"I can't be the active mum I wanted to be"* and *"It has changed life choices. I really wanted kids [but] I wouldn't be able to give them what is needed."* Their future is then expressed through their capacity to cope with the challenges of life with IH. Expressions such as *"I really don't think much about the future with IIH and what could happen … I'm trying to just live each day and deal with things as they happen"* demonstrate how pwIH manage by focusing on the present rather than the future.

Smilges (2023) contends that multiple futures and choices are necessary for nurturing collective dreams, suggesting that if not for the medical framework that holds pwIH to endless cycles of treatment and the push for recovery/remission/cure, then pwIH may have broader (and more positive) future imaginaries. People with IH express uncertainty about their future with IH. In addition to the dynamic and unpredictable nature of IH, their negativity often arises from frustration with the medical system and their healthcare providers, including a lack of understanding of the cause of IH and a lack of reliable treatment options. For pwIH, the collective dream is for the condition and their experience of it to be better understood: *"It's a daily struggle with many symptoms that aren't understood"* and *"I'm constantly sick. I haven't had a day without some semblance of a headache since I was 16 … IIH is a serious condition and it shouldn't be discounted."* Although pwIH demonstrate a rich understanding of their condition and the heterogeneity of lived experiences means there is no straightforward solution, they are clear that their future imaginaries are not simply framed in curative terms.

Conclusion

The overwhelming crip negativity expressed by participants was clear, with participants expressing their lived experience as *"nightmarish"* and a *"living hell"*. Sheppard (2022) contends that in moving in crip time, we find more spacetime for the joyful experience of non-normative lives/futures, which they term 'crip joy', yet participants in this study contend that this is far from what they experience or necessarily seek. They stress that their lived experiences are anything but joyful, and living beyond normative time structures adds to the burden of their lived experience. Despite this, their resilience and determination is also evident. Through their 'crip negativity' (Smilges, 2023), they can also find ways to manage and adapt despite the pain, challenges, and negative impacts of life with IH. Participants emphasised the importance of living in the present. Although they express it in variable ways, in this slowing down of life, expressions of 'crip joy' can be seen to develop over time, with some noting they develop a value and appreciation for the *"small things"* and increased empathy for others. While Sheppard sees crip time as an active statement of self-worth—one that relies on accepting and embracing a disabled present and future, we must also understand the challenges associated with doing so—and recognise those who experience crip joy as a form of self-care while also acknowledging and supporting those who actively reject it. Framing IH in a way that embraces the grief and bitterness of the temporalities of the lived experience will, therefore, enhance the overall understanding of this uncommon chronic illness.

Matters of time and temporality in the context of IH are experienced as a time in flux, disrupting normative ideals of past and future selves. There is a clear tension between IH as medical time and a desire to embrace crip time, which significantly impacts the present and future narratives for people with IH. Grounded in notions of crip time, we show that those living with IH express a sense of temporal dissonance characterised by ambient uncertainty. Life with IH is deeply entwined with a medical perspective that creates temporal experiences framed by normative expectations for health and wellness. This generates a sense of deep ambivalence—highlighted by mixed feelings and contradictory perspectives about their future. While expressing hope for a cure/remission and desire to lead a life they consider 'normal', participants also demonstrated strong negativity and hopelessness about their future with IH. I contend that by embracing crip negativity, the future imaginaries of IH can be reframed by the lived experience. The future narratives of people living with IH highlight the need for greater awareness, understanding, and support for individuals living with uncommon chronic illness-disability. While this chapter focuses on the case study of Intracranial Hypertension, many of the aspects of chronic illness-disability I have highlighted are shared experiences of chronic illness more broadly.

A disability-focused, time-aware approach informed by my emic understanding of IH was key in facilitating high levels of engagement and interpreting the deep narrative expressions. The concept of 'crip labour' advocates for inclusive research that is flexible and open-ended in terms of what the research looks like and what it is expected to produce (Inoue, 2023, Ch. 3). The impairment effects of chronic illness are often unapparent to others, leading to disbelief and disregard (Evans et al., 2023). This is problematised in the ways chronic illness is understood, influenced and shaped by sociocultural meanings ascribed to health and illness (Pieri, 2023, p. 18). Being open to the ways people with chronic illness know and understand their lived experiences and meaningfully engaging them in the research about them while being attentive to their temporal needs is crucial in redressing the invalidation and epistemic injustice experienced by this population. Re-evaluating our perspectives on time and temporality in the context of chronic ill-health and disability is therefore essential to develop more inclusive and comprehensive research and supports.

Acknowledgements This research would not be possible without the support of the Intracranial Hypertension community on Facebook and the significant contributions from members of the 'IH Voices Research Discussion Group', in particular, Rachel Ivey (USA) and Yvonne Porter (Aus), who provided critical feedback on the content of this chapter.

The author acknowledges the support and guidance of her supervisory team, Professor Mike Kent (Curtin University), Dr Sky Croeser (Curtin University), and Dr Shafiiq Gopee (Curtin Mauritius). I am also grateful for the advice and feedback from this chapter's reviewers and the editors of this collection.

Competing Interests The author is supported by an Australian Government Research Training Program Scholarship. There are no conflicts of interest to declare relevant to this chapter's content.

Ethics Declaration This study was performed in line with the principles of the Declaration of Helsinki and the requirements described in the National Health and Medical Research Council's (NHMRC) National Statement on Ethical Conduct in Human Research (2007). Approval was granted by the Curtin University Human Research Ethics Committee (Approval number: HRE2022-0037). Informed consent was obtained from all individual participants.

References

Bê, A. (2016). Disablism in the lives of people living with a chronic illness in England and Portugal. *Disability & Society, 31*(4), 465–480. https://doi.org/10.1080/09687599.2016.1181048

Benness, B. (2019). Welcome to no end in sight on medium. *No end in sight.*. https://medium.com/no-end-in-sight/welcome-to-no-end-in-sight-on-medium-da153e8c7f55

Brown, A. (2018). *The lived experiences of managing uncertainty in chronic illness*. Walden University.

Bury, M. (1997). *Health and illness in a changing society*. Psychology Press.

Carel, H., & Kidd, I. J. (2014). Epistemic injustice in healthcare: A philosophical analysis. *Medicine, Health Care and Philosophy, 17*(4), 529–540. https://doi.org/10.1007/s11019-014-9560-2

Charmaz, K. (1991). *Good days, bad days: The self in chronic illness and time*. Rutgers University Press.

Charmaz, K. (1995). The body, identity, and self: Adapting to impairment. *The Sociological Quarterly, 36*(4), 657–680.

Chen, M. Y., Kafer, A., Kim, E., & Minich, J. A. (Eds.). (2023). *Crip genealogies*. Duke University Press.

Cluley, V., Burton, J. O., Hull, K. L., & Eborall, H. (2024). The paradox of haemodialysis: The lived experience of the clocked treatment of chronic illness. *Health Sociology Review, 0*(0), 1–19. https://doi.org/10.1080/14461242.2024.2319189

Evans, B., Allam, A., Hale, C., Pereira, A. B., Rose, M., & Ruddock, A. (2023). *Disbelief and disregard: Gendered experiences of healthcare for people with energy limiting conditions*. http://disbeliefdisregard.uk/

Fricker. (2007). *Epistemic injustice: Power and the ethics of knowing*. Oxford Academic.

Grech, O., Mollan, S. P., Wakerley, B. R., Alimajstorovic, Z., Lavery, G. G., & Sinclair, A. J. (2020). Emerging themes in idiopathic intracranial hypertension. *Journal of Neurology, 267*(12), 3776–3784. https://doi.org/10.1007/s00415-020-10090-4

Hale, C. (2021). *What are energy impairment and ELCI?* Chronic Illness Inclusion. https://chronicillnessinclusion.org.uk/2021/04/28/what-are-energy-impairment-and-elci/

Hermes, S. M., Miller, N. R., Waslo, C. S., Benes, S. C., & Tanne, E. (2020). Mortality among patients with idiopathic intracranial hypertension enrolled in the IH Registry. *Neurology, 95*(7), e921–e929. https://doi.org/10.1212/WNL.0000000000009312

Inckle, K., Brighton, J., & Sparkes, A. C. (2023). Who is "Us" in "Nothing About Us Without US"? Rethinking the politics of disability research. *Disability Studies Quarterly, 42*(3–4), Article 3–4. https://doi.org/10.18061/dsq.v42i3-4.7947

Inoue, A. B. (2023). *Cripping labor-based grading for more equity in literacy courses*. The WAC Clearinghouse; University Press of Colorado. https://doi.org/10.37514/PRA-B.2023.2203

Jowsey, T., Yen, L., & W, P. M. (2012). Time spent on health related activities associated with chronic illness: A scoping literature review. *BMC Public Health, 12*, 1044. https://doi.org/10.1186/1471-2458-12-1044

Kafer, A. (2013). *Feminist, queer, crip*. Indiana University Press. http://www.jstor.org/stable/j.ctt16gz79x

Kitchin, R. (2000). The researched opinions on research: Disabled people and disability research. *Disability & Society, 15*(1), 25–47. https://doi.org/10.1080/09687590025757

Larsson, A. T., & Grassman, E. J. (2012). Bodily changes among people living with physical impairments and chronic illnesses: Biographical disruption or normal illness? *Sociology of Health & Illness, 34*(8), 1156–1169. https://doi.org/10.1111/j.1467-9566.2012.01460.x

Lehman, C. A. (2003). Idiopathic intracranial hypertension within the ICF model: A review of the literature. *Journal of Neuroscience Nursing, 35*(5), 263–269.

Linton, S. (1998). *Claiming disability: Knowledge and identity*. NYU Press. https://nyupress.org/9780814751343/claiming-disability

Lupton, D. (1997). Foucault and the medicalisation critique. In *Foucault, health and medicine*. Routledge.

Mason, J. (2011). Facet methodology: The case for an inventive research orientation. *Methodological Innovations Online, 6*(3), 75–92. https://doi.org/10.4256/mio.2011.008

McCluskey, G., Doherty-Allan, R., McCarron, P., Loftus, A. M., McCarron, L. V., Mulholland, D., McVerry, F., & McCarron, M. O. (2018). Meta-analysis and systematic review of population-based epidemiological studies in idiopathic intracranial hypertension. *European Journal of Neurology, 25*(10), 1218–1227. https://doi.org/10.1111/ene.13739

Mills, M., & Sanchez, R. (Eds.). (2023). *Crip authorship: Disability as method*. New York University Press. https://doi.org/10.18574/nyu/9781479819386.001.0001

Miserandino, C. (2003). *The spoon theory*. But you dont look sick. https://butyoudontlooksick.com/articles/written-by-christine/the-spoon-theory/

Mollan, S., Hemmings, K., Herd, C. P., Denton, A., Williamson, S., & Sinclair, A. J. (2019). What are the research priorities for idiopathic intracranial hypertension? A priority setting partnership between patients and healthcare professionals. *BMJ Open, 9*(3), e026573. https://doi.org/10.1136/bmjopen-2018-026573

Mollan, S. P., Grech, O., & Sinclair, A. J. (2021a). Headache attributed to idiopathic intracranial hypertension and persistent post-idiopathic intracranial hypertension headache: A narrative review. *Headache: The Journal of Head and Face Pain, 61*(6), 808–816. https://doi.org/10.1111/head.14125

Mollan, S. P., Mitchell, J. L., Ottridge, R. S., Aguiar, M., Yiangou, A., Alimajstorovic, Z., Cartwright, D. M., Grech, O., Lavery, G. G., Westgate, C. S. J., Vijay, V., Scotton, W., Wakerley, B. R., Matthews, T. D., Ansons, A., Hickman, S. J., Benzimra, J., Rick, C., Singhal, R., et al. (2021b). Effectiveness of bariatric surgery vs community weight management intervention for the treatment of idiopathic intracranial hypertension: A randomized clinical trial. *JAMA Neurology, 78*(6), 678–686. https://doi.org/10.1001/jamaneurol.2021.0659

Morrigan, C. (2017). Trauma time: The queer temporalities of the traumatized mind. *Somatechnics, 7*, 50–58. https://doi.org/10.3366/soma.2017.0205

Parsons, T. (1951). Illness and the role of the physician: A sociological perspective*. *American Journal of Orthopsychiatry, 21*(3), 452–460. https://doi.org/10.1111/j.1939-0025.1951.tb00003.x

Pieri, M. (2023). *LGBTQ+ people with chronic illness: Chroniqueers in Southern Europe*. Springer Nature.

Price, M. (2016). *Moving together: Toward a theory of crip spacetime*. National Women's Studies Association. https://margaretprice.files.wordpress.com/2011/01/smith-talk-4-17-17.docx

Price, M., & Kerschbaum, S. L. (2016). Stories of methodology: Interviewing sideways, crooked and crip. *Canadian Journal of Disability Studies, 5*(3), Article 3. https://doi.org/10.15353/cjds.v5i3.295

Samuels, E. (2017). Six ways of looking at crip time. *Disability Studies Quarterly, 37*(3), Article 3. https://doi.org/10.18061/dsq.v37i3.5824

Shaia, J. K., Sharma, N., Kumar, M., Chu, J., Maatouk, C., Talcott, K., Singh, R., & Cohen, D. A. (2024). Changes in prevalence of idiopathic intracranial hypertension in the United States between 2015 and 2022, stratified by sex, race, and ethnicity. *Neurology, 102*(3), e208036. https://doi.org/10.1212/WNL.0000000000208036

Sheppard, E. (2020). performing normal but becoming crip: Living with chronic pain. *Scandinavian Journal of Disability Research, 22*(1), 39–47. https://doi.org/10.16993/sjdr.619

Sheppard, E. (2022). *Crip time and crip joy* [YouTube]. Challenging disbelief and disregard. https://www.youtube.com/watch?v=360ir9gUFDQ

Smilges, J. L. (2023). *Crip negativity*. University of Minnesota Press. https://www.jstor.org/stable/10.5749/j.ctv2zfjd4z

Thaller, M., Homer, V., Hyder, Y., Yiangou, A., Liczkowski, A., Fong, A. W., Virdee, J., Piccus, R., Roque, M., Mollan, S. P., & Sinclair, A. J. (2023). The idiopathic intracranial hypertension prospective cohort study: Evaluation of prognostic factors and outcomes. *Journal of Neurology, 270*(2), 851–863. https://doi.org/10.1007/s00415-022-11402-6

Toshniwal, S. S., Kinkar, J., Chadha, Y., Khurana, K., Reddy, H., Kadam, A., & Acharya, S. (2024). Navigating the enigma: A comprehensive review of idiopathic intracranial hypertension. *Cureus*. https://doi.org/10.7759/cureus.56256

Wendell, S. (1996). *The rejected body: Feminist philosophical reflections on disability*. Routledge. https://doi.org/10.4324/9780203724149

Williams, G. (1984). The genesis of chronic illness: Narrative reconstruction. *Sociology of Health & Illness, 6*(2), 175–200. https://doi.org/10.1111/1467-9566.ep10778250

Williams, S. (2000). Chronic illness as biographical disruption or biographical disruption as chronic illness? Reflections on a core concept. *Sociology of Health & Illness, 22*(1), 40–67. https://doi.org/10.1111/1467-9566.00191

Witry, M., Kindler, C., Weller, J., Linder, A., & Wüllner, U. (2021). The patients' perspective on the burden of idiopathic intracranial hypertension. *The Journal of Headache and Pain, 22*(1), 67. https://doi.org/10.1186/s10194-021-01283-x

Woodard, C. (2022). The value and significance of ill-being. *Midwest Studies in Philosophy*. https://doi.org/10.5840/msp202212130

Wyckoff, M. M. (2007). *Living with intracranial hypertension: A phenomenological inquiry* [Ph.D., Barry University School of Nursing]. https://www.proquest.com/docview/304717356/abstract/5A09CC6302094EC9PQ/1

Yiangou, A., Mollan, S., & Sinclair, A. (2023). Idiopathic intracranial hypertension: A step change in understanding the disease mechanisms. *Nature Reviews, Neurology, 19*(12), 769–785. https://doi.org/10.1038/s41582-023-00893-0

Part IV

Temporal Recursivity

12

Multiple Temporalities of Lifestyle Change

Martine Robson and Sarah Riley

As non-communicable diseases become the leading cause of death worldwide, encouraging healthy lifestyle behaviours has become a global goal (WHO, 2023). Health promotion often presents lifestyle change as a simple process. Yet adherence to lifestyle change is low, indicating that it is neither easy nor simple, and thus research is needed to explore subtle processes involved in patterns of adoption, adherence, and resistance (Kotseva et al., 2019; Theis & White, 2021). To do this, we start by questioning linear models of time that are an under-examined, taken-for-granted element underpinning healthy lifestyle advice, and which implicitly imagine individuals progressing through sequential timescales as they implement new behaviours with the promise of future states of stable health. We propose instead Deleuze's philosophy of time, which conceptualises multiple, subjective temporalities which have important implications for health

M. Robson (✉)
Department of Psychology, Aberystwyth University, Aberystwyth, UK
e-mail: mtr1@aber.ac.uk

S. Riley
School of Psychology, Massey University, Wellington, New Zealand
e-mail: s.riley@massey.ac.nz

K. Kenny et al. (eds.), *Timescapes of Health, Illness and Care*,
https://doi.org/10.1007/978-981-96-7055-0_12

promotion and lifestyle advice (Robson & Riley 2019). We use this chapter to provide empirical support for our use of Deleuze's concepts through a poststructuralist analysis of how time was evoked within 35 longitudinal interviews with 22 people who were in long-term relationships where one partner had been newly diagnosed with coronary heart disease. In so doing, we show shifting temporalities that afforded a range of practices that could work for, as well as against, engagement in lifestyle change. We conclude that time is a powerful but under-theorised element in research relating to lifestyle change, and that drawing on Deleuze's philosophy of time to recognise how multiple, fluid, non-linear timescales shape lifestyle identities and behaviours can offer new, more affirmative directions for health promotion and healthy lifestyle advice.

Theorising Time in Health Subjectivities

Dominant health discourses construct health as a stable state, produced through adherence to a healthy lifestyle that, once achieved, must be maintained (Hansen & Easthope, 2007; Lupton, 2014). Within these discourses, time is absent, or only implicitly present in notions of becoming more or less healthy through reversible changes in lifestyle (e.g. the UK Better Health, formerly Change4life, campaign[1]). Although socio-cognitive approaches to lifestyle behaviour change have developed to include a wider range of individual and social 'factors' (Hagger et al., 2017; Leventhal et al., 2011) and produced some successful interventions and valuable insights (Rhodes et al., 2019), overall, government health promotion policies based on socio-cognitive models have had limited effectiveness at reducing unhealthy lifestyle behaviours (Hackett et al., 2018; Theis & White, 2021). We suggest that poststructural concepts offer a framework for exploring the more complex and subtle processes that underlie apparently straightforward decision-making and behaviours and propose that time forms an under-examined aspect of lifestyle change. We argue that considering the complexity of time in relation to health and lifestyle offers insights into factors that may enable or

[1] https://www.nhs.uk/healthier-families/

challenge people's ability to achieve and sustain lifestyle change (Fothergill et al., 2016; Kotseva et al., 2019; Robson & Riley, 2019).

Time is implicit in the linearity of common socio-cognitive approaches to lifestyle advice that conceptualise behaviour change as a response to health information (Mentrup et al., 2020). Cause-and-effect relationships between stimulus and motivation to action assume linear, unitary, and sequential temporal processes. Understandings of linear, unitary time also underpin individualistic advice predicated upon a present self who is flawed and needs to make lifestyle change in line with expert advice to achieve an ideal future self. Motivation is further provided through a feared future self who fails to follow such advice and who suffers ill-health and premature death as a result. Anxiety about the future thus shapes present experience (Adams et al., 2009).

Lifestyle change is thus conceptualised as a linear, agentic, rational process that individuals engage in. The logic of responsibility and therefore blame is also reinforced through these 'causal and deterministic time frames' (Robson & Riley, 2019). Abject bodies and identities are constructed for people who do not achieve or maintain weight loss, for example (Meleo Erwen, 2015; Tischner & Malson, 2012). The absence or assumed simplicity of temporal processes involved in healthy lifestyle behaviours further discounts lived experience of lifestyle change as effortful and non-linear and reinforces stigma for those whose lifestyles are constrained by individual and wider social factors, such as poverty (Warin et al., 2015; Williams, 2011). The assumed stability of a state of health achieved through engagement in healthy lifestyle also creates an absence of representations of death as natural or inevitable (Robson & Riley, 2019) or of the innate fluidity and fragility of health in the context of ageing (Garland-Thomson, 2011).

Mainstream academic literature dealing with patients' experience also rarely addresses issues of time (Stronge, 2012). In contrast, there is a limited but important literature applying poststructuralist theories of time to health (Coleman, 2008, 2010; Jowsey, 2016; Warin et al., 2015). For example, Annemarie Mol (1999) drew on Deleuze' theories to conceptualise patients' experiences of time in the context of anaemia, proposing that multiple, coexisting and distinct realities of disease 'are different versions, different performances, different realities that co-exist in the present'. This concept of parallel timescales has also been applied to health screening, which 'involves a dense multiplicity of durations' of past, present, and future health and illness that can 'trade places, blur, slide into one another, and occasionally come into conflict in an unending and fluid process' (Stronge, 2012). Similarly, in her study of temporalities of dieting, Coleman (2010) argued that different parts of dieting websites create multiple understandings of dieting that have clear temporal dimensions. For example, websites attempt to bring the future desired self/body temporally closer to the present self, while acknowledging that dieters will make multiple attempts to lose weight. In this way, such websites implicitly recognise and normalise fluid, multiple temporalities of diet and weight loss as people begin, abandon, and recommence their diets.

Although limited and scattered, poststructuralist-informed work, particularly that which draws on Deleuze's notion of multiple realities and temporalities of health, provides a useful framework for examining the multiple time frames in health-related sense making (McLeod, 2017). For example, Annemarie Mol (1999) argued that Foucault's assertion of the performativity and situatedness of reality is also predicated upon multiplicity, since 'if reality is done, if it is historically and culturally located, then it is also multiple'. Multiplicity involves many relations between conflicting or interdependent realities, accounting for complexity and unpredictability. Recognition of multiplicity thus affords a mapping of phenomena such as lifestyle change in the context of multiple time frames, including the trajectory of illness, diagnosis, treatment, and recovery, as well as people's lifespan and other disease and ageing processes.

Deleuze's theory of time is integrated into his metaphysics, but key features of his philosophy of time as multiple, parallel, subjective, and embodied affords a framework for understanding the complexity of lived experience of health, illness, and change (Deleuze, 1988; Duff, 2014; Robson & Riley, 2019; Williams, 2011). Drawing on Bergson's (1946, 2007) concept of duration, Deleuze challenged unitary, linear notions of time as an external force within which life is lived. In his concept of duration, Bergson (1921, 1999) conceptualised time as the unfolding of human subjectivity and experience, the process of becoming—'unceasing creation, the uninterrupted upsurge of novelty' (Bergson, 1946, 2007,

p. 16). Bergson thus also accounts for the coexistence of multiple temporalities, as multiple experiences and subjectivities unfold simultaneously. Traditional understandings of time are 'spatialised'—the past, present, and future are imagined as linear, unitary segments that succeed each other unidirectionally. Past, present, and future, rather than separated spatially, coexist in Deleuze's conceptualisation of a 'living present' in which past and future are experienced physically and affectively (Deleuze, 1988, 1994; Grosz, 2000; Loewen Walker, 2014). Fear of future illness or hope of future health, for example, are ways in which different futures are embodied in the present, a model of human experience of time as subjective, unfolding, embodied and affective. The different subjectivities that these multiple temporaries produce may account for parallel, different, and not mutually exclusive levels of engagement in lifestyle change.

The Study

Moving away from individualist approaches to health and health education that decontextualise the subject, our study took account of the social context of participants who were in long-term relationships and who had recently received a diagnosis of coronary heart disease. After NHS ethical approval was obtained, 35 longitudinal interviews were conducted at monthly intervals over three months with 22 people in long-term cohabiting relationships. The longitudinal design allowed for a mapping of participants' talk and experiences over time. Relationship length ranged from 15 to 50 years. Participants' ages ranged from early 50s to early 80s with a mean age of 63 years. All but three were of white British descent, which reflects the demographics of the recruitment area in West Wales. Audio-recorded interviews lasted between 30 and 90 minutes. Recordings were transcribed verbatim, with short or longer pauses indicated by (.) or (…), and anonymised, including using pseudonyms. Our analytic method used a combination of Foucauldian-informed discourse analysis and a Deleuzian 'mapping' (Alvermann, 2000; Riley et al., 2021; Ringrose, 2011). During this process we considered affect and assemblage in relation to what was enabled or blocked during interactions and recounted experiences. We noted and coded sections where participants talked about time, and the apparent contradictions and discontinuities in their talk, in relation to illness, recovery, aging and death. We then identified what ways of being or modes of experience were afforded by those temporalities (Brown et al., 2011). This was complicated by the different ways a topic was talked about, often in the same interview. For example, a participant might construct death as fearful, and their diagnosis and treatment as a lucky escape, which warrants their engagement in lifestyle change. But when considering their lifespan and balancing the value of rigorous adherence to a healthy lifestyle, death might offer a more accepting, fatalistic standpoint, from which an anxious concern with avoiding pleasurable but risky food seemed futile. These apparent contradictions would have been difficult to resolve into a unitary narrative of health identity, but Bergson and Deleuze's concepts allowed us to make sense of the multiple temporalities in participants' talk, and attempt to capture their vivid evocations of the coexistence of present, past, and future, virtual and actual, and multiple durations of subjective experience, such as distinct but parallel time-frames of illness, recovery, and aging.

Analysis

Participants described their experience of time in relation to health and illness, through three discourses: lifestyle change as multiple, unfixed and unfolding; recovery as involving temporal selves and plural time frames of recovery; and that death comes to us all. Below, we examine how couples' talk in these discourses constructed fluidity and uncertainty against a backdrop of wider discourses of health and healthy living as stable and controllable. We connect this analysis to Deleuze's argument for the coexistence and accessibility of past and future when he wrote that 'there is no present that is not haunted by a past and a future, by a past that is not reducible to a former present, by a future that does not consist of a present to come' (2005, p.36). This concept of time affords a recognition of coexisting and distinct realities of disease as 'different versions, different performances, different realities that co-exist in the present' (Mol, 1999, p.79), and provides a framework for thinking about the ways that participants drew on past, present, and future selves in their negotiations of lifestyle change.

Lifestyle Change: Multiple, Unfixed, and Unfolding

Participants made time salient in the way that they constructed lifestyle change as inherently short term and unsustainable. But time was also an element in the fluidity with which they switched between different constructions as they negotiated contradictory understandings of lifestyle change as simultaneously effortful and easy, valuable and futile, negative but also affirmative. Participants adopted and resisted these conflicting discourses over an interview or series of interviews, and even sometimes in the same interchange. From a Deleuzian standpoint, the dynamism of participants' health interactions can be understood as an unfolding of novel relations rather than a predictable pattern of behaviour. An example of this dynamic can be seen in the extract below that focused on the sustainability of joint and individual engagement in exercise that represented a pattern in the data set of participants talking positively about the value of exercise in opening up new capacities and ways of being, but simultaneously constructing it as effortful, not fully within their control, and ultimately short term and unlikely to be sustained. When asked whether they would continue to attend the classes after the end of the exercise programme, this ambiguity, multiplicity, and fluidity was reflected in the following equivocal reply:

George:	I think probably so um
Susan:	yeah (.) oh yes I should imagine so I mean how how long we
George:	whether we do it twice a week or
Susan:	um (.) um sense of gratefulness on your part to have come through it and the sense of um wanting to exercise parts of our body through repetition movements will carry us to further along the road I don't know (.) uh I I I'd like to think we do
George:	mm
Susan:	we would do it
George:	it does get
Susan:	yeah
George:	a little boring

Above, George and Susan (mid-60s, retired public service workers) negotiate negative and positive formulations of exercise in their considerations of continued attendance. Lifestyle change is necessarily future oriented (Hansen & Easthope 2007) and above, this future orientation encompassed hopes and fears that created ambivalence about the sustainability of their engagement in exercise. In their reflection on whether they would continue to attend, there was uncertainty shown in their hedging 'I think probably so', and 'I should imagine'. In these imaginings, George and Susan's future selves moved in and out of the gym as they spoke; they wavered between motivators such as gratitude, a sense of duty, the hope of greater physical capacities, and the demotivating admission that they experienced exercise regimes as boring. An admission that ultimately offered the possibility to not continue with the exercise. The coexistence of both negative and positive evaluations of lifestyle change thus had implications for the sustainability of activities such as the exercise class, and is an example of how the productive, affirmative experiences of cardiac rehabilitation can coexist with its disciplinary and sometimes oppressive dimensions. In her study of a cardiac rehabilitation clinic in the United States, Wheatley (2005), for example, reported how patients negotiated their own desires and priorities alongside the regime of the clinic, producing fluid positions and practices, as well as power relations.

Deleuze's concept of dynamic assemblages and multiplicity accounts for the fluid, ephemeral, and apparent contradictions and inconsistencies that were traceable in our participants' talk about health. Material elements of assemblages of health and lifestyle, such as the weather, and the negative as well as positive affective experiences of the rehabilitation class, food and eating habits all contributed to lifestyle as a complex, unpredictable, and ever changing; in contrast to public health campaigns that construct lifestyle change as simple to achieve and maintain. Talk of illness and recovery and lifespan also formed fluid but distinct time frames as we explore below.

Temporal Selves: Plural Time Frames of Recovery

Participants referred to multiple timescales in relation to recovery, ageing and other disease processes and diagnoses which coexisted in dynamic relation to each other, and facilitated management, acceptance, stoicism, and the assertion of values other than the narrow pursuit of health through healthy lifestyle. Temporalities of recovery and aging could be affirmative, though these affirmative constructions were complicated by parallel discourses of ageing and loss of function. Carl (late 60s retired office worker), for example, had been extremely active throughout his life; he cycled, walked, and worked on his house and garden, and had even been 'told off' for over-exerting himself in the cardiac rehabilitation class. In the following extract, Carl reflected on his recovery, fitness, and health, drawing on his past and present, as well as his hopes for the future:

Carl: well I the concern is you (...) there doesn't seem to be an end stop on what you can do er (.) for me er erm and so there is a danger you've still got old age there there is a danger you can (.) over do it which I would probably be guilty of lots of stuff but erm (...) er that that's the only thing you you you do have to remember you're 65 or whatever it is and er (.) but er you know (.) generally speaking I've got er so much more energy than I ever well probably ever had

Int: really

Carl: I was gonna say or should I say ever can remember ((laughs)) that's probably nearer the mark I I don't feel I've lost anything from when I was young er that's how it is (.) er you feel as though you've got a new engine unburstable and er off you go you know see what happens (...) on the negative side (.) I I do still feel tired sometimes or quite quite I'll say quite often you know erm but that probably is the old age thing recovery takes longer when you're older and as you will find out ((Laughter))

Carl talked about old age and its capacities in fluid and apparently contradictory ways, oscillating between affirmative affects of increased powers, in which his physical capabilities had not diminished from his youth to more conventional discourses of old age as marked by risks and deficits. He began with an affirmative statement of the fluid possibilities of old age, echoing Deleuze's sense of the body's possibilities and powers 'there doesn't seem to be an end stop to what you can do', but after this statement he equates old age with risk in his repetition of the 'danger' of over-exertion. His drawing on a normative, moral framework to such overdoing, 'I would probably be guilty of', reinforced the boundaries of age-appropriate behaviour that he contravened in the exercise class. He then immediately contradicted such age-related norms when he asserted that his energy levels exceeded those of his youth, which was counterbalanced with his joke about his memory, which again asserted a more stereotypical association of old age with deficit. Switching back to his more affirmative standpoint, Carl then repeated his claim to have experienced no decline in his physical powers, with his striking, powerful construction of his mended heart as an 'unburstable engine'. This claim to increased capacities thus troubled notions of time and the ageing processes as linear and tending towards deficit and loss. Yet Carl followed this with a statement about his concurrent, embodied experience of tiredness, which he normalized in his attribution of tiredness to 'the old age thing'.

As we have shown above, Carl continuously switched between coexisting realities that would usually be considered conflicting or mutually exclusive. His experience of ageing encompassed a chronological age in his mid-60s, but a sense that his capacities were the same as a younger man, a dissonance he bridged by asserting that old age is a time when powers can be undiminished, and that he still possessed the physical capacities of his youth. Bergson and Deleuze's theories of time offer a resolution for these apparently contradictory experiences and constructions. They proposed that time can be thought of as the unfolding of subjective experience. The multiplicity of experience therefore produces distinct 'durations' that coexist, a fluidity that people then negotiate, as Carl's extract demonstrated.

The participants' talk about health also indicated more ineffable ways in which processes of aging as well as recovery shaped engagement with lifestyle change. This included patterns of ambivalence around recovery and increasing vitality. Such multiplicity and unpredictability in couples' health interactions were also present in Catherine and Henry's (mid-60s, semi-retired skilled and retired office worker) three interviews. Their interactions appeared gentle and supportive. Catherine was intimately involved in Henry's health, and monitored and managed his dietary changes, though she had limited mobility and was unable to take part in his exercise classes. As he recovered, however, and talked about his improving fitness, Catherine repeatedly responded with talk about her past as an athlete and sports coach, contrasting this with and emphasising Henry's lack of physical capacity or sporting prowess. For example, when Henry was talking about his exercise class, which he enjoyed and felt was benefiting his health:

Henry:	I just get a a a bit of a sweat on so it's obviously doing some good
Catherine:	I find Henry gets treder now he he's slowed down quite a bit to when I first er worked with him years ago

Henry equated physical exertion with improving health in his vivid evocation of his strength and physicality as he worked up a sweat during exercise. Catherine countered Henry's positive, embodied experience with a claim about his tiredness and physical decline in comparison with his past physical capacities; and referred to her own past as a sports coach invoking her strength and equality at a time when she 'worked with' him.

MacLean et al. (2014) reported an unexpected finding that some women were ambivalent about their male partner's weight loss, anxious that their newly slim and fit partner might be attracted by or attractive to other women. Developing this work, we account for such patterns by drawing on Deleuzian notion of assemblages as made up of virtual as well as actual components, exemplified in the drawing out of a virtual self in Catherine's affective response. The self who cannot take part in the exercise class coexisted in her account with the powerful athlete and teacher. Henry and Catherine's interchanges indicated the unpredictable, multiple affective flows within the assemblage of Henry's health. He was at once the patient who had a life-threatening cardiac event, necessitating dietary change and caution with physical activity which Catherine anxiously monitored, but also the attender of cardiac rehabilitation and gym classes which had opened new capacities for him. His exercise regime highlighted and widened the gap between their relative physicality; he was clearly fitter than her now, and his engagement in cardiac rehabilitation illuminated deficits and differences as well as new strengths and possibilities, which they had to negotiate. Catherine oriented to his physical strength as a troubling disparity in their physical capacities, a gap which she worked to equalize or diminish by bringing the past into the present.

In their last interview, however, there was a break in the pattern of Catherine's affective responses to talk of Henry's physicality. Catherine recounted a recent family walk to a nearby beach and hill. Henry and the younger members of the family climbed the hill, and Catherine made her first acknowledgement of Henry's recovery and regained capacities:

Catherine: we went went down on our favourite all of our favourite the whole family er always used to go to [the beach] and the younger ones erm Henry walked up the top you know and erm (.) onto the beach er (.) and he managed ok didn't you

Her account of Henry's successful climb positioned him with the 'younger ones', but despite this categorisation, her use of 'all', 'whole family', and 'we' also created a sense of unity and togetherness. With this acceptance of his recovery, Catherine also acknowledged her own more limited capacities:

Catherine: I used to go up there I don't go up there now [...] yeah we the rest of us the old crocks down at the bottom sat there waving and they were waving back you know

The emotions implicit in and evoked by Catherine's positioning of herself among the 'old crocks' at the bottom of the hill, waving to the younger and fitter members of the family were fluid and multiple. There was both a poignant sense of loss, but also of acceptance of changing times and capacities in the balance of 'I used to go up there I don't go up there now', and the disdainful but also humorous designation of herself and her siblings as 'old crocks'. However, the space between the younger and older people was bridged by affection and communication, as Catherine 'sat there waving and they were waving back', her use of 'you know' signalling the normality of this situation. This extract is illustrative of the multiplicity and complexity of such embodied, affective experiences and temporalities that were present across the data, and which resisted clear categorisations and evaluations. Our participants constructed health as a moving horizon in their recovery from their diagnosis and treatment of CHD. They drew on multiple temporalities in their accounts, constructing past experiences and capacities as affecting their present functioning and future hopes. The joint endeavour of couples' health (Robson et al., 2023) compounded this complexity, as participants negotiated the fluidity of their own and their partner's experiences and expectations of recovery, lifestyle, and health. Participants also constructed affirmative temporalities relating to lifespan and death, perhaps surprisingly in the context of our cultural fear of dying. As we show below, these accounts transformed health advice and discourses that invoke fear of death to motivate adherence to lifestyle change.

Death Comes to Us All

A focus on health brings its corollary and a greater sense of jeopardy (Bauman, 2000; Crawford, 2006), especially in health promotion that confines any references to illness and death to fear-evoking warnings (Lupton, 2014; Petersen & Wilkinson, 2008). In dominant health discourses, death is the antithesis of life, the endpoint against which people struggle, which creates fearful, deficit discourses of aging and death. Yet our participants oriented to more than just this deficit discourse of death. Their diagnoses of heart disease brought awareness of mortality, and they acknowledged fear and distress. But death was also constructed in affirmative ways, offering a perspective on life, issues and problems (including those relating to lifestyle change), wisdom and acceptance. For Deleuze, death is part of life, not its opposite, it is 'coextensive with life … living is inseparable from the partial deaths that it goes through' (Colombat, 1996). Deleuze also argued that even when we die, 'one is nonetheless affirmed as an individual'. In life, because death is always ahead of us, it is 'a virtual that never gets accomplished—we are always in the process of but never complete dying' which is 'essential to the creation and proliferation of life and thought' (ibid., p. 242). Such a concept of death affords a mapping of the creative and affirmative evocations of death in participants' accounts, such as when awareness of death was used to warrant a zest for living, and a hedonistic rather than a puritan way of life, we return to George and Susan below for an example:

George: yeah I'm happy to do moderation I'm not happy to cut things out (..) I'm still not happy about those absent fried breakfasts I mean we'll occasionally have them
Susan: yeah occasionally
George: we stayed in one of these Premier Hotels
Susan: oh gosh and tuck into them like there's you know no tomorrow
George: eat as much as you like breakfast …
Susan: oh a real treat yeah and that's it it's moderation
George: I know I won't cut it out completely I'm not going to be a puritan about it I don't see the point because it's something in life I actually enjoy and I mean if it has to be written on his tombstone you know he continued to eat the occasional fried breakfast ((laughter)) then I'll settle for that but I'm not going to ((laughing)) (…) I don't care that's fine erm (…) having survived this long (…) you know (…)

In this extract, shifting temporalities afforded different and contradictory constructions and practices of dietary management. Initially, George adopted the discourse of moderating rather than eliminating unhealthy items from one's diet, but immediately qualified his statement that he's 'happy to do moderation', when he expressed his unhappiness at the deprivation of the 'absent fried breakfasts'. They were still desired, and their absence was fluid; they were still indulged in 'occasionally'. Susan and George vividly evoked the pleasure they both took in such breakfasts through their laughter and emotive exclamations 'oh gosh' and 'oh a real treat'. The temporality that allowed such abandonment of restraint was a present disconnected from future consequences, 'tuck into them like there's you know no tomorrow'. This hedonism was a temporary line of flight away from dominant understandings of certain foods as risky and in need of control, but it was soon fenced in with time-related modifiers, 'occasionally' and 'it's moderation' in a reassertion of health promotion values of self-discipline. But George also referred to his future death, what will be 'written on his gravestone', to provide a perspective on the self-denial of the present. In a cost–benefit analysis, at that moment George came down on the side of hedonism and pleasure, an acceptance of risk, and freedom if not from judgement, at least from anxiety about such a judgement, 'I'll settle for that … I don't care'.

Death was also invoked in ways that afforded peace of mind amid the anxieties of ill-health. Deleuze conceptualised this position as a 'third axis' that coexists with Foucauldian conceptualisations of power and knowledge and which allows a resolution, however brief, of their impasses and power relations, 'the place where a sense of serenity would finally be attained and life truly affirmed' (Deleuze, 2006, p. 80). At points, some participants appeared to access such serenity and acceptance, as in the extract below, where Louise (late 60s, self-employed professional) deterritorialised the limitations and unfulfilled promise of health injunctions:

Louise: yeah I always yell at my husband about you need to eat three times a day you need to exercise at least three times a week you need to go to bed at a regular hour you need to get up at a regular hour you need to take care of yourself (.) and then who winds up with a heart attack and so it's like what did I do and the first thing I started to cry the other day when I was with [nurse] and I said what did I do wrong she says you didn't do anything wrong she says Louise if this is genetics you did nothing it just happened just like it's you know trees get leaves trees lose leaves trees get leaves trees lose leaves one branch might grow bigger than the other branch it's part of the tree and and it's the same thing with me and as long as I can stay on top of that thought I'm okay

Louise's extract started with her past practices in line with dominant understandings of a linear, causal relationship between lifestyle and CHD. She had imposed all the 'rules' on herself and her husband, so her illness left her questioning an understanding of disease that positioned her as responsible and culpable. In her adoption of the tenets of healthy living, she could not get outside of the discourse, and was trapped in the painful logic of causality and culpability, 'I started to cry ... what did I do wrong?'. The nurse's reassurance offered her an alternative conceptualisation of health and illness that constructed them as cyclical, natural, unpredictable, and uncontrollable. When she equated herself with trees that gain and lose leaves, her illness, and by implication, her eventual death, became inevitable, a natural phenomenon, removed from the distress of causality or blame. Louise's peace of mind was fragile, lasting only 'as long as I can stay on top of that thought', but however briefly, this acceptance of natural, cyclical processes and her lack of agency in them calmed her guilt and anxiety, and produced a serene perspective.

Discussion

A mapping of Deleuzian concepts of time showed that in patients' and partners' talk about lifestyle change, multiple temporal selves were constructed within plural time frames of recovery, including histories and imagined futures. These shifting temporalities afforded multiple subject positions and legitimised a range of practices that could work both for and against engagement in lifestyle change. These patterns of adoption and resistance demonstrated a temporal complexity that is largely absent in health promotion and lifestyle advice, and illuminated how people can be oppressed by linear discourses of healthy living whose logic of blame produces spoiled identities and abject bodies. However, the multiplicity and non-linearity of participants' experienced also opened up new possibilities and hopeful affects, such an acceptance of illness, ageing, and death as natural processes, which buffered against fear, self-blame, and uncertainty.

In contrast to healthy living discourses that promote health as simple, achievable, and sustainable through rationally chosen lifestyle behaviours that achieve a stable state (Stronge, 2012), couples in this study negotiated healthy living as fluid, effortful, and ultimately, short term. An inability to maintain diets or exercise regimes can evoke blame, guilt, and frustration as individuals perceive this as a failure which reflects on their own identity. In contrast we suggest that health and healthy living can be understood as fluid and unfolding rather than predictable and controllable. And that acceptance of uncertainty, rather than producing passive or fatalistic disengagement (Adams et al., 2009), can increase capacities and positive, hopeful affects (Massumi, 2003; Vogel & Mol, 2014), such as serenity, self-acceptance, and pleasure from eating and exercise. In our data, death, rather than being a feared endpoint, could provide a perspective on life, a philosophical standpoint from which excessive concern about the minutiae of daily lifestyle habits may not be prioritised. Other positions and practices become more valued from this viewpoint. Acceptance, resignation, and hedonism are all put forward as appropriate responses to the contemplation of death, all of which may work against a conscientious adherence to lifestyle change and rigorously healthy living.

Deleuzian concepts afforded a mapping of the multiplicity and fluidity of participants' accounts which were full of ephemerality and change. Such complexity is not so chaotic as to be impervious to study and understanding, however, and conceptualising the multiplicity, unpredictability, and dynamism of lifestyle-related health interactions can account for the affirmative as well as negative ramifications of lifestyle advice. There are implications for health promotion and clinical practice that encompass the complexity of embodied and affective experiences of time. For example, although the focus of this study was not on patient-clinician communication, there were examples of affirmative interactions between health-care professionals, such as when the cardiac nurse's acknowledgement of health and illness as natural processes functioned to lift Louise's burden of guilt and anxiety over the cause of her heart disease.

Our findings demonstrate that time is very salient in people's lived experience of adopting and resisting lifestyle change, and this finding sits in contrast to lifestyle advice where time is rarely considered. By illuminating how reductive traditional, linear, notions of time limit understanding of processes involved in lifestyle change, Deleuze's conceptual framework points to new and more affirmative directions for health promotion and future research that encompass the temporal as well as social, physical, and emotional complexity of health behaviours.

Acknowledgments This chapter draws on work completed and submitted as part of Martine Robson's PhD thesis at Aberystwyth University.

Competing Interests The authors have no conflicts of interest to declare that are relevant to the content of this chapter.

References

Adams, V., Murphy, M., & Clarke, A. (2009). Anticipation: Technoscience, life, affect, temporality. *Subjectivity, 28*(1), 246–265. https://doi.org/10.1057/sub.2009.18

Alvermann, D. (2000). Researching libraries, literacies, and lives: A rhizoanalysis. In *Working the ruins: Feminist poststructural theory and methods in education*. Routledge.

Bauman. (2000). *Liquid modernity*. Polity Press.

Bergson, H. (1921). *Duration and simultaneity, with reference to Einstein's theory*. Clinamen Press.

Bergson, H. (1946). *The creative mind: An introduction to metaphysics*. Dover Publications Inc..

Bergson, H. (1999). *Duration and simultaneity, with reference to Einstein's theory*. Clinamen Press.

Bergson, H. (2007). *The creative mind: An introduction to metaphysics*. Dover Publications Inc..

Brown, S., Cromby, J., Harper, D., Johnson, K., & Reavey, P. (2011). Researching "experience": Embodiment, methodology, process. *Theory & Psychology, 21*(4), 493–515. https://doi.org/10.1177/0959354310377543

Coleman, R. (2008). "Things that stay": Feminist theory, duration and the future. *Time & Society, 17*(1), 85–102. https://doi.org/10.1177/0961463X07086303

Coleman, R. (2010). Dieting temporalities: Interaction, agency and the measure of online weight watching. *Time & Society, 19*(2), 265–285. https://doi.org/10.1177/0961463X10368918

Colombat, A. P. (1996). November 4, 1995: Deleuze's death as an event. *Man and World, 29*, 235–249. https://doi.org/10.1007/BF01248435

Crawford, R. (2006). Health as a meaningful social practice. *International Journal of Health Services, 10*(3), 401–420. https://doi.org/10.1177/1363459306067310

Deleuze, G. (1988). *Bergsonism*. Zone Books.

Deleuze, G. (1994). Difference and repetition. (P. Patton, Trans.). Columbia University Press.

Deleuze, G. (2005). Cinema 2: The time-image. (H. Tomlinson, & R. Galeta, Trans.). Continuum.

Deleuze, G. (2006). *Two regimes of madness: Texts and interviews 1975–1995*. Columbia University Press.
Duff, C. (2014). *Assemblages of health: Deleuze's empiricism and the ethology of life*. Springer. https://doi.org/10.1007/978-94-017-8893-9
Fothergill, E., Guo, J., Howard, L., Kerns, J., Knuth, N., Brychta, R., et al. (2016). Persistent metabolic adaptation 6 years after "The Biggest Loser" competition. *Obesity, 24*(8), 1612–1629. https://doi.org/10.1002/oby.21538
Garland-Thomson, R. (2011). Misfits, A feminist materialist disability concept. *Hypatia, 26*(3), 591–609. https://doi.org/10.1111/j.1527-2001.2011.01206.x
Grosz, E. (2000). Deleuze's Bergson: Duration, the virtual and the politics of the future. In I. Buchanan & C. Colebrook (Eds.), *Deleuze and feminist theory*. Edinburgh University Press.
Hackett, R., Moore, C., Steptoe, A., & Lassale, C. (2018). Health behaviour changes after type 2 diabetes diagnosis: Findings from the English longitudinal study of ageing. *Scientific Reports, 8*(1), 16938. https://doi.org/10.1038/s41598-018-35238-1
Hagger, M., Koch, S., Chatzisarantis, N., & Orbell, S. (2017). The common sense model of self-regulation: Meta-analysis and test of a process model. *Psychological Bulletin, 143*(11), 1117–1154. https://doi.org/10.1037/bul0000118
Hansen, E., & Easthope, G. (2007). *Lifestyle in medicine*. Routledge.
Jowsey, T. (2016). Time and chronic illness: A narrative review. *Quality of Life Research, 25*(5), 1093–1102. https://doi.org/10.1007/s11136-015-1169-2
Kotseva, K., et al. (2019). Lifestyle and impact on cardiovascular risk factor control in coronary patients across 27 countries: Results from the European Society of Cardiology ESC-EORP EUROASPIRE V registry. *European Journal of Preventive Cardiology, 26*(8), 824–835. https://doi.org/10.1177/2047487318825350
Leventhal, H., Leventhal, E. A., & Breland, J. (2011). Cognitive science speaks to the "common-sense" of chronic illness management. *Annals of Behavioral Medicine, 41*(2), 152–163. https://doi.org/10.1007/s12160-010-9246-9
Loewen Walker, R. (2014). The living present as a materialist feminist temporality. *Women: A Cultural Review, 25*(1), 46–61. https://doi.org/10.1080/09574042.2014.901107
Lupton, D. (2014). "How do you measure up?" Assumptions about "obesity" and health-related behaviors and beliefs in two Australian "obesity" prevention campaigns. *Fat Studies, 3*(1), 32–44. https://doi.org/10.1080/21604851.2013.784050

MacLean, A., Hunt, K., Gray, C., Smillie, S., & Wyke, S. (2014). How do men's female relatives feature in their accounts of changing eating practices during a weight management programme delivered through professional football clubs? *International Journal of Men's Health, 13*(2), 121. https://doi.org/10.1186/1471-2458-14-50

Massumi, B. (2003). *An interview with Brian Massumi* (M. Zournazi, Interviewer) Retrieved from The Open University Research Projects http://www.theport.tv/wp/pdf/pdf1.pdf

McLeod, K. (2017). *Wellbeing machine: How health emerges from the assemblages of everyday life*. University of Tasmania. https://hdl.handle.net/102.100.100/539362

Meleo Erwen, Z. (2015). Shape carries story: Navigating the world as fat. *M/C Journal, 18*(3) http://journal.media-culture.org.au/index.php/mcjournal/article/view/978

Mentrup, S., Harris, E., Gomersall, T., Köpke, S., & Astin, F. (2020). Patients' experiences of cardiovascular health education and risk communication: A qualitative synthesis. *Qualitative Health Research, 30*(1), 88–104. https://doi.org/10.1177/1049732319887949

Mol, A. (1999). Ontological politics. A word and some questions. *The Sociological Review, 47*(1), 74–89. https://doi.org/10.1111/j.1467-954X.1999.tb03483.x

Petersen, A., & Wilkinson, I. (2008). Health, risk and vulnerability: An introduction. In A. Petersen & I. Wilkinson (Eds.), *Health, risk and vulnerability*. Routledge.

Rhodes, R., McEwan, D., & Rebar, A. (2019). Theories of physical activity behaviour change: A history and synthesis of approaches. *Psychology of Sport and Exercise, 42*, 100–109. https://doi.org/10.1016/j.psychsport.2018.11.010

Riley, S., Robson, M., & Evans, A. (2021). Foucauldian-informed discourse analysis. In M. Bamburg, C. Demuth, & M. Watalawik (Eds.), *Cambridge handbook of identity* (pp. 285–303). Cambridge University Press.

Ringrose, J. (2011). Beyond discourse? Using Deleuze and Guattari's schizoanalysis to explore affective assemblages, heterosexually striated space, and lines of flight online and at school. *Educational Philospphy and Theory, 43*(6), 598–618. https://doi.org/10.1111/j.1469-5812.2009.00601.x

Robson, M., & Riley, S. (2019). A Deleuzian rethinking of time in healthy lifestyle advice and change. *Social and Personality Psychology Compass, 13*(4), e12448. https://doi.org/10.1111/spc3.12448

Robson, M., Riley, S., Gagen, E., & McKeogh, D. (2023). Love and lifestyle: How 'relational healthism' structures couples' talk of engagement with lifestyle advice associated with a new diagnosis of coronary heart disease. *Psychology & Health, 38*(12), 1606–1622. https://doi.org/10.1080/08870446.2022.2033240

Stronge, P. (2012). A confusion of tenses: Health screening and time. *Health, 17*(4), 340–357. https://doi.org/10.1177/1363459312460700

Theis, D. R., & White, M. (2021). Is obesity policy in England fit for purpose? Analysis of government strategies and policies, 1992–2020. *The Milbank Quarterly, 99*(1), 126–170. https://doi.org/10.1111/1468-0009.12498

Tischner, I., & Malson, H. (2012). Deconstructing health and the un/healthy fat woman. *Journal of Community and Applied Social Psychology, 22*(1), 50–62. https://doi.org/10.1002/casp.1096

Vogel, E., & Mol, A. (2014). Enjoy your food: On losing weight and taking pleasure. *Sociology of Health and Illness, 36*(2), 305–317. https://doi.org/10.1111/1467-9566.12116

Warin, M., Zivkovic, T., Moore, V., Ward, P., & Jones, M. (2015). Short horizons and obesity futures: Disjunctures between public health interventions and everyday temporalities. *Social Science and Medicine, 128*, 309–315. https://doi.org/10.1016/j.socscimed.2015.01.026

Wheatley, E. (2005). Discipline and resistance: Order and disorder in a cardiac rehabilitation clinic. *Qualitative Health Research, 15*(4), 438–459. https://doi.org/10.1177/1049732304273044

Williams, J. (2011). *Gilles Deleuze's philosophy of time*. Edinburgh University Press.

World Health Organization. (2023). Non-communicable diseases. https://www.who.int/health-topics/noncommunicable-diseases#tab=tab_1

13

Haunting Diagnosis: Identity, Temporality, and Futures in Light of ADHD

Sebastián Rojas-Navarro and Samanta Alarcón-Arcos

Diagnoses wield significant power, capable of profoundly influencing how we perceive ourselves, interact with others, and navigate our futures. While they offer valuable insights into our experiences and struggles, they can also distance us from our social environments and relationships. This is particularly true for children, who are especially sensitive to the impact of diagnoses (Merten et al., 2017). The potential detrimental consequences of labelling children with mental health conditions have

S. Rojas-Navarro (✉)
Faculty of Education & Social Sciences, Universidad Andrés Bello, Santiago, Chile

Millennium Institute for Care Research (MICARE), Santiago, Chile
e-mail: sebastian.rojas.n@unab.cl

S. Alarcón-Arcos
Instituto de Sociología, Pontificia Universidad Católica de Chile, Santiago, Chile
e-mail: salarcon2@uc.cl

K. Kenny et al. (eds.), *Timescapes of Health, Illness and Care*,
https://doi.org/10.1007/978-981-96-7055-0_13

contributed to a certain reluctance in Western societies to pursue such diagnoses for the young. This hesitancy stems from concerns that exposure to these labels and categories at an early age may distort children's life experiences, ultimately shaping their futures in ways that might be unanticipated or unintended (Rojas-Navarro & Rojas, 2021).

In this chapter, we delve into the hauntological role of mental health diagnoses for children attending Chilean schools, using the case of the diagnosis of Attention Deficit/Hyperactivity Disorder, or ADHD. We turn to the notion of hauntology as this concept proves particularly useful to examine themes of temporality and spectrality in relation to health, illness, diagnoses, and care. Hauntology reveals that care is never straightforward, but rather imbued with profound ambivalence, haunted by the spectres of what once was or what never came to be (Broom et al., 2020; Harrison et al., 2024; Rojas-Navarro et al., 2024).

Our intention is to explore how hauntological thinking can provide an alternative framework for understanding how the ADHD diagnosis haunts the child in different ways, eventually pushing forward a sense of identity stagnation regarding the diagnosed child. We argue that ADHD, as a diagnosis, entails a reconfiguration of temporal experience—an enmeshment with time that is marked by a specific form of temporal recursiveness. These modifications have significant implications for diagnosed children's health trajectories and their possibility to be cared for. By altering the perception and management of time, the diagnosis potentially influences how children's developmental paths are understood and addressed, impacting both their immediate care and long-term well-being. We argue for the importance of understanding the myriad forces and contextual dynamics shaping the spectre of ADHD diagnosis in Chilean schools, and the relevance of incorporating these ghosts and hauntings to create something unique and transformative.

We begin by surveying pertinent literature on diagnoses, their impact, and the evolving societal perspectives surrounding them. Our focus then narrows to a specific and contentious diagnosis: Attention Deficit/Hyperactivity Disorder (ADHD), a subject of much debate in Chile and globally. We examine the diagnosis before delving into hauntological literature to shed light on particular dimensions of ADHD, namely its temporality and its link to identity. Subsequently, we introduce our fieldwork, contextualizing it within the framework of the Chilean educational system. This sets the stage for an analysis of vignettes, where we explore how hauntology offers a valuable perspective on their interpretation and circulation. We conclude by advocating not for the abandonment of diagnoses altogether but for their reorientation to amplify the voices of the ghosts and spectres that haunt the child through the diagnosis. We argue that paying attention to and caring for the forces and dynamics that drive, shape, and imbue the diagnosis, and accompany the child, is also an ethical and political positioning. It is a way of recognizing and attuning to issues that require care and attention.

Disclosing the Many Facets of Mental Health Diagnoses

Scholars and lay people have engaged in extensive discussions regarding the profound implications of medical diagnoses (Armstrong, 2011; Jutel & Nettleton, 2011; Rose, 2013). According to Jutel (2019), diagnoses stand as formidable tools within the domain of medicine, possessing the transformative capacity to reshape the dynamic between the subject undergoing diagnosis and the expert wielding diagnostic authority. This transformative potential extends beyond the systematic organization and categorization of diverse illnesses to include both the reconfiguration of bodily experience and the facilitation of access to essential resources and therapeutic interventions.

Amidst the myriad conditions and ailments that may prompt a diagnosis, mental health disorders have garnered significant attention. Their prevalence and societal visibility appear to have surged in recent decades, leading to profound transformations in our everyday experiences (Rose, 2018). Yet, their prevalence in contemporary discourse has come with increasing scrutiny. Brinkmann (2016) posits that these diagnoses have assumed a cultural intermediary role, serving as tools through which professionals, experts, and laypersons navigate and interpret their own experiences and those of others in everyday life. Interestingly, for Brinkmann and other scholars, such a Nikolas Rose (2013), the examination of the current role of mental health diagnoses necessitates a departure from traditional modes of critique.

While traditional critical approaches focus primarily on how biomedicine and mental health diagnoses can foster coercion and control, current modes of critique also highlight the multifaceted nature of our interactions with mental health categories. Rather than viewing diagnoses solely as problems to be disciplined or corrected by the medical apparatus, these contemporary approaches allow us to recognize how diagnoses also enable modes of sociality (Bradley, 2021), citizenship and political action (Rose & Novas, 2007), and care (Rojas-Navarro et al., 2023) through everyday and shared practices.

However, some resistance has been reported on mental health diagnoses for children, since it might lead to stigma (Ohan et al., 2011; Iudici & Faccio, 2013), labelling, and even exclusion (Singh, 2004; Blum, 2015, Fried & Plotkin-Amrami, 2023), all of which may meaningfully impact their futures. A substantial body of literature has examined the potential drawbacks associated with diagnosing children with mental health conditions (Mukolo et al., 2010). Moreover, evidence suggests a pervasive increase in the prevalence of mental health conditions, prompting concerns about potential overdiagnosis, particularly regarding conditions such as ADHD, often driven by demands from educational institutions for academic purposes (Kazda et al., 2021; Rojas-Navarro et al., 2018a, 2018b). While this may happen, a diagnosis may also serve as crucial tool for understanding, supporting, and caring for children and helping them attain their own best possible futures.

The Case of Attention-Deficit Hyperactivity Disorder

The heightened interest in ADHD within discussions of the global circulation of biomedical diagnoses stems from multiple and complex reasons. The increasing prevalence of ADHD has raised concerns among social scientists, who argue that standardized models, such as those outlined in the Diagnostic and Statistical Manual of Mental Disorders (DSM), impose culturally specific norms onto diverse local communities (Jain & Orr, 2016). They contend that this process reshapes both medical and public perceptions of specific behaviours and conduct (Rojas-Navarro & Filipe, 2023). However, evidence also reveals that outside the United States, different communities have adopted the diagnosis while transforming and adapting it to various cultural settings (Smith, 2017). On an individual level, debates surrounding the diagnosis centre on what Singh has termed the 'ambiguous nature' of its core symptoms and the ethical considerations surrounding its pharmaceutical treatment (Singh, 2004).

Notably, others argue that the real challenge lies not in the diagnosis itself, but in the behaviours and cultural perceptions associated with it, particularly in settings like schools (Muller et al., 2012). Despite these differing views, there is a consensus that reframing these behaviours and traits as medical issues, rather than moral or personal flaws, may foster more supportive and constructive interactions between children and their communities (Hawthorne, 2010; Singh, 2011; Rojas-Navarro & Rojas, 2019).

While we acknowledge the complexities of these debates, our analysis focuses on the temporal effects of an ADHD diagnosis. Following Brady (2014), we explore how the concept of the 'ADHD child' becomes stabilized via diagnostic processes as a singular, unchanging entity, devoid of the capacity to surprise us by evolving or diverging from expectations. In this regard, we contend that hauntology offers a potent framework for contemplating the challenges inherent in envisioning an opening toward transformation in diagnosed children, for novelty to emerge, as they find themselves ensnared in a recursive temporality. This recursive temporality creates a fixed biomedical imaginary of ADHD diagnosis, leading educational institutions to consistently perceive the child as disorderly, thereby trapping them in a temporal and spatial sameness. This unchanging view hinders the potential for embracing alternative futures for the child. In contrast, a more caring approach to diagnosis could open up possibilities for addressing the diagnosis and its effects as dynamic and contextually influenced. By doing so, it allows for different ways of understanding and caring for the child, thus opening pathways for the child to become different and to transcend the limiting perceptions imposed by traditional diagnostic frameworks.

Hauntology and Its Potency for Thinking about Mental Health Diagnoses

As previously mentioned, hauntology has recently garnered increasing interest among social scientists as a conceptual framework for exploring a diverse range of topics (Broom et al., 2020; Good, 2019; Gordon, 2008; Lincoln & Lincoln, 2015). It has become so influential that it has spurred the emergence of a distinct field of study known broadly as 'spectrality studies', particularly within cultural, film, and literature studies (Blanco & Peeren, 2013). This interdisciplinary approach examines phenomena as continually intertwined with time and the echoes of the past, enriching our understanding of various aspects of human experience.

Originally introduced by French philosopher Jacques Derrida in his work 'Spectres of Marx' (1994), hauntology offers a framework to comprehend how the past continues to exert influence on the present. The term itself, 'hauntology', is a fusion of 'haunting' and 'ontology', reflecting the notion that the present is permeable to the lingering presence of entities and phenomena that have ceased to exist but persist as ghosts and spectres. While Derrida initially applied hauntology to investigate the enduring legacy of Marxism and its spectral presence following the perceived ascendancy of capitalism and neoliberalism globally, scholars have since utilized the concept to explore various facets of human experience. Hauntology provides insights into how the remnants of the past can still shape and inform our current reality, highlighting the enduring resonance of history in shaping our present existence, and the strangeness that this can produce.

The conceptual framework of hauntology, particularly its exploration of time and space, has been further developed by philosopher Karen Barad (2010). Her timely emphasis on the necessity to engage affectively and politically with hauntings resonates with what has been termed the 'politics of haunting' (Hollan, 2019). Barad proposes a dynamic understanding of time, rejecting its characterization as a static entity and instead portraying it as an ongoing process, a continuous entanglement that reshapes and articulates what exists and what may emerge in various forms. According to Barad, time is not merely a backdrop but the result of material forces, actively producing temporalities and imbuing coherence upon events and entities. But hauntings, she argues, are not solely material; they possess an affective dimension, manifesting in embodied experiences and producing tangible effects by perpetually folding the past into the future. However, hauntings are not confined to subjective encounters; they are integral to the inherent indeterminacy of time and existence, giving rise to diverse encounters, associations, and emergences (Barad, 2017).

In relation to issues of health, illness, and care, the concept of hauntology illuminates how 'the real' possesses an illusory character, perpetually influenced by the past and by what seemingly no longer exists yet still lingers. As Hodkinson (2019) mentions, revealing these ghosts and allowing them to enter enables us to tell 'the real story of the real'. This approach provides a more complex, situated, and enriched understanding of phenomena such as health and illness. In this context, care is seen as a privileged method for addressing these ghosts and spectres, integrating them as actors in the real (Rojas-Navarro et al., 2024). Hauntology thus helps us understand that temporality in health and illness is neither linear nor stable. Instead, it is imbued with history, future possibilities, and virtuality, all of which flood the present and produce various effects and affects. Consequently, a diagnosis can blur the temporal boundaries of what will come, what was, and what the present is (Broom et al., 2020).

In our fieldwork with children diagnosed with ADHD in Chilean schools, an approach based on hauntology allows us to explore how the diagnosis exhibits a temporality that connects the child not only with their present but also captures their past and future. This perspective reveals how the diagnosis creates a temporal disjunction in the school setting, disrupting or altering the linearity of time and producing a variety of effects. The considerations surrounding hauntology provide a framework to examine how schools serve as unique arenas where past experiences and emotions are continually reintroduced into the present, shaping the future trajectories of children.

Locating the Research: Contexts and Methods

Our research was conducted in Chile, where the public education system has undergone significant restructuring since Pinochet's dictatorship, aligning with neoliberal principles of accountability while facing resource constraints (Sisto, 2019). This new framework has compelled schools to compete for funding, driving processes of standardization and ongoing inspection under a voucher scheme (Chumacero et al., 2016). In this scheme, the state allocates subsidies to schools based on the number of enrolled students, fostering a competitive environment where innovation and differentiation must be included to attract more students. If a student transfers from one school to another, the voucher moves with them (Sapelli & Aedo, 2001).

In terms of the inclusion of Special Educational Needs (SEN), the enactment of 'Decree 170' (Ministerio de Educación, 2010) increased subsidies for children requiring special support, through the School Integration Program (PIE, for its Spanish name).[1] For a school to benefit from this subsidy, a child must undergo a diagnostic process. Since schools do not have mental health experts, such as psychiatrists or neurologists, on-site, they typically ask parents to take their children to external mental health centres for examination and diagnosis. Once diagnosed, parents must return the completed forms from these experts to the school for submission to a funding platform. Voucher schools receive funding on a per-child basis, and for diagnosed children, this amount is increased.

The mechanism described above has faced criticism from Chilean experts, particularly for its potential to lead to over-diagnosis, especially in cases like ADHD. This is due to ADHD being considered a more flexible diagnosis, with symptoms that are open to professional interpretation—a point that has sparked considerable debate among national experts (Rojas-Navarro et al., 2018a; Sir et al., 2019). While we have previously delved into how this educational model influences the

[1] It is not compulsory for schools to count with a special educational needs programme, although it is encouraged.

production of diagnoses like ADHD[2] from a hauntological perspective (Rojas-Navarro et al., 2024), and also from the perspective of the caring arrangements that the diagnosis can entail (Rojas-Navarro et al., 2023), in this chapter, we focus on effects of these processes on the everyday practices of sense-making and identity formation regarding diagnosed children. Over a span of three years, we engaged in interviews with medical professionals responsible for diagnosing children for educational purposes, conducted ethnographic research within two schools, and observed the daily experiences of diagnosed children aged nine to ten within these environments. In total, we interviewed ten psychiatrists who at the moment worked diagnosing children, six educational psychologists, eight professionals hired to support diagnosed children (such as speech therapists or psychopedagogues[3]), and nine teachers related to subjects that include the accompaniment of support professionals for students with special educational needs. The research was approved by the ethics committee hosting this research under Protocol ID 190322004.

We approached the study of this diagnosis under the idea that its production and circulation is an entanglement of affective, relational, cultural, institutional, and discursive dimensions (Rojas-Navarro et al., 2023). Furthermore, we understood that diagnoses are not only effects of these forces but also have their own agency, which modifies the practices of those with whom they relate. By focusing on the hauntological, we were able to understand a particular dimension of analysis: how time and space are affected by the diagnosis, impacting the possibilities of the diagnosed child to move through different identities. We engage with ghosts and hauntings while transcribing and coding interviews, analysing fieldwork, and reflecting upon the dynamic influence of diagnoses and mental health conditions on daily life.

[2] ADHD is defined by the Ministry of Education as a Transitory Special Educational Needs, that needs to be reaffirmed every year by a specialist.

[3] In the case of Chile, a Psychopedagogue is a Professional that is prepared to work in the educational field, supporting the evaluation and intervention or accompaniment of all special educational needs.

Stagnated in Time: Hauntological Aspects of the ADHD Diagnosis in Chilean Schools

The Chilean context presents specific characteristics that have led national researchers to exercise caution regarding ADHD diagnoses in schools. While not all schools are financially dependent on these incentives, there is a belief that some schools may overemphasize the need for diagnoses to secure additional funds, as outlined in the previously mentioned scheme (Santana-Vidal et al., 2020). This finding underscores the environment in which ADHD diagnoses may arise in Chilean school institutions—amid uncertainties and pressures. However, this does not necessarily imply a lack of genuine concern for children, as expressed by some of our interviewees:

> Sometimes schools hire external services to assess students for the School Integration Program (PIE). I remember feeling pressure from the school, as if they were telling me, "find something diagnosable in him." It's a bit perverse in that sense because if I said, "I don't really think he has ADHD," they would respond, "no, but he has something; I've seen it here," and then describe his behaviour (...) Since ADHD is the most well-known diagnosis, there's a tendency to fit everything into that category.
>
> Jose, child psychiatrist

> At the beginning of the year, schools have to register children in these programmes, so they call you and ask. "Hello, I'm...", any name, it's just an example, "I'm X, the psychopedagogue of such-and-such school, or of a chain of schools. We have 135 children that we need to register before April. These children already had a diagnosis in previous years, and it needs to be renewed. We have their records and past exams from other doctors. Can you come to our centre for a whole day, see the 135 patients, we'll pay you X amount per patient, and you renew the certificate?" (...) I haven't done it yet, but I know colleagues who have.
>
> Juan, child psychiatrist

This type of practice often results in the diagnosis being used primarily as a means of securing additional funds. To comply with regulations and obtain the extra funding for each diagnosed child, some interviewees suggest that the diagnostic processes lack thoroughness and are not followed necessarily by appropriate follow-up care. The vignette presented above illustrates how these diagnostic procedures can be driven more by institutional pressures than by the actual needs of the child. Moreover, the process often focuses on reaffirming a previous diagnosis as problematic for the student's development. Due to this careless production, the diagnosis can fail to unfold in a manner that genuinely addresses the child's needs.

Understanding the forces and dynamics described above is crucial for grasping the hauntological process of diagnoses in schools. As Gordon (2008) argues, investigating a haunting compels us to reflect on the economic, political, and sociocultural factors that make this phenomenon possible. In this context, we argue schools can turn into spaces where diagnoses acquire a ghostly presence. This spectral condition has tangible effects on the daily life of the school. The issue is not necessarily the diagnosis itself but rather the way it is summoned within the school environment—sometimes with little regard for its impact, while at other times invoked to highlight and address specific forms of relationality and their effects on the identity of children.

For Alejandra, an educational psychopedagogist working with diagnosed children in primary education, this poses a significant challenge. She notices that the diagnosis is not just used by the school, as commonly believed, to interpret children's actions in class. As shown below, parents and family members also incorporate the diagnosis into their explanations in the school setting. The child gets stuck in a repetitive cycle, where current events cannot break free from past ones, hindering understanding or attributing their actions to anything else. The ADHD diagnosis, like a veil, seems to obscure their future possibilities, preventing anything different from emerging:

> It's everywhere, all the time—the diagnosis just keeps cropping up. It's constant, relentless. You hear phrases like 'oh, it's just that my child has ADHD', or 'sorry, he just can't seem to focus', or 'oh, it's just that kid has this or that condition'. So, essentially, there's this continual resurgence of this belief that he'll never be able to achieve anything. And, from what I

> observe, that belief lingers and becomes infectious. When you have someone constantly feeding you that narrative, just imagine the impact.
> Alejandra, psychopedagogist.

Alejandra highlights a critical aspect of living with a diagnosis: the persistence and stickiness of the diagnostic label once it is established within the school setting, and its potential consequences for the child's identity. This diagnosis becomes a recurring framework for interpreting the past, present, and future behaviour and emotions of the diagnosed child. Just as reports of a ghost sighting gain momentum once confirmed, a diagnosis reshapes not only the daily life of the diagnosed individual but also how others perceive and interpret their actions and emotions. This phenomenon spreads among those in positions of authority within the community, creating an environment ripe for haunting experiences to take hold.

As Mark Fisher (2012, 2014) explains, haunting occurs when a space is imbued with the remnants of a past temporality, which has been forgotten or buried. This present-focused approach further suppresses alternative modes of existence in the classroom, with teachers playing a pivotal role. However, responses to this can vary. For instance, in cases like ADHD diagnoses, uncertainty about what constitutes 'difference' may exacerbate exclusionary practices or, conversely, lead to efforts to counter them.

Ministerial guidelines suggest a series of steps for the diagnostic evaluation of ADHD—such as conducting an anamnesis, pedagogical evaluation by the classroom teacher, interviews with the family members, review of school records, and application of tests like the Conners Test or TOCA-RR (Bello Sanchez, 2022). But our interviewees indicate that these steps are often not followed in practice. Many schools use versions of the Conners scale that have been adapted by teachers themselves. This test consists of an evaluation scale applied to teachers and parents to assess the child's behaviour. The Conners test is widely used in Chilean schools when ADHD is suspected, and increasingly abbreviated and simplified versions of it can be found in online teacher forums, highlighting the lack of time and budget to conduct the original evaluation (Peña Ochoa et al., 2015).

This is significant because it ends up shifting diagnostic expertise to teachers. They conduct the initial screening and suggest that parents consult with a mental health expert, who then receives a report suggesting a diagnosis. However, this expertise does not come from formal training in diagnosis and often must be combined with academic pressures and time constraints. In this context, their past experiences become crucial for navigating the present, as expressed by Maria during an interview:

> It's usually teachers, who are most present in the classroom who … who come with certain information. Sometimes the class teachers also say, 'well, this kid seems a bit odd to me, I don't know, he's having trouble adapting,' or 'he's not responding, he doesn't understand.' But, you know, there's not a … we don't have a strict observation guideline, it's more like a gut feeling, you know? But it's based on our past experiences.
>
> Maria, school psychologist

In his account of hauntology, Fisher (2013) stresses how cultural artifacts of technologies play a pivotal role in bringing the past into the present, therefore blurring the line between the two. As a biomedical technology, diagnoses play a similar role. It is not merely that past actions of diagnosed children create an unchanging framework for understanding their future behaviour, or that teachers' prior experiences limit room for new interpretations and surprises. The spectral nature of the diagnosis seems to merge these elements, animating them within the school's spaces and times. Even when professionals like María strive to resist the temptation of hastily concluding that what they are witnessing is a relic from the past, this process still identifies the spectre of ADHD within this scene, albeit with an effort to avoid being overwhelmed by it:

> When I see a child who moves around during class and seems to be inattentive, I don't immediately jump to the conclusion that they have ADHD. But it's clear that we need to address the situation somehow. I'm unsure of how to approach the child during class. I feel like we need to consider the situation from various angles and not rush to conclusions. Let's observe what's happening with the child in class. Perhaps they learn at a different pace or in a different way than other kids, but that doesn't necessarily mean they have ADHD.

Delia, school psychologist

For professionals like Alejandra and Delia, the ADHD diagnosis serves as a conduit to past experiences, challenging the perception of the present by suggesting that what unfolds is merely a reverberation from history. However, Delia's perspective introduces a fresh avenue for inquiry. It encourages us to explore these ghosts with curiosity, delving into the forces and narratives that underpin these hauntings. Rather than dismissing what haunts us, her approach illuminates the possibility of engaging with classroom dynamics in a different light. This endeavour requires unearthing alternative modes of reflection on how the present is constructed, reevaluating the components that shape our current reality. Such a stance resonates with Barad's (2010) notion of time and space as active agents imbued with affective significance, encapsulated within a framework that urge political and ethical response-ability for the ongoing construction of our reality, for the choices we make, and the entities we bring into existence each day.

According to Rahimi (2021), hauntings result from unresolved injustices, silenced realities, or different forms of past violence resurfacing to be acknowledged. Alejandra perceives this ongoing recurrence of the diagnosis and its capacity to explain and distress the present due to unresolved conditions, while Delia manages to go beyond that point, asking, even tangentially, if things could be understood differently.

Unveiling the Silenced Past: Embracing New Possibilities in the Present through Ghosts and Spectres

Hauntings produced by the interplay between the school institution and diagnoses can manifest in various ways. If we understand a ghost as a remnant of the past that exerts influence in the present, we can see the spectral nature of a diagnosis as the reactivation of a past problem that reverberates, seeking resolution. In this sense, we can identify a second layer at which these hauntings occur within schools: not only as the persistent return of the diagnosis, anchoring the child to a fixed identity rooted in the past and restricting their ability to evolve, but also on a more intimate level, as a relationship between the child (and their environment) and a version of themselves that demands attention, continually resurfacing to be reworked. On this alternative level, we observe that the diagnosis holds meaning for our interviewees:

> The school usually responds with something like, "Thank you very much, doctor. We'll discuss this with the school integration team and request the support you've recommended for the child." You can often sense whether the diagnosis will actually lead to meaningful action. If I continue to monitor the situation and the parents or the child tells me, "Yes, the teacher is now helping me with this or that," or "They take me out once a week to work with a specific teacher," and then I see improvements in the child's grades—or even if the grades don't improve, but there are positive changes in interactions—you know the process is bearing fruit.
>
> Pedro, child psychiatrist

As Spooner-Lockyer and Kilroy-Marac (2021) argue, hauntings blur the boundaries between what is and what was, revealing that these divisions are ultimately artificial. They suggest that to account for these hauntings, we must take responsibility for the pasts they bring into the present—even when those pasts are difficult or unsettling, disrupting our current reality and future prospects. In this sense, attending to these hauntings becomes a repetitive act of care that propels us toward the future. In the context of diagnoses, this haunting allows us to reflect on the circuit activated by the diagnosis in the relationship between the diagnosed child and a troubled past—a past discomforting enough to necessitate reframing through the diagnosis. Pedro's reflection aligns in this direction. It suggests that when a diagnosis is carefully articulated, its ability to bridge the past and present can help address discomforts and discontents, creating a form of reconciliation that opens new pathways for the future.

The educational process implemented by schools is inherently forward-looking, always aiming toward future development. As a result, children are immersed in various practices designed to foster the acquisition of academic skills and, depending on the school's orientation, also certain socio-emotional and value-based competencies. So, if we take Rahimi's (2021) consideration seriously, what kind of realities are being cast aside, and what kind of injustices are being displayed? This unease is a topic of reflection widely shared among the different interviewees, and it also emerged in spontaneous conversations during the ethnographic research. Antonia, a primary school teacher, shares the following with us:

> I used to see it differently before, but now my perspective has shifted. Previously, I viewed it as each child having their own unique way of learning. In a system that heavily emphasizes academics and direct instruction from teacher to student, some children inevitably lag behind, leading to the emergence of special educational needs. This may occur because certain children require alternative learning methods. Nowadays, I believe that the standardized nature of the education system encourages the development of these educational needs in children who might not have exhibited them otherwise (…) Therefore, I perceive that these transient educational needs arise because the system, particularly the public system, fails to accommodate every child's unique learning style.
>
> Antonia, schoolteacher

Antonia's reflection sheds light on a crucial aspect, revealing not only the prevalence of the diagnosis but also the underlying dynamics that sustain it. According to her perspective, the real issue lies not solely in the diagnosis itself but rather in how the Chilean education system is constructed upon the remnants of otherness, effectively erasing and marginalizing differences. In this context, the diagnosis is not merely a reflection of an unchangeable reality or a natural condition. Instead, it persists due to the system's actions and mechanisms. This viewpoint doesn't negate the material circumstances facilitating the diagnosis but rather underscores why its emergence often triggers confusion and can be unsettling. Essentially, the diagnosis signifies the resurgence of what should have no place, of something that is out of time: a haunting spectre of difference lingering among students, frequently unaddressed by the educational institution. This viewpoint is also shared by Karen, when arguing the following:

> I say all children have different learning styles, and a first-grade child, I mean we're talking about 5–6-year-olds, so these are children who obviously have a lot more energy, who need dynamic learning experiences, and sitting them alone at a desk, in front of the chalkboard, changing that whole dynamic from preschool where they're in groups doing more playful activities, it's quite powerful.(...) all children are active. I worry if the children remain still and don't move. But of course, they are generally children who don't allow the "normal" [quotation marks] activity of the educational system.
>
> Karen, Special Educational Needs expert.

Perspectives like Karen's prompt us to recall insights from authors like Good (2021), who suggest that ghosts and hauntings can serve as forms of memory resistance—ways in which forgotten elements strive to resurface and reclaim attention. From this perspective, it seems reasonable to interpret these hauntings as instances where diagnosed children are not only surrounded by an aura that evokes lost modes of understanding the school environment and its participants but also as attempts to disrupt the stagnation of generating novelty. While we've argued elsewhere that diagnoses can foster care and guide new actions (Rojas-Navarro et al., 2023), the accounts shared by our interviewees suggest that such efforts remain limited and are primarily viewed as exceptions rather than common practice. In this context, there is a sense that the current educational system, as it interacts with diagnoses, can foster neglect and forgetfulness toward many diagnosed children. Karen and other interviewees suggest that alternatives to this approach typically emerge from individual efforts. It is specific individuals, driven by their commitment or an emotional connection with these children, who manage to attune themselves to these ghosts and, from this place of understanding, advocate for their care and attention.

However, there is potential for change. Even within the constraints of today's school environment, reflecting on the past can provide valuable insights for the present—insights that should not be dismissed, but rather acknowledged and understood. When this reflective approach is embraced, everyday interactions and situations within schools can lead to alternative outcomes. Let us revisit Alejandra's perspective to explore this idea further:

> Recently, something happened at school that really struck me. I was assigned to work with a remarkable child [diagnosed with ADHD]. He's truly exceptional. But during tests, he gets incredibly nervous… and as a result, he misreads the questions and gives the wrong answers. He shines in class, yet his test scores don't reflect his potential. So, he sought help, and I began to evaluate him based on input from teachers and the available information we have about his class, and feedback from his parents. But with me, it's different. He engages in my classes, reads perfectly, and thrives.
> Alejandra, psychopedagogist.

What does it truly mean for a child to thrive? It prompts a critical pause, inviting us to ponder deeply. On one front, we might approach this notion with scepticism, viewing it as merely ensuring the diagnosed child's integration into the educational system. However, another perspective, echoing Alejandra's insights, suggests a more profound narrative. Thriving involves a shared agency among the diagnosis, the child, and the educational environment, which must be open to embracing alternative actions and perspectives. Alejandra emphasizes that it is the child who seeks support. The focus should be on fostering environments where identities are seen not as burdens but as dynamic constructs, capable of evolving and reshaping in ways that honour the individuality and potential of each child. For a diagnosis to be truly caring and generous, it must address both the child's unique situation and the ways in which the diagnosis interacts with the educational space, considering its capacity to support diverse behaviours, emotions, and experiences. In this way, a diagnosis like ADHD not only identifies the outer boundaries of "typical" behaviours but also highlights the shortcomings of environments that fail to adapt sufficiently to enable children with ADHD to thrive.

Interrogating the Haunting Power of the Diagnosis: Living with Ghosts

What alternatives can we make use of to understand mental health diagnoses differently in schools, their power, and consequences? In this chapter, we have delved into these inquiries through the lens of hauntology, a concept that offers a unique vantage point for examining the complexities of diagnoses. By embracing hauntology, we are encouraged to transcend the surface of diagnoses and delve into their deeper implications, considering the intricate interplay between past, present, and future. This perspective illuminates the multifaceted relationships between spaces and times, unveiling the intricate tapestry of experiences that shape the lives of children diagnosed with conditions like ADHD, and indeed, those with various other diagnoses as well. Through hauntology, we come to understand that the temporalities experienced by these children are not static entities but dynamic forces that permeate their daily lives within the school environment.

If we indeed inhabit a culture saturated with diagnostics (Brinkmann, 2016), and if diagnoses themselves are imbued with spectral qualities (Rojas-Navarro et al., 2024), what are the political implications of these hauntings? As Hollan (2019) astutely observes, while hauntings may be commonplace, they truly gain significance when they impact individuals in positions of authority within a community. If such is the case, how do we elevate their importance? How do we transform them into issues that capture the attention and concern of others? Presently, we posit that reframing these diagnoses not as static, natural phenomena, but as dynamic and spectral forces, constitutes an initial stride toward unsettling them, allowing their voices to resonate and be heard.

In line with the thinking introduced by Mark Fisher (2014), we argue that the issue lies not solely with mental health diagnoses themselves, but rather with the societal forces that have led to their widespread presence in our schools and society. Reflecting about the music industry, Fisher argues that its main problem is not music per se, but it's inability to produce novelty beyond mere repetition of past styles. In a similar vein, we argue that the issue lies not in diagnoses themselves, but in their occasional use by institutions to suppress difference and stifle novelty. Diagnoses are tools woven into the fabric of our society, and they can also become instruments in articulating alternative narratives for those diagnosed and their relations with their environments.

Diagnoses like ADHD, with their spectral qualities, serve as a lens through which we can uncover and address the silences and omissions that haunt these institutional spaces. It is crucial to shed light on how our interviewees perceive their roles within these broader dynamics—dynamics that, according to their accounts, often foreclose difference. Yet, within these same systems, there exists the potential to engage with these hauntings in ways that foster care and attention otherwise neglected. The spectral reverberations of ADHD diagnoses echo through the present, shaping current practices and understandings. When these haunting effects are not properly acknowledged, they risk perpetuating the very diagnostic histories they seek to address, obscuring alternative pathways that could lead to more inclusive and compassionate outcomes.

Acknowledgements We thank the interview participants for their generous contributions to this research. This article was written with support of the Millennium Institute for Care Research (MICARE), Santiago, Chile, supported by the ANID Millennium Science Initiative Program (ICS2019_024).

Competing Interests This study was funded by Agencia Nacional de Investigación y Desarrollo (ANID), Fondecyt Regular, project number N°1231796 and Proyecto Fondecyt Iniciación 11190285. *The authors have no conflicts of interest to declare that are relevant to the content of this chapter.*

Ethics Approval The research was approved by the ethics committee hosting this research under Protocol ID 190322004.

References

Armstrong, D. (2011). Diagnosis and nosology in primary care. *Social Science & Medicine, 73*(6), 801–807. https://doi.org/10.1016/j.socscimed.2011.05.017

Barad, K. (2010). Quantum entanglements and hauntological relations of inheritance: Dis/continuities, spacetime enfoldings, and justice-to-come. *Derrida Today, 3*(2), 240–268. https://doi.org/10.3366/drt.2010.0206

Barad, K. (2017). No small matter: Mushroom clouds, ecologies of nothingness, and strange topologies of spacetimemattering. In A. Tsing, H. Swanson, E. Gan, & N. Bubandt (Eds.), *Arts of living on a damaged planet* (pp. G103–G120). University of Minnesota.

Bello Sánchez, O. (2022). Infancias, diagnósticos y salud mental: discursos sobre el trastorno por déficit de atención e hiperactividad en la región de Los Lagos, Chile. *Salud Colectiva, 18*. https://doi.org/10.18294/sc.2022.4233

Blanco, M. P., & Peeren, E. (Eds.). (2013). *The spectralities reader: Ghosts and haunting in contemporary cultural theory*. Bloomsbury Academic.

Blum, L. (2015). *Raising generation Rx: Mothering kids with invisible disabilities in an age of inequality*. NYU Press.

Bradley, B. (2021). From biosociality to biosolidarity: The looping effects of finding and forming social networks for body-focused repetitive behaviours. *Anthropology & Medicine, 28*(4), 543–557. https://doi.org/10.1080/13648470.2020.1864807

Brady, G. (2014). Children and ADHD: Seeking control within the constraints of diagnosis. *Children & Society, 28*(3), 218–230. https://doi.org/10.1111/chso.12069

Brinkmann, S. (2016). *Diagnostic cultures: A cultural approach to the pathologization of modern life*. Routledge.

Broom, A., Kenny, K., & Kirby, E. (2020). Entangled and estranged: Living and dying in relation (to cancer). *Sociology, 54*(5), 1004–1021. https://doi.org/10.1177/0038038520918853

Chumacero, R., Gallegos, J. A., & Paredes, R. (2016). Competition pressures and academic performance in Chile (December 6, 2016). *Estudios de Economía, 43*(2). Available at SSRN: https://ssrn.com/abstract=2881579

Derrida, J. (1994). *Specters of Marx: The state of the debt, the work of mourning, and the new international*. Routledge.

Fisher, M. (2012). What is hauntology? *Film Quarterly, 66*(1), 16–24. University of California Press. https://doi.org/10.1525/fq.2012.66.1.16

Fisher, M. (2013). The metaphysics of crackle: Afrofuturism and hauntology. *Dancecult, 5*(2), 42–55. https://doi.org/10.12801/1947-5403.2013.05.02.03

Fisher, M. (2014, May 30). *Ghosts of my life: Writings on depression, hauntology and lost futures*. Zero Books.

Fried, T., & Plotkin-Amrami, G. (2023). Not all diagnoses are created equal: Mothers' narratives of children, ADHD, and comorbid diagnoses. *Social Science & Medicine* (1982), 323, 115838. https://doi.org/10.1016/j.socscimed.2023.115838

Good, B. (2019). Hauntology: Theorizing the spectral in psychological anthropology. *Ethos, 47*(4), 411–426. https://doi.org/10.1111/etho.12260

Good, B. (2021). Afterword: Haunted histories and the silences of everyday life. *History and Anthropology*. https://doi.org/10.1080/02757206.2021.1954635

Gordon, A. (2008). *Ghostly matters: Haunting and the sociological imagination.* University of Minnesota Press.

Harrison, M., Smith, A. K. J., & Adams, S. (2024). Matters of time in health and illness. *Health Sociology Review, 33*(1), 1–9. https://doi.org/10.1080/14461242.2024.2319943

Hawthorne, S. C. C. (2010). Institutionalized intolerance of ADHD: Sources and consequences. *Hypatia, 25*(3), 504–526. http://www.jstor.org/stable/40928635

Hodkinson, A. (2019). The unseeing eye: Disability and the hauntology of Derrida's ghost. A story in three parts. *Qualitative Inquiry*. https://doi.org/10.1177/1077800419847429

Hollan, D. (2019). Who is haunted by whom? Steps to an ecology of haunting. *Ethos, 47*(4). https://doi.org/10.1111/etho.12254

Iudici, A., & Faccio, E. (2013). The conflict at school: Clinical implications and mediation interventions. *Procedia - Social Behavioral Sciences, 89*, 901–905. https://doi.org/10.1016/j.sbspro.2013.08.953

Jain, S., & Orr, D. M. (2016). Ethnographic perspectives on global mental health. *Transcultural Psychiatry, 53*(6), 685–695. https://doi.org/10.1177/1363461516679322

Jutel, A. (2019). 'The expertness of his healer': Diagnosis, disclosure and the power of a profession. *Health, 23*(3), 289–305. https://www.jstor.org/stable/26652475

Jutel, A., & Nettleton, S. (2011). Towards a sociology of diagnosis: Reflections and opportunities. *Social Science & Medicine, 73*(6), 793–800. https://doi.org/10.1016/j.socscimed.2011.07.014

Kazda, L., Bell, K., Thomas, R., McGeechan, K., Sims, R., & Barratt, A. (2021). Over diagnosis of attention-deficit/hyperactivity disorder in children and adolescents: A systematic scoping review. *JAMA Network Open, 4*(4), e215335. https://doi.org/10.1001/jamanetworkopen.2021.5335

Lincoln, M., & Lincoln, B. (2015). Toward a critical hauntology: Bare afterlife and the ghosts of Ba Chúc. *Comparative Studies in Society and History, 57*(1), 191–220. https://doi.org/10.1017/S0010417514000644

Merten, E. C., Cwik, J. C., Margraf, J., & Schneider, S. (2017). Overdiagnosis of mental disorders in children and adolescents (in developed countries). *Child and Adolescent Psychiatry and Mental Health, 11*, 5. https://doi.org/10.1186/s13034-016-0140-5

Ministerio de Educación. (2010). *Decreto 170. Fija normas para determinar los alumnos con necesidades educativas especiales que serán beneficiarios de las subvenciones para educación especial.* https://especial.mineduc.cl/wp-content/uploads/sites/31/2018/06/DTO-170_21-ABR-2010.pdf

Mukolo, A., Heflinger, C. A., & Wallston, K. A. (2010). The stigma of childhood mental disorders: A conceptual framework. *Journal of the American Academy of Child and Adolescent Psychiatry, 49*(2), 92–198. https://doi.org/10.1097/00004583-201002000-00003

Müller, A. K., Fuermaier, A. B. M., Koerts, J., & Tucha, L. (2012). Stigma in attention deficit hyperactivity disorder. *ADHD Attention Deficit and Hyperactivity Disorders, 4*(3), 101–114. https://doi.org/10.1007/s12402-012-0085-3

Ohan, J., Visser, T., Strain, M., & Allen, L. (2011, February). Teachers' and education students' perceptions of and reactions to children with and without the diagnostic label "ADHD". *Journal of School Psychology, 49*(1), 81–105. https://doi.org/10.1016/j.jsp.2010.10.001

Peña Ochoa, M., Rojas Navarro, P., & Rojas Navarro, S. (2015). ¿Cómo diagnosticar a un niño? Diagnóstico del Trastorno de Déficit Atencional con Hiperactividad desde una perspectiva discursive crítica. *Athenea Digital, 15*(1), 91–110. https://doi.org/10.5565/rev/athenea.1304

Rahimi, S. (2021). *The hauntology of everyday life.* Palgrave Macmillan.

Rojas Navarro, S., & Filipe, A. M. (2023). Situer la vie sociale des TDAH: entre le médical, le local et le global. In L. Caliman, Y. Citton, & M. R. Prado (Eds.), *L'attention médicamentée: La Ritaline à l'école* (pp. 57–76). PUR.

Rojas-Navarro, S., & Rojas, P. (2019). Subjetivaciones farmacológicas: Déficit atencional, psicoestimulantes y prácticas escolares en dos colegios de Santiago, Chile. *Athenea Digital, 19*(3), 21–28. https://doi.org/10.5565/rev/athenea.2465

Rojas-Navarro, S., Alarcón-Arcos, S., & Tabilo-Prieto, I. (2023). Care entanglements: Upholding difference through the uses of mental health diagnosis in Chilean schools. *Sociology of Health & Illness, 45*(6), 1317–1333. https://doi.org/10.1111/1467-9566.13506

Rojas-Navarro, S., Alarcón-Arcos, S., & Tabilo-Prieto, I. (2024). Spectralities of ADHD: hauntological diagnosis amidst agency, politics and pedagogies. *Health Sociology Review, 33*(1). Matters of time in health and illness. https://doi.org/10.1080/14461242.2024.2316736

Rojas-Navarro, S., & Rojas, P. (2021). Re-entangling childhoods: Post-essentialist approaches to children's everyday lives. In R. Machin Suarez (Ed.), *New waves in social psychology.* Palgrave Macmillan. https://doi.org/10.1007/978-3-030-87406-3_7

Rojas-Navarro, S., Rojas, P., Castillo-Sepúlveda, J., & Schöngut-Grollmus, N. (2018b). Reensamblando la medicalización: hacia una pluralización de las explicaciones del TDAH en Chile. In E. Bianchi & S. Faraone (Eds.), *Medicalización, salud mental e infancias* (pp. 335–367). Teseo.

Rojas-Navarro, S., Rojas, P., & Peña, M. (2018a). From problematic children to problematic diagnosis: The paradoxical trajectories of child and adolescent ADHD in Chile. In M. Bergey, A. Filipe, P. Conrad, & I. Singh (Eds.), *Global perspectives on ADHD: Social dimensions of diagnosis and treatment in 16 countries* (pp. 310–331). Johns Hopkins University Press.

Rose, N. (2013, June). *What is diagnosis for? DSM-5 and the future of psychiatric diagnosis*. Institute of Psychiatry.

Rose, N. (2018). *Our psychiatric future: The politics of mental health*. Polity.

Rose, N., & Novas, C. (2007). Biological citizenship. In A. Ong & S. J. Collier (Eds.), *Global assemblages*. https://doi.org/10.1002/9780470696569.ch23

Santana-Vidal, P., Gatica-Ferrero, S., & Valdenegro-Fuentes, L. (2020). Evidencia de sobrediagnóstico en el TDAH en base a evaluación neuropsicológica: un estudio en escolares chilenos. *Psicogente, 23*(44), 1–20. https://doi.org/10.17081/psico.23.44.3587

Sapelli, C., & Aedo, C. (2001). El sistema de vouchers en educación: una revisión de la teoría y evidencia empírica para Chile. *Estudios Públicos, 82*, 35–82.

Singh, I. (2004). Doing their jobs: Mothering with Ritalin in a culture of mother-blame. *Social Science & Medicine, 59*(6), 1193–1205. https://doi.org/10.1016/j.socscimed.2004.01.011

Singh, I. (2011). A disorder of anger and aggression: Children's perspectives on attention deficit/hyperactivity disorder in the UK. *Social Science & Medicine* (1982), *73*(6), 889–896. https://doi.org/10.1016/j.socscimed.2011.03.049

Sir, H., Castañeda, I., & Radiszcz, E. (2019). Excess of attention. The construction of a disorder in Chilean schools. *Práxis Educacional, Vitória da Conquista, 15*(36), 131–153. https://doi.org/10.22481/praxisedu.v15i36.5882. Disponível em: Acesso em: 10 ago. 2024. https://periodicos2.uesb.br/index.php/praxis/article/view/5882

Sisto, V. (2019). Inclusion "in the Chilean way": School inclusion in a context of advanced neoliberal policies. In *Education policy analysis archives* (Vol. 19). Políticas de Inclusión y Extensión de la Obligatoriedad Escolar. https://doi.org/10.14507/epaa.27.3044

Smith, M. (2017, November). Hyperactive around the world? The history of ADHD in global perspective. *Social History of Medicine, 30*(4), 767–787. https://doi.org/10.1093/shm/hkw127

Spooner-Lockyer, K., & Kilroy-Marac, K. (2021, October 18). Ten things about ghosts and haunting. *Anthropology News website*.

14

Troubling Time in the Face of Life-Limiting Illness

Jianni Tien, Roberta Pala, Katherine Kenny, and Alex Broom

One of the most poignant aspects of experiencing illness is an altered sense of time. While this is the case to greater or lesser degrees given the particularities of illness, treatment options and available care, an altered timescape is especially acute in experiences of living with life-limiting illnesses like cancer. Perhaps because of the centrality of survival statistics to both its discursive construction and lived experience, cancer involves constant prognostication against temporal horizons made uncertain by illness. Time bends, stalls, quickens, is rearranged, reconfigured, and made strange when encountering cancer, especially for those who *outlive* their prognosis and thus wade beyond the projected mortal shores and into the uncertain waters of living on 'borrowed time'. What happens to one's sense of self, underpinned as it often is by an orientation towards the future, when it is foreshortened by the certainty of impending

J. Tien • R. Pala • K. Kenny (✉) • A. Broom
Sydney Centre for Healthy Societies, The University of Sydney, Sydney, NSW, Australia
e-mail: katherine.kenny@sydney.edu.au; jianni.tien@sydney.edu.au; roberta.pala@sydney.edu.au; alex.broom@sydney.edu.au

K. Kenny et al. (eds.), *Timescapes of Health, Illness and Care*,
https://doi.org/10.1007/978-981-96-7055-0_14

mortality, or even mortality that is now 'overdue'? What temporal landscapes come into view, which recede, and what futures are imposed upon one's present against the backdrop of cancer? What are the specific contours of living on 'borrowed time' and how does terminality imbue the time remaining of one's journey through life?

Drawing on in-depth qualitative interviews with 80 people living with cancer and 50 carers (including 49 patient/carer dyads) that were conducted as part of a larger programme of research into contemporary experiences of cancer survivorship, we examine the complex experience of living with cancer and the temporal and relational reconfigurations that ensue. In particular, we examine how time, troubled by cancer, is revealed as far more complex than the linear march of clock time that implicitly structures much 'well' time, even if it carries with it many of the same normative orientations. As we will show, our participants' reflections on their temporal experiences testify to the ways in which 'the present' both demands full commitment to the treatment and management of their cancer—but also a conviction to live to the fullest whatever time one has left.

Troubling Time

Living with poor cancer prognosis disrupts the temporal continuity and coherence that is often taken for granted in the untroubled passage of daily living. From the moment one is diagnosed with cancer, the experience of time shifts in disorienting ways. The past is abruptly loaded with new affective intensity that forces one to wonder not only about what is yet to come, but also what has passed in the life lived until then.

In this chapter, we turn to Karen Barad's work on troubling time to make sense of the experience of living with cancer on 'borrowed time'. We engage with Barad's (2010, 2013, 2014) analysis that challenges the pervasive ways time is understood as a linear progression of successive and determinate moments. For Barad, the three fundamental dimensions of existence—space, time and matter—do not exist separately from one another in a configuration of smooth unfolding, as is frequently assumed in popular imaginings of linear time. Instead, Barad introduces the term 'spacetimemattering' to emphasise how space, time and matter are fundamentally entangled in a process of continuous becoming. As she explains:

> It is not merely that the future and the past are not 'there' and never sit still, but that the present is not simply here-now. Multiply heterogeneous iterations all: past, present, and future, not in a relation of linear unfolding, but threaded through one another in a nonlinear enfolding of spacetimemattering, a topology that defies any suggestion of a smooth continuous manifold. (Barad, 2013, p. 18)

For Barad, space, time and matter are inescapably entangled, featuring *intra-action*, or the iterative co-constitution of being/becoming in relation to other beings/things rather than the commonly presumed *inter*-action between distinct things playing out across a unidirectional singular timeline. As a result, the past that has been, and the future to come, cannot be relegated to 'elsewhere' but are constantly threaded through each present moment. As Barad explains (2010, p. 240), 'entanglements result in a dis/orienting experiences of the dis/jointedness of time and space, entanglements of here and there, now and then, that is a ghostly sense of dis/continuity'. On such an understanding, the bodily experience of living with cancer can be seen as always entangled with both the past and the future, with ghosts of the past and apparitions of the future, which iteratively unfold in non-linear ways, across time troubled by cancer.

Throughout this chapter, we explore such temporal re-patternings and forms of dis/continuity, drawing on qualitative semi-structured interviews with people living with cancer (N = 80) and nominated carers (N = 50). These interviews were conducted as part of a larger programme of research focused on the landscapes of cancer 'survivorship'. Ethics approval was gained through a large metropolitan hospital on the east coast of Australia. Participants were initially approached by a clinician/researcher and, if they expressed interest in the study, contacted via phone to schedule an interview. In-depth interviews of between 30 and 90 minutes were conducted with individual patients and, separately, with their nominated carer (if a carer was nominated) at the patient's home, in a private hospital room or a quiet location of the participant's choosing. Interviews were digitally recorded and transcribed in full. Our analysis of the interviews draws on interpretive and inductive traditions in qualitative social research using an in-depth exploratory approach to data collection to explore the full range of complex, sometimes contradictory, subjective experiences of the respondents (Charmaz, 1990; Clarke, 2003), who are identified throughout using pseudonyms and their designation as either 'patient' or 'carer' for clarity.

In the following sections, we detail our findings of three major threads that make up the unsettling timescapes of terminality. First, cancer disrupts the presumed linear unfolding of a life's trajectory, resulting in narrative *incoherence*, a state of temporal and relational disorientation. Second, that living in the anticipatory space of prognostic time is unsettling, with cancer a constant 'haunting' of the day-to-day, often experienced acutely in relation to various forms of 'waiting'. Finally, future-making continues, even in the face of a terminal diagnosis, but is carried out in such a way that reveals the complicated diffraction of past, present, and future, for example, in practices of making (good) memories in anticipation of future absence, and in the normalisation of the *universal* experience of impending mortality and the capriciousness of fate, articulated through the common trope that any of us could 'be hit by a bus' at any time, thereby also disrupting the unfolding of whatever future was imagined—with cancer or otherwise.

Narrative Incoherence and Dis/Continuity

Across the interviews it was clear that living with advanced cancer was a complex, unfolding, and relational processes, in which unsettling temporal tensions impacted and challenged the normative construction of temporally coherent and smoothly unfolding narratives, resulting even in what has been termed 'narrative wreck' (Frank, 2013). This played out across the interviews as participants struggled to create a coherent narrative around the dis/continuity caused by cancer. Stories typically reference a certain linearity, involving a 'beginning', middle', and 'end', which are mapped temporally on to 'past', 'present', and 'future'. When thinking about the pervasive way in which time is lived and understood as a linear and continuous progression, Barad (2013) argues that 'we know this story well, it is written into our bones, in many ways we inhabit it and it inhabits us' (p. 25). Stories, and narratives in general, are a primary method through which we attempt to tame the unruliness of our intra-active entanglements with the world. In particular, autobiographical narratives—the stories we tell ourselves to make sense of our world—tend to smooth over uncertainties in favour of narrative coherence, searching for patterns, meaning, and continuity.

Social science scholars have engaged closely with the importance of narrative coherence in people's conceptions of self (Neimeyer, 2000; Singer, 2004; McAdams, 2006). Others, though, have engaged with the issue of narrative *incoherence*, where those whose lived experiences that lie outside of normative linearity—such as those with illness—are marginalised, leading to various affects of uncertainty, distress, and unease (Bury, 1982; Brockmeier & Carbaugh, 2001; Frank, 2013; Kenny et al., 2017; Voorhees, 2023; Rushforth et al., 2021). In particular, scholars have emphasised the disruption that illness catalyses in normative orientations towards the (chronological and linear) future (Broom et al., 2018; Kenny et al., 2017; Williams, 2000). Such normative orientations treat time as singular and calibrated towards a projected future that unfolds predictably and become troubled when one's experience of time becomes entangled with the unpredictability of illness. What happens when the narrative and temporal continuity of one's life is disrupted by an advanced cancer diagnosis? How does the temporal order of self-narrative adapt to the spectre of death in one's immediate to mid-range future? As we see below, those with advanced cancer must grapple with a certain narrative *incoherence* as the temporal registers of the future are called into question and orientation towards the future is disrupted, leading to feelings of both temporal and existential disorientation. Following Barad (2007), we note the ways in which these self-making practices and experiences of time are troubled and undone not only at a discursive level but at a material and embodied one, too.

Cancer flies in the face of linear temporal unfolding presenting an unsettling, disorienting, and uncertain disruption, instead (see Bury, 1982; Harrop et al., 2017; Mathieson & Stam, 1995). The chronology of past, present, and future is continuously threatened when the speculative and promissory horizons of the future are made void, replaced with the uncertainty of 'how much' time one has remaining. Across the interviews the impact of temporal dis/continuity was made apparent, as participants struggled to 'make sense' of how their lives were unfolding and to make decisions about their futures. These were experienced in the existential register around questions of mortality, but also at the level of day-to-day decision making about seemingly mundane future-oriented action. As Daniel (patient) explained, in relation to deciding whether or not to buy a car

> … I think, 'I've got to buy a new car.' I'm thinking, 'No, I can't actually go and get a new car because that might be irresponsible unless I get a car that my wife's happy to drive when I have to stop driving again.' I have these funny thoughts. Again, at the same time, you have these good thoughts and you think, 'Well no. Wait until you're actually allowed to sit behind the wheel before you actually worry about things like that. Don't get too far ahead. Don't get carried away because then you'll go in and you'll find some bad news and it will put you two steps back. Don't try and push it too much. … You've got to be very, very careful not to slip. (Daniel, patient)

The unfolding of Daniel's future is disrupted by uncertainties brought by cancer, complicating everyday decision-making and imposing a degree of incoherence on his plans. Daniel explains his frustration at being mired in an uncertain present, disoriented and unbalanced, being 'careful not to slip', cautious not to 'push' or get 'carried away'.

Cancer is 'an experience rife with contradiction and confusion' in which 'prognosis appears as a concrete scientific fact' in a time and place rife with uncertainty (Jain, 2007, p. 79). This played out across the interviews as many turned to the 'numbers game' of prognosis, searching for certainty by drawing on the framework of statistics to counterbalance the narrative incoherence and temporal dislocation they experienced. As one patient explained:

> … around 3% will live for five years, but 80% have got 18 months to two years as a life expectancy from diagnosis to death. Some people might look at it as, geez, that's bad, but I'm going to be one of the 3%. That's the way I've always looked at it. There's 3% of people that go to five years, well, I'm going to be one of the 3% and that's just how it is. (Miranda, patient)

Here, Miranda reveals the tension between the flattening of statistics and the specificity of lived experience as she distances herself from the '80%' who have only 18 months to two years to live, asserting her own agency and orienting towards a future of the 'lucky' 3% who will live to five years. This forceful orientation was echoed by Cathy (patient):

> I've got a five-year plan, which is now a four-year plan. I don't have to be their three-year prognosis. I want to be a five-year plan.

As the excerpts from Miranda and Cathy demonstrate, a focus on numbers, statistics, and 'years left' was front of mind for many participants as they sought to tame the temporal unruliness of their oncological and prognostic landscapes.

While prognosis may provide structure—a temporal container for the terminal future in which one may 'live life to the fullest'—what happens when one's survival 'overspills' the temporal categories provided? The orientation and desire for 'more time' expressed by Miranda and Cathy above was held in tension with the experience of others, for whom 'more time' created further confusion and incoherence as they grappled with outliving their prognosis. This was especially the case for those providing care for people living with cancer. The tensions of 'extra' time played out in the excerpt below, as told by Sarah, a carer for Justin:

> … you're told, 'Statistically speaking, based on his prognosis with the prognostic markers, we suspect he's got a 50–50 two to three year.' So, I suppose, for the first 12 months we were fine. Getting through the emotional bit was the hard part. In terms of the timeframe, we were fine … Because we were busy and we still knew—Well, we had a whole year. It's been now, since January this year, the 18 month mark. When he had the seizures in January we both thought, 'This is it,' … Now, who knows? We're sort of hitting the two-year mark now. So this two to three year window is still going to be hell. (Sarah, Carer)

The on-going dis/orientation that Sarah and Justin experienced reveals how prognostic attempts to contain uncertainty can become problematic and even distressing. Dealing with the 'nonlinear enfolding' (Barad,

2013) and dis/continuity of time means dealing with the materialisation of different temporalities at once. Justin's embodied sense of self is called into question by the problem of 'outliving' temporal estimations of mortality, a tension that was echoed by Melinda (patient):

> I watched my mum when she was dying. She put a circle on the calendar <laughter>, which was bloody stupid .... And then she got past the circle and got pissed off ... She got really annoyed, yeah, because she'd had enough. No, I don't think it's [numbers] useful, but I think you'd need some sort of a ballpark. Brian and I are currently travelling as much as we can and spending our retirement money. Well if nobody gives you any idea you don't know whether to do it or not ... I think you deserve some sort of a vague idea. (Melinda, patient)

Melinda identifies how calendars operate as temporal containers, as particular dates circled, in an attempt to contain and tame uncertainties about the future. At the same time, the limits of these temporal containers are made clear in Melinda's mothers' frustration that the 'tamed' future has broken free from attempts to contain it, and from Melinda's assertion that while numbers are not useful, that you still 'need' a ballpark.

Prognostic time can work to reassure people living with advanced cancer, creating the semblance of narrative coherence, as we saw with the examples above. At the same time, temporal estimations of mortality are imperfect, unpredictable, and encompass vastly different ranges of time, as expressed by Rowan (patient): 'the doctors gave to me a life expectancy of 12 months to 10 years. So a massive window.' Prognosis, then, is both 'stunningly specific' and 'bloodlessly vague' (Jain, 2007, p. 78), raising questions about how to 'keep on keeping on' against such temporal dis/continuities.

The complex temporalities of advanced cancer engender narrative and material incoherence, which persisted despite participants' attempts to grapple with and tame the unruly temporalities of living with a terminal diagnosis. As we detail above, temporal uncertainties overspilled attempts at containment and led to uncomfortable feelings of temporal and relational disorientation for those we interviewed. In the next section, we detail how such uneasy temporal disorientations also lead to a type of ontological 'haunting', in which those with cancer live in the uncertain prognostic space of *waiting*.

Waiting and Clinical Hauntings

Rapid developments in cancer care and promises of technological innovations in cancer treatment are further producing conditions under which cancer patients wait. Living with terminal prognoses inevitably means living in a state of anticipation and waiting. Social sciences scholars have explored the many ways in which health care practices are entangled with the act of waiting (Baraitser et al., 2024; Anucha et al., 2021; Salisbury et al., 2023). Waiting is an embodied and social experience, affecting the ways in which illness is perceived to intervene on people's lives and their relations with others. Waiting operates within structures of power and expertise, within medical discourses that condition the legitimacy of knowledge claims around sickness and wellness, hope and hopelessness, and ideas of what a life worth living looks like. Waiting renders cancer something discrete and separate, out of one's control. Patients wait to see what 'it' does. In this sense waiting does not require an intention, rather it is perceived as passive. However, there is something productive in waiting, and we follow Barad's insistence on the ways in which time and matter are inevitably entangled, emphasising how the temporal instability of waiting produces and materialises different lives and futures.

Different from simple uncertainty, which is an epistemological tension towards knowledge, waiting is an affective temporal relation where the present and the future become unclear. Where time proceeds but, in the background, is synchronised around the possibility of an event. This event could be the progression of the disease, the next scan or test, feeling better or worse, surviving or not. Waiting is a temporal condition that is reconfigured and experienced physically, relationally, and affectively.

As Sarah, Justin's carer, reflected on the emotional experience of waiting, especially in the time between scans or in the absence of disease progression, and the arresting affect it has on people's agency and ability to take ownership of their lives:

> The watch and wait is shocking. It's the timeframe that I'm struggling with the most. It's the whole unknown. You can't organise anything. You can't do anything. It's like your life is just now in this constant limbo. It's our anniversary in October and for 15 years we've always gone away. We can't

> book anything until the scan … because we might have to jump into treatment or something. It's this constant living by these three-month windows, living by when the seizures happen. It's controlling our lives. It really is. It's just taken over, this prognosis of time. (Sarah, carer)

As we see from this quote, for this family waiting is a form of affective precarity that folds the future into 'three-months windows', during which people feel stuck, unable to know and make decisions on what to do. Waiting becomes not only a temporal condition but a spatial one as well, a physical limbo that constrains movements and planning.

Dealing with troubled times also means dealing with troubled and uncertain possibilities of history and accountability (Barad, 2010). For those living in the liminal space of cancer survivorship, waiting is an affective and material reality of everyday life. As Mac (patient), expressed, the experience of waiting involves a daily encounter with fear that never leaves him, emphasised by the daily reminder of his medication:

> The sudden diagnosis, all that happened six-and-a-half years ago. It's a long time ago now and I've lived with this for so long, I've lived with stability for so long. But even in those years of living with that, I think not a day goes by that I don't remember it. I still think of it because I still take the medication, right? I still take the tablets every day. It's at the back of the mind all the time that it could, at any time, be resistant and it could progress. …And every time you go for a scan, it's still that fear of recurrence that never, ever goes away, I don't think. (Mac, patient)

For Mac the interplay of waiting and bodily surveillance produced by the medications complicated the affective tensions around the omnipresence of disease—of its constancy 'at the back of the mind', its presence 'always there' and the struggle to just be. The spectre-like character of the prognosis, the way in which incurability makes itself a constant presence that never goes away, further qualifies waiting in this context as the experience of being haunted, as being stuck in-between the time 'borrowed' from a life that takes away your ability to live it, and the terminal prognosis. The impossibility to move outside these time frames becomes a form of clinical haunting.

In characterising time as spectral phenomenon, Barad (2010, 2013, 2014) argues that time is diffractive and distinctions between past, present, and future collapse in an entangled coexistence. Time is therefore indeterminate. We can see the folding of past, present, and future in the lived experience of waiting in cancer survivorship, when one tries to resume their past lives (such as going to the ballet, as in the quote below) while dealing with the constant reminder of cancer in one's own body and the very tangible way in which thoughts of, possibilities and hopes for a future that is ever so close take over one's present. As Julia (patient) described:

> That's why I say I never think too far ahead. Never think, 'Oh, maybe I won't see this happen,' or, 'Maybe I won't see that happen.' I look forward to things. I'm going to the ballet next week and looking forward to that. I've been to the ballet a few times. One time I wasn't extremely well, but I was there. I was there at the ballet. I had a little bit of pain so I just took some painkillers and I was fine. But the last couple of times I've been to the ballet I have enjoyed myself.... This week I'm really looking forward to the ballet. So I'm not thinking, 'Oh, I hope I live long enough to see the ballet.' I think that's pointless. (Julia, patient)

Julie's attempt to explain her own experience of time clearly illustrates the struggle to live in this temporal dis/continuity. One can look only so much forward and those affective practices of planning, hoping, and making sense that go together with linear understandings of the future, of life and its progression, are felt as pointless but also constantly creeping in, unescapably entangled.

Barad (2013) considers the haunting quality of time as the moment in which this indeterminacy collapses into a determinate state. The temporal indeterminacy of waiting and not being able to discern present from the future while waiting, is suddenly very tangible when all one's life gravitates around a determinate and single event like medical scans or the progression of cancer.

This spectre-like presence of cancer and terminality, even when indeterminate in the impossibility of breaking out of it, becomes clearly distinct when synchronised around, for example, eight-week windows, as Ben (patient) expressed:

> I don't want to know. I've never asked [my doctor] how long and I never will. … That's why you should never ask and no one should ever tell you. I think they take a guess half the time and when you go past what they've said they go, 'Oh gee, I've done a good job.' It's just something I've never asked or need to know. …I stopped chemo last June I think it was, and I haven't had any since. It's not that far away to June again. At the moment it's good. But I try and just concentrate on eight weeks to eight weeks to eight weeks. If you think too far ahead you're going to think the worst. There's a part of me that knows I'm not going to live forever. I may not see my kids get married, but while I'm here then I'll make the best of it. There is days. There is days that I've had where I'll sit down and put my face in my hands and cry and asked the question, 'Why me?' But you get over that and you get on with it again. (Ben, patient)

There's a sense in which waiting, eight weeks to eight weeks, makes the life you have left both possible and impossible. In the quote above, Ben explains his attempt to maintain some control over his waiting time by refusing to subscribe to the temporal estimation of his prognosis. Inevitably though, he is stuck in the daunting and haunting experience of a timeline that folds onto itself, taking with it his ability to plan to live beyond eight week windows of time.

The struggle that comes from these temporal and even logical disjunctures, of living while incurable, of living while terminal, are affective and embodied experiences that take an extreme toll on both people with cancer and their carers. This quote from carer Sarah speaking of Justin's reaction when they thought 'this is it' but then it wasn't 'It', evocatively frames the experience of these impossibilities as a pressure cooker.

> [He] went into an emotional basket case. He's a very strong, very robust, like he's a chef and he's worked in kitchens with people yelling at each other and abusing each other and it's water off a duck's back because of the environment that he's worked in. …This pressure, he just said, 'It's like the pressure cooker is different,' because it's his own life. With the last seizures …we thought it was over, and he was fine and we held it together, he

> held it together… until the doctor came in and said, 'No, your scan's still stable. We think this is just a medication blip.' … He just went to pieces. (Sarah, carer)

The concentrated and affective energy that is produced in the lived-experience of this indeterminate waiting and anticipation reaches a breaking-point around determinate events, such as the return of the seizures for Justin and the doctor's news that his time had not actually arrived yet. Everything becomes oriented around these distinct moments, when all the practices that one has engaged in to make sense of their time left, of their life and death, suddenly collapse.

Despite the troubling effects of these clinical hauntings, our participants demonstrated the need to recreate some form of continuity around borrowed time by 'making memories' or 'putting things in order', as we show in the next section.

Terminal Orientations Towards the Future

Orientations towards the future are embedded in the ways we make sense of our lives and understand ourselves. Living with terminal cancer—where speculative horizons of the future are unceremoniously cut short—is to live with ontological insecurity (Giddens, 1991) and temporal disjointedness (Barad, 2017), a disruption of the 'anticipatory regimes' (Adams et al., 2009) that govern orientations towards our futures. As the following section explores, participants' responses to such insecurities, estrangements, and disruptions were to *return* to future-orientating behaviours, albeit in modified ways. This return to ontological futuring played out in a variety of ways, including the need to 'optimise' one's future as a 'good' cancer citizen (even in the context of impeding death); the anticipation of one's own absence in the making of (good) memories, and finally, in the embracing of the *universal* inevitability of death (and by extension, a minimising of the difference between those with a terminal cancer diagnosis, and those without), as anybody can 'be hit with a bus tomorrow'.

Anticipatory regimes underpin the relational dynamics of 'good' cancer citizenship (see Kenny et al., 2017; Steinberg, 2015), where moral imperatives to 'make the most' of remaining time and to 'stay positive' are often imposed upon, or self-imposed on, those living with terminal cancer. This played out across the interviews as participants described their use of time left to put their affairs 'in order', as Daniel (patient) described:

> … it was a definite shock and there were some things going through, not just my mind, but my wife's mind as well, the things that we needed to tidy up. So, in one respect, I'm grateful for the time that I have had since the diagnosis, that I've had the time to put things in order, so to speak, finances and things like that that need to be taken care of. And if you're run over by a bus you don't get that opportunity. But we've had that opportunity to sort things like that out that I'm grateful for. (Daniel, patient)

This was echoed by Agnes (patient):

> I think it is a bit of a wake-up call to get your life in order and do what you want to do and get rid of all the rubbish that you've collected, scale things down and focus on what's important. (Agnes, patient)

The 'shock' and 'wake-up call' of Daniel and Agnes' terminal diagnosis is presented here as a welcome intervention, where time 'given' by a terminal diagnosis (as opposed to other, swifter modes of death) 'allowed' Daniel and Agnes to 'tidy up', to get their lives 'in order' and to 'get rid of all the rubbish' they've collected. Daniel and Agnes' framing of their diagnosis as a catalyst to effectively organise themselves for death demonstrates the persistence of anticipatory regimes that require a focus on the 'positives' of terminal cancer and the imperative to return to 'order', with all of its linear associations.

The endurance of anticipatory orientations toward an orderly and continuous future played out again in participants descriptions of their relational others:

Christy: … My stepdad and that says, 'You'll be fine. You'll live another 30 years.' and I go, 'Well no, I won't. That's just ridiculous. I won't.'
Interviewer: Why do you think they're saying things like that?
Christy: Because the thought of losing me is harder, I suppose. We'll just pretend that's not happening. It's easier. <laughter>
Interviewer: How do you feel when people do that?
Christy: I just think, 'Whatever.' I let a lot of things go these days. It makes them feel better, but, really, I prefer the reality of it all, really. 'Okay, this is going to happen. Let's deal with it.' It's just sad, really. Where my sadness comes, really, is looking at my children and my granddaughter, I suppose, not being there. But I can't dwell on that. I just have to live in the moment and have as much good time as I can with them. (Christy, patient)

Here, Christy (patient) describes the tensions of 'good' cancer citizenship, where the imperative to look towards the future is prioritised over Christy's own emotions, who would prefer the 'reality of it all' but who instead doesn't 'dwell', instead choosing to 'live in the moment' and 'have as much good time' as she can with her family. Christy's desire to make memories is an anticipation of her *own* absence in the future, focusing once more on her relational others. The urge to 'make memories', then, is another example of the anticipatory regime toward a speculative future where one is no longer there, putting pressure on the present to unfold in particular ways that would be remembered fondly.

Another example of the pull towards ontological futuring played out in participants' embracing of their terminal diagnosis as 'no different' from conceptions and fear of death in those without cancer or other terminal illnesses:

> … We're all on borrowed time anyway, in a sense, aren't we? So, I suppose, it's just perspective and how you look at it and try and make the most. (Agnes, patient)

> … I think I'm getting more at peace with the idea that everybody dies and it's not a scary thing, it's just part of life… Coming to accept that everybody dies, its fine, don't be scared of it, it's nothing to be scared of. (Ella, patient)

> … it's something that's going to happen to all of us at some point. We are all going to die. Basically, none of us really know when, and I don't know when either. I've got a disease, but I still can't say that I'm going to die tomorrow, I'm going to die in five years' time, I'm going to die in three years' time. I don't look at it as much as … It hasn't changed the way I look. I didn't know when I was going to die before I was diagnosed. (Miranda, patient)

As Agnes, Ella, and Miranda express, living simultaneously in the uncertainty of prognostic time (exactly 'how much' time remaining) and the certainty of terminal diagnosis (that time, will inevitably 'run out') is arguably no different to the ontological registers we all must live in, knowing that death will come for us, but not when. As Agnes poignantly noted, 'we're all on borrowed time'; the difference for those with terminal cancer, however, lies in the knowing of *how*, as Mac (patient) described:

> … this central part of how I think I live is not any different to anyone else because no one actually knows. You don't know whether you're to be hit by a bus or whether you'll have a heart attack tomorrow. We don't know. But I think most people won't dwell on one event. They won't go, 'Will I be hit by a bus tomorrow?' … That's right, most people don't … But, for me, it's 'It could be that bus. That could be that bus.' … That one thing, that the bus is coming for you. (Mac, patient)

Whilst the anticipation of certain death is one that we all experience, this universalising falls short of fully encapsulating the phenomenology of waiting in terminal cancer diagnosis. For Mac, while we could all 'be hit by a bus tomorrow' the knowledge that 'the bus is coming' is a deviation from normative orientations to the future (and the inevitability of death that the future implies) because the *mode* of death is certain. Once again, for those with terminal diagnosis, the speculative horizon of the future collides with the certainty of terminal diagnosis.

Across the interviews, the analogy of the bus was returned to, time and time again:

> It's like the bus comes down the road and if it hits you, it hits you. You can't do something about that. (Ashley, patient)

> Because people walk down the street, they get hit by a bus. Yeah, I think I've learnt to accept that a little bit more .... So, I think a lot of it is got to do with your attitude. (Miranda, patient)

> ... I don't so much think about time, I don't think, 'I could die any time.' Death doesn't bother me at all. It will upset the kids. For me, it doesn't bother me really because everybody will die at some stage. At least they have warning. I say to the kids, 'I could be hit by a bus, you've got no warning.' They are prepared. (Rebecca, patient)

The bus, as a metaphor of routine, normalcy, community, and travel, along paved and pre-determined roads, operates to normalise the experience of anticipating death. Here, the unsettling nature of ontological insecurity, the disruption of anticipatory futures, and the complexity of terminal timescapes can, for a short while, be swept away by the fundamental uncertainty that all of us, terminal or not, must live with—the idea that we could 'be hit by a bus tomorrow'.

Temporal and ontological incoherence emerge in these experiences of living with, or outliving, terminal cancer, as the spectre of the past and the future haunt the present, in which the 'finality' of a terminal diagnosis is complicated by the vast temporal ranges of prognostic uncertainty. As we have detailed above, the imperative toward future orientation was a common response to the anxieties of terminal diagnosis, playing out in participant's desires to enact 'good' cancer citizenship, preparing and getting their lives 'in order' in anticipation of a future in which they were no longer there.

Conclusion

Living with a terminal prognosis has the dis/orienting effect of shattering time as it is normally understood: a time that is continuous and unilinear, where only one moment exists at a time, and where each moment falls continuously and predictably after another. Drawing from Barad's work on the nature of time as diffractive and material, we suggest that the embodied experience of advanced cancer troubles such linear understandings of time. Thinking of time as diffractive means troubling the experiences that stabilise one's sense of self: a clear sense of one's history, how it causally leads to the present and the open potentiality of a yet undecided future.

Living on borrowed time illustrates how who one was before the cancer diagnosis, who one is with cancer and who one will be (gone/healthy again) are enacted within the present in complex and dis/orienting ways. This troubled sense of time informs the affective experience of living with cancer—where feelings of hope, gratitude but also dread, distress, grief, are constantly entangled, often incoherently, re-patterning any overarching meaning or sense of time. For those living with cancer, the future is anticipated with a new and heavy emotional weight—as time folds onto itself, partitioned by scans, tests, and the progression of the disease, all while simultaneously demanding that things are 'put in order'. Not only did participants have to navigate the biomedical environment that abruptly started synchronising their life through scans, tests, and disease progression; they were also caught in the crosshairs of past memories, the pressing present, and future imaginaries and plans. People with advanced cancer must build their own story around impossible uncertainties, calibrating their time around their illness and away from other future imaginaries. Following Barad, the entanglement between matter and time means that dealing with cancer is not only about the embodied experience of malignancy but also about the unsettling of the lived experience of time that normally sustains one's meaning-making practices and a coherent sense of self.

Despite these temporal disruptions, or because of them, people living with cancer re-turn—in Barad's sense of materialising new temporalities—to future orienting narratives to somehow stabilise their present living on borrowed time and resist the turmoil of a diffracted time. People living with terminal cancer live in new temporal landscapes of cancer chronicity, rather than survivorship, which stretch time and effectively locate them in a categorical liminality between curable and palliative. We focused on the affective temporal relations that shape what can and cannot be done, imagined and felt, when living with incurability. The ontological insecurity of this condition led most of our participants to reflect on the universal condition of anticipating death, when we can all be 'hit by a bus tomorrow', and the ways in which living haunted by this anticipation enacts new affective relations with others, oneself and their bodies in space and time.

Living through troubled times is the dis/orienting experience of blurring the boundaries between past, present, and future. It means living haunted by disrupted binaries, between self and other and between life and death. One's sense of self is constantly done and undone, diffracted through one's experience of multiple times interfering. The way in which the bodily encounter with cancer produces confusing, affectively dense and multiple realities of time is evocatively exemplified in our interviews with people with terminal cancer.

Acknowledgements The authors gratefully acknowledge the contributions of research participants who generously shared their experiences and stories with us. This Open Access chapter was published with financial support from the University of Sydney.

Competing Interests This research was funded by an Australian Research Council Discovery Grant (DP150100414), and Katherine Kenny is supported by an Australian Research Council DECRA Fellowship (DE220101498). The authors have no conflicts of interest to declare that are relevant to the content of this chapter.

References

Adams, V., Murphy, M., & Clarke, A. E. (2009). Anticipation: Technoscience, life, affect, temporality. *Subjectivity, 28*(1), 246–265.

Anucha, K., Baraitser, L., Davies, S., Flexer, M. J., & Robinson, D. (2021). Investigating waiting: Interdisciplinary thoughts on researching elongated temporalities in healthcare settings. In *Temporality in Qualitative Inquiry*. Taylor & Francis.

Barad, K. (2007). Meeting the universe halfway: Quantum physics and the entanglement of matter and meaning. Duke University Press.

Barad, K. (2010). Quantum entanglements and hauntological relations of inheritance: Dis/continuities, spacetime enfoldings, and justice-to-come. *Derrida Today, 3*(2), 240–268.

Barad, K. (2013). Ma(r)king time: Material entanglements and re-memberings: Cutting together-apart. In P. R. Carlile, D. Nicolini, A. Langley, & H. Tsoukas (Eds.), *How matter matters: Objects, artifacts, and materiality in organization studies* (p. 0). Oxford University Press.

Barad, K. (2014). Diffracting diffraction: Cutting together-apart. *Parallax, 20*(3), 168–187.

Baraitser, L., Anucha, K., Catty, J., Davies, S., Osserman, J., Salisbury, L., Flexer, M., & Moore, M. (2024). (Un)timely care: Findings from the Waiting Times project [version 1; peer review: 1 approved with reservations]). *Wellcome Open Research, 9*, 490. https://doi.org/10.12688/wellcomeopenres.22556.1

Barad, K. (2017). Troubling time/s and ecologies of nothingness: re-turning re-membering and facing the incalculable. *New Formations 92*(92), 56-86.

Brockmeier, J., & Carbaugh, D. A. (Eds.). (2001). *Narrative and identity*. John Benjamins.

Broom, A., Kenny, K., & Kirby, E. (2018). On waiting, hauntings and surviving: Chronicling life with cancer through solicited diaries. *The Sociological Review, 66*(3), 682–699.

Bury, M. (1982). Chronic illness as biographical disruption. *Sociology of Health & Illness, 4*(2), 167–182.

Charmaz, K. (1990). 'Discovering' chronic illness: Using grounded theory. *Social Science & Medicine, 30*(11), 1161–1172.

Clarke, A. E. (2003). Situational analyses: Grounded theory mapping after the postmodern turn. *Symbolic Interaction, 26*(4), 553–576.

Eisikovits, Z., & Koren, C. (2010). Approaches to and outcomes of dyadic interview analysis. *Qualitative Health Research, 20*(12), 1642–1655.

Frank, A. W. (2013). *The wounded storyteller: Body, illness & ethics*. University of Chicago Press.

Giddens, A. (1991). *Modernity and self-identity*. Stanford University Press.

Gordon, A. F. (2011). Some thoughts on haunting and futurity. *Borderlands, 10*, 1–21.

Harrop, E., Noble, S., Edwards, M., et al. (2017). Managing, making sense of and finding meaning in advanced illness. *Sociology of Health & Illness, 39*(8), 1448–1464.

Jain, S. L. (2007). Living in prognosis: Toward an elegiac politics. *Representations, 98*(1), 77–92.

Kenny, K., Broom, A., Kirby, E., Wyld, D., & Lwin, Z. (2017). Terminal anticipation: Entanglements of affect and temporality in living with advanced cancer. *Subjectivity, 10*(4), 374–392.

Mathieson, C. M., & Stam, H. J. (1995). Renegotiating identity. *Sociology of Health & Illness, 17*(3), 283–306.

McAdams, D. P. (2006). The problem of narrative coherence. *Journal of Constructivist Psychology, 19*(2), 109–125.

Neimeyer, R. A. (2000). Narrative disruptions in the construction of the self. In R. A. Neimeyer & J. D. Raskin (Eds.), *Constructions of disorder* (pp. 207–242). American Psychological Association.

Rushforth, A., Ladds, E., Wieringa, S., Taylor, S., Husain, L., & Greenhalgh, T. (2021). Long COVID–the illness narratives. *Social Science & Medicine, 286*, 114326.

Salisbury, L., Baraitser, L., Catty, J., Anucha, K., Davies, S., Flexer, M. J., & Osserman, J. (2023). A waiting crisis? *The Lancet, 401*(10375), 428–429.

Singer, J. A. (2004). Narrative identity and meaning making across the adult lifespan: An introduction. *Journal of Personality, 72*(3), 437–460.

Steinberg, D. (2015). The bad patient. *Body & Society, 21*(3), 115–143.

Voorhees, H. L. (2023). 'I was literally just not myself': How chronic pain changes multiple frames of identity. *Health Communication, 38*(8), 1641–1653.

Williams, S. (2000). Chronic illness as biographical disruption or biographical disruption as chronic illness? Reflections on a core concept. *Sociology of Health & Illness, 22*, 40–67.

Part V

Afterword

15

Between Deep Time and Indigenous Wellbeing

Susie Anderson

> last time I looked for stars
> I saw what was lit up
> four made a simple cross
> pattern I'd been taught not
> what was between I felt
> expansive knowledge bigger
> held within sky

I grew up hearing stories about how the snake ate the sun and the emu in the sky. In year eight our English class was on an excursion in Gariwerd and went to the Aboriginal cultural centre Brambruk. Peeling off from the group and I looked at pictures of local people who lived at Ebenezer, the Lutheran mission in the Wimmera. My great-grandmother had been born there, and I saw her in the pictures of the exhibit, my middle name the same as hers. Afterwards, we were assigned to write our own dream-time story.

"A deep time awareness might help us see ourselves as part of a web of gift," said Robert Macfarlane, writing in *Underland* (2019), "inheritance

S. Anderson (✉)
Glenisla, VIC, Australia

K. Kenny et al. (eds.), *Timescapes of Health, Illness and Care*,
https://doi.org/10.1007/978-981-96-7055-0_15

and legacy stretching over millions of years past and millions to come". He sensed the the multilinear nature of our existence. And, too, the inadequacy of Western spiritual practices. In Australia, First Peoples are holders of the deep time knowledge that I believe Macfarlane is referring to. He describes field research for the book, putting a hand out to an ochre handprint painted in a cave and feeling the connection to humans from another time. It's this deep time awareness, long held inheritance and legacies that could soften existential anguish of today's fears: our climate emergency, the COVID-19 pandemic and ongoing colonisation.

Deep time awareness is a foundational part of the knowledge systems of Aboriginal and Torres Strait Islander communities often called Dreamtime or Dreaming. It relates to the past, present and future, interweaving understanding of people, place and time. Christine Nicholls (2014) offers this definition by Jeannie Herbert Nungarrayi (2002) in her article for The Conversation, referring to it as "an all-embracing concept that provides rules for living, a moral code, as well as rules for interacting with the natural environment. The philosophy behind it is holistic – the Jukurrpa[1] provides for a total, integrated way of life.... The Dreaming isn't something that has been consigned to the past but is a lived daily reality."

My understanding of the practical, interwoven nature of Dreaming expanded during a research trip to Tiwi Islands, as part of my work for Museum of Contemporary Art Australia. During research interviews for the 2015 exhibition *Being Tiwi*, I met artists Pedro Wonaeamirri, Timothy Cook, Maria Josette Orsto and others who shared the significance of their personal symbology or Dreaming. They explained it was integrated far beyond their visual arts practice into seasonal cycles, ceremony, dance, food production and more. Totemic animals or constellations, might be generally referred to as their 'Dreaming' but the way they interact with it happens on multiple levels in a holistic way. As Nicholls writes,

[1] Jukurrpa a word used in Central Australian Aboriginal communities as opposed to the English 'Dreaming'.

> Unfortunately, since colonisation, this multiplicity of semantically rich, metaphysical word-concepts framing the epistemological, cosmological and ontological frameworks unique to Australian Aboriginal people's systems of religious belief have been uniformly debased and dumbed-down – by being universally rendered as "Dreaming" in English – or, worse still, "Dreamtime".

When I was younger, I thought everything was lost, that I needed to create something new, and writing the Dreamtime story for class affirmed it. It was an education that didn't create space for my identity and culture, housed within a system flattening what it means to be Aboriginal. It needed to forget and remove our complexity in order to continue the work of colonisation. My English teacher was encouraging and I liked her, but my story tumbled out like an episode of Blinky Bill. A bush forum headed by a noble kookaburra and a troublesome kangaroo that led to the creation of thunder and lightning.

Regular fixtures in Wergaia stories are two cheeky brothers Bram. Possums and spiders guarding lakes on Country, getting up to mischief. Though I know it wasn't my teacher's fault or her intention, the distance I felt from our cultural knowledge was the intention of the colonial project and reinforced by the education system. Cycles of removal and disconnection moving down through the years from my ancestors until it reached me.

Stories of Country relate to past, present and future, interweaving understanding of people, place and time. They may seem like simple metaphorical fables but they are full of meaning. Knowledge of caring for Country, seasonal knowledge of places to find food in abundance or camp safely. Ambelin Kwaymullina explains the interconnectedness in her poem 'Holism' (2020, p. 23):

> Ask an Indigenous thinker
> to explain a hill
> they might speak
> about the river that runs past it
> the plants and animals
> to whom it is home

about the earth below
the turning stars above
about the Ancestor
who is hill
the Ancestor hill
who is family

I grew up on Country where Wergaia stories and language had been spoken long before I came and will remain long after I go. From the hefty presence of Gariwerd, shouldering almost all of Western Victoria, mountains even out into wide golden expanses and desert towards the South Australian border. Occasionally the surprise of enormous lakes, pink saltwater and freshwater, emerging billabongs and rivers. The barenji gadjin (flowing waters) of the Wimmera river is the artery that feeds them, loping up to Guru (Lake Hindmarsh). Country is wiser than me, is alive with knowledge of deep time, could speak many memories and true stories.

Yet I feel the confines of existential dread, compacting and minimising me into the pinprick of my brief timeline. Even though I am a storyteller, crafting words and building worlds, it doesn't feel authentic enough, doesn't feel like it is built from the land. I've wondered whether conscious reconnection to Aboriginal mythological knowledges and spiritualities will give me the sense of ease that is missing from my life. If I knew all the cultural stories of my ancestors, would I feel at ease because I know I am connected to stories of deep time?

The health and wellbeing challenges and inequalities that face First Nations people across communities are well understood as having their roots in colonisation. To disconnect us from Country and our knowledges creates a despairing, vulnerable people for whom a carefree life and wellbeing is a foreign concept. Kingsley, Townsend, Henderson-Wilson and Bolam note that this "lack of control, stress and social gradient [has] been shown to effect peoples' health outcomes across all population groups, this disconnect from Country may contribute an extra layer to this distress and inequality" (2013, p. 683). While there is a growing understanding of how nature and the environment has a positive impact on wellbeing, "they are still often overlooked in scientific arenas … local

Aboriginal environmental narratives and knowledge should be accorded similar standing to scientific information".

The distance I felt from my cultural knowledge was intentional and continued the work of colonisation that settlers began. The disconnection from our place on Country resulted in trauma that still impacts on Aboriginal people today, playing out in a myriad of mental health challenges. Yet through making art, it is possible to soothe the legacies of this disconnection. "To reclaim spirituality [through arts practice] is to reclaim identity and to develop resilience in the face of generational trauma" (Poroch et al., 2009, p. 2).

Recently the honey scent of wattle called me up the mountain. Urging me higher. I put my hand out to the boulders jutting out of the base. Ochre layers teaching the story of deep time. Speaking the same language as it always has.

Acknowledgement This essay was originally published in 2021 as part of The University of Melbourne exhibition Emu Sky at Old Quad, curated by Zena Cumpston.

Competing Interests The author has no conflicts of interest to declare that are relevant to the content of this chapter.

References

Kingsley, J., Townsend, M., Henderson-Wilson, C., & Bolam, B. (2013). Developing an exploratory framework linking Australian Aboriginal peoples' connection to country and concepts of wellbeing. *International Journal of Environmental Research and Public Health, 10*(2), 678–698.

Kwaymullina, A. (2020). *Living on stolen land.* Magabala Books.

Macfarlane, R. (2019). *Underland: A deep time journey.* Penguin UK.

Nicholls, C. (2014, January 23). 'Dreamtime' and 'The Dreaming'—An introduction. *The Conversation.* https://theconversation.com/dreamtime-and-the-dreaming-an-introduction-20833

Nungarrayi, J. (2002). Introduction. In Museum of contemporary Art (Hg.): Dancing up country. The Art of Dorothy Napangardi, Sydney 2002, Ausst. Kat., ISBN 1875632824. https://www.aboriginal-art.de/EN/Literatur_Info_MCA_2002_469.htm#Kla

Poroch, N., Arabena, K., Tongs, J., Larkin, S., Fisher, J., & Henderson, G. (2009). Spirituality and aboriginal people's social and emotional wellbeing: A review. Discussion Paper No. 11, Cooperative Research Centre for Aboriginal Health, Darwin, pp. 1–54.

Index[1]

[1] Note: Page numbers followed by 'n' refer to notes.

K. Kenny et al. (eds.), *Timescapes of Health, Illness and Care*,
https://doi.org/10.1007/978-981-96-7055-0

Kolibri 360 GmbH
Ferdinand-Jühlke-Straße 7
99095 Erfurt, Deutschland
produktsicherheit@kolibri360.de